Oxford Clinical Practice Series

HANDBOOK OF BENIGN PROCTOLOGICAL DISORDERS

T0177766

The Oxford Clinical Practice series covers an array of resources providing essential evidence-based, up-to-date information and key clinical references that will enhance the clinical knowledge of healthcare practitioners and medical students across the globe.

Oxford Clinical Practice Series

HANDBOOK OF BENIGN PROCTOLOGICAL DISORDERS

Authored by
Pravin Jaiprakash Gupta
MS, FICS, FAIS, FASCRS, FACS

Director, Fine Morning Hospital and Research Centre,
Nagpur, India

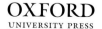

OXFORD
UNIVERSITY PRESS

Oxford University Press is a department of the University of Oxford.
It furthers the University's objective of excellence in research, scholarship,
and education by publishing worldwide. Oxford is a registered trademark of
Oxford University Press in the UK and in certain other countries.

Published in India by
Oxford University Press
2/11 Ground Floor, Ansari Road, Daryaganj, New Delhi 110 002, India

First Edition published in 2017

Second impression 2018

ISBN-13: 978-0-19-947221-5
ISBN-10: 0-19-947221-1

Typeset in Helvetica Neue LT Std 7.5/9.5
by Tranistics Data Technologies, Kolkata 700 091
Printed in India by Rakmo Press, New Delhi 110 020

To my parents
and
my wife Alka

Contents

Abbreviations

ADSC	adipose-derived stem cell
AIDS	Acquired Immune Deficiency Syndrome
AIN	anal intraepithelial neoplasia
BTX	Botulinum toxin
CCB	calcium channel blocker
CMV	Cytomegalovirus
DGHAL	doppler-guided haemorrhoid artery ligation
EAS	external anal sphincter
EMG	electromyography
ESR	erythrocyte sedimentation rate
FAP	Familial adenomatous polyposis
FFS	flexible fibreoptic sigmoidoscope
GI	gastrointestinal
GTN	glyceryl trinitrate
HAART	highly active anti-retroviral therapy
HeLP™	haemorrhoidal laser procedure
HIV	Human Immunodeficiency Virus
HPV	Human Papillomavirus
HRA	high-resolution anoscopy
IAS	internal anal sphincter
IBD	inflammatory bowel disease
IRC	infrared photocoagulation
JV	juvenile polyp
LAS	levator ani syndrome
LIFT	ligation of inter-sphincteric fistula tract
MPFF	micronised purified flavonoid fraction
MRAP	maximum resting anal pressure
MRI	magnetic resonance imaging
MRP	maximum resting pressure
Nd:YAG	neodymium-doped yttrium aluminium garnet
OPD	outpatient department
PACD	perianal Crohn's disease
PCR	polymerase chain reaction
PNTML	pudendal nerve terminal motor latency
PPH	prolapsing haemorrhoid
RBL	rubber band ligation
RFA	radiofrequency ablation
SCJ	squamous-columnar junction
STARR	stapled transanal rectal resection procedure
STD	sexually transmitted disease
TCA	trichloroacetic acid

THE	thrombosed external haemorrhoid
TEMS	transanal endoscopic microsurgery
VAAFT	video-assisted anal fistula treatment
VRM	volume rendering mode

×

Preface

Not long ago, the anorectal ailments were considered a matter of shame and were discussed in hushed tones. Those suffering from such ailments used to resort to home remedies without success. The patients, more particularly females, continued to suffer in silence. Even family physicians were not consulted.

Admittedly, the general practitioners, also fondly known as family doctors, are the core group attending to patients with myriad issues. Those suffering from anorectal ailments form a large chunk of these patients. These physicians could guide the patients by suggesting appropriate diagnostic tests to arrive at a conclusion as to the treatment modality needed in each case. This book, based on the literature available on the wide variety of known benign procotological pathologies and, most importantly, on hands-on experience attempts to summarize the available treatment options at one place and in a nutshell. The book is primarily aimed as a handbook of proctology for ready reference of the family physicians. The surgeon fraternity may also find this handy in their practice.

A galaxy of physicians over centuries clinically and ethically researched the ailments involving the colorectal region and had advanced diverse treatment modalities based on their studies for the benefit of the ailing humanity. The edifice of the advanced techniques that are in vogue today stands on the solid foundation laid by those luminaries. I owe a great deal to all of them in constructing the text of this book.

My thanks are due to my anaesthetists, hospital staff, and my wife Alka who were always the source of help and inspiration to me. I am indebted to all the researchers, journals, and publishers whose abstracts and write-ups have been referenced in this book to provide the latest concepts in the diagnosis and management of various diseases of the anorectum.

Last but not the least, my publishers deserve special thanks for presenting the content in this form.

Acknowledgements

My regards are due to my teachers and colleagues who have guided me from time to time to bring this book to the present shape. My particular thanks to my father Jaiprakash, who has edited and compiled the entire manuscript.

Author

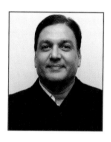

Dr Pravin Jaiprakash Gupta, MS, FICS, FAIS, FASCRS, FACS, is a surgeon-proctologist. He is the Director at Fine Morning Hospital and Research Centre in Nagpur, India. Having completed his postgraduation in Surgery, Dr Gupta underwent formal training in proctology from various centres in India and abroad. He has the honour of being selected as International Fellow of the American Society of Colon and Rectal Surgeons in June 2011, Fellow of the American College of Surgeons in October 2013, and Fellow of the International Society of Coloproctology in January 2014. He is a National Board Member of Global Practice in Piles Management, India, which works for patient education and awareness on haemorrhoids, setting up practice parameters for the management of haemorrhoids in the Indian scenario. An extensive writer in his area of specialisation, Dr Gupta has to his credit more than 103 research papers published in various peer-reviewed indexed international journals, more than 450 articles in various national and international health magazines, and four books on anorectal diseases and haemorrhoids. He has also contributed chapters to *Emerging Infectious Diseases in India, Principal and Practice of Anal Fistula*, and *A Comprehensive Guide to Proctology*. In addition, he has authored five books in Indian languages on various health topics. A much sought after speaker in the international community of doctors, he has travelled the globe, sharing his techniques with fellow doctors around the world. His presentation was awarded as the best podium presentation at the annual meeting of the American Society of Colon and Rectal Surgeons at Vancouver, Canada in May 2011. He was invited to deliver the 'Menda and Muragami Oration' at the Asia Pacific Federation of Coloproctology meeting in Thailand in 2011. He has presented more than 65 papers in about 32 international colorectal congresses abroad. He is an editorial board member of seven international medical journals and reviewer for more than 40 surgery journals. Organizing many surgical workshops in proctology in different parts of the country, he has trained hundreds of surgeons from India and abroad in his specialised technical field. The famous American company Ellman International Inc. named a surgical device 'Radio wave gun handle' after him as 'Pravin Gupta Procto Gun'. A pioneer in an innovating procedure using radiofrequency surgery in various anorectal conditions, Dr Gupta is contributing immensely to the field of anorectal surgery.

Chapter 1

History of proctology

Proctology is a branch of medicine that deals with the structures and diseases of anus, rectum, and sigmoid colon.

The word 'proctology' is probably derived from the Greek words πρωκτός ('Proktos'), meaning anus or hind parts and λόγος ('Logos'), meaning science or study. Since ancient times, the surgical interventions of anorectal lesions were performed by barbers and surgeons; with time, proctology has become a well-defined and recognised surgical speciality today.

'No one knows who was the first doctor to examine the rectal orifice of the human frame', said Charles Elton Blanchard in *The Romance of Proctology* (1938). The history of proctology is illustrated by some legends and events: St. Fiacre Felix was the surgeon who operated on King Louis XIV's fistula and the acutely thrombosed haemorrhoidal prolapse of Napoleon.

A cursory review of the history of medicine reveals that for many centuries, proctology has generated some interest. The earliest illustrations of the study of 'rectal diseases' have been found in the 'Code of Hammurabi', written around 2200 BC. It includes instructions to a patient to the effect that he should 'pay the doctor five shekels for healing a diseased bowel'. The 'haemorrhoids' are mentioned more particularly in the famous *Ebers Papyrus*, *c.* 1700 BC, which gives 33 prescriptions or recipes for the treatment of anorectal diseases, including ointments, suppositories, liniments, and enemas. The *Beatty medical papyrus* of the twelfth–thirteenth centuries BC consists of methods and remedies for many colon and rectal diseases. These medications mainly comprised honey, myrrh, flour, ibex fat, and rectal injections containing honey and sweet beer. The *Beatty papyrus* contained more than 40 prescriptions that were used to treat pruritus ani, thrombosed haemorrhoids, and rectal prolapse. It is said that the Hindus had a clinical knowledge of haemorrhoids and fistula as early as 1000 BC.

Until towards the end of the last century, the occurrence and pathology of the many diseases affecting the lower part of the bowel were not understood and the treatment suggested was simplistic and unscientific. It was not until this time that any serious and orderly consideration of them was undertaken. A considerable impetus was given to these studies by Dr Joseph Mathews of Louisville, who has been considered the 'Father of Proctology'. He was the first medical person in the world to limit his practice to this field. He preferred being called a rectal specialist rather than being referred to by any other complicated terminology. Since his time, there has been a continued and progressive advancement in the knowledge of these diseases.

In 1938, Charles Elton Blanchard, a renowned proctologist who wrote over a dozen books on the subject, published *The Romance of Proctology*. It was the story of the history and development of this much-neglected branch of medicine from its earliest times to the time when it was written, and included brief biographical information and photographs of the pioneers in the field. The previous year, Blanchard had released a more practical volume titled *A Handbook of Ambulant Proctology,* offering the latest developments of methods and technic for doing proctologic work by office practices.

HIPPOCRATES AND PROCTOLOGY

Hippocrates, the traditional 'Father of Medicine', remains an elusive, shadowy character. He was a physician and teacher. He was born in Cos in Greece and lived in the latter part of the fifth and early part of the fourth centuries BC. An extensive collection of 70 books, *The Corpus Hippocraticum* was attributed to him for many centuries. However, philologists studying the differences in the style, dialect, and the 1966 study by Wake suggested that only four of the principal works had a famous author. It is, of course, impossible to prove that this author was Hippocrates. The two books of particular interest here are *On Fistulae* and *On Haemorrhoids*. The book on fistula starts with a brief section on their aetiology: 'Fistulae are produced by contusions and tubercles; they are also caused by rowing or riding on horseback when blood accumulates in the nates near the anus.' The tubercle is probably used here to refer to an inflammatory swelling because the author goes on to describe the parts as going putrid and spreading until the tubercle breaks and discharges below at the anus.

In the case of contusions produced by a fall, blow, a wound, or riding or rowing, a haematoma forms, which suppurates, and the course is as described for tubercles. The ideal treatment is to 'cut it open while still unripe before it suppurates and burst into the rectum'.

The second method is perhaps more common. A slender thread of raw lint is folded and wrapped around with horsehair and attached to a tin director with an opening at its extremity. Then, it suggests to 'introduce the head into the fistula and, at the same time, enter the index finger of the left hand in the anus; and when the director touches, the finger brings it out'. The ends of the threads are then twisted and knotted, and the patient is sent about his business. Whenever the thread is loosened owing to the fistula becoming putrid, it is to be tightened and twisted.

The book *On Haemorrhoids* is probably as much a tribute to the patients of antiquity as to the surgeons. As usual, the author begins by describing the engorged veins, bruised by faeces passing out so that they squirt out blood. He remarks, '… as all of us might have done in our time, that "cutting, excising, sewing … to the anus, all of them appearing to be very dangerous things, and yet, after all, they are not attended with mischief"'.

The first way of treatment recommended is the cautery—lay the patient on his back with a pillow under the breech, force out the anus with the fingers, and burn the pile with red-hot irons. To help the surgeon, a note has been inserted in this portion of technique: 'The patient's head and hands should be held so that he may not shake, but he should cry out, for this will make the rectum project the more.' It is followed with the instructions for dressings, diet, and baths.

Another method is to truncate the extremities of the haemorrhoids: here, bleeding or ligature is not mentioned. The next two chapters deal with a lesion that must probably be adenomatous polypi, as it mentions 'there grows upon the weeping condyloma, a protuberance like the fruit of the mulberry'. It was performed by placing the patient in the kneeling position and whipping away the condyloma with a finger—no more difficult, we are assured, than skinning a sheep. It was added that 'this should be accomplished without the patient's knowledge while he is kept in a conversation'.

Just like the Egyptians and the Greeks, the Romans did not contribute much to the practice of proctology and were following the methods of treatments as laid down by the others. Since the beginning, two topics beyond all others have engaged the attention of rectal surgeons, namely fistula and piles.

Aulus Cornelius Celsus matured in the golden age; that is to say, in the reigns of the Emperors Augustus and Tiberius. He has been called the 'Latin Hippocrates'. He possessed a diversity of talent. He framed works on the military art, rhetoric, and agriculture, as well as medicine. Celsus also suggested the gradual division of a fistula-in-ano by a thread passed through the tract and gradually tightened. He recommended that the patient should 'walk about and attend to his business as if in perfect health', thus assuming the modern method of getting the patient up early. The difficulties and dangers of operating upon a fistula with a high internal opening were appreciated 19 centuries ago. The dictum of Celsus holds true in essence even in the present day.

Many centuries passed without registering any particular record pertaining to this field of medicine before Paul Aegina, a seventh-century surgeon of the Byzantine period, gave an excellent description of the procedures of haemorrhoids and anal fistula. Under the Arabs, only Maimonides (AD 1135–1204) wrote a treatise on haemorrhoids, in which he recommended light diet and sitz baths.

During the Middle Ages, sufferers from most diseases had a patron saint whom they could invoke. St. Fiacre, a middle-era acolyte, was the patron saint of gardeners and eventually became the patron saint of haemorrhoid sufferers. He must be a favourite saint; an inn in Paris was named after him and it featured a statue of the saint.

Fourteenth-century surgeon John Arderne of Newarkon-Trent, whose *De arte phisicali et de cirurgia* was a widely influential treatise on the treatment of numerous ills both inner and outer, was born in AD 1307. He is acclaimed as the 'Father of British Proctology'. Arderne was the first to describe and practise what is virtually the modern operative treatment for fistula-in-ano (Figure 1.1). He was of the view that the treatment of fistula-in-ano had fallen into disrepute because of being a troublesome condition that brought little credit to surgeons, although it required long and patient treatment. He recognised ischiorectal abscess as the cause of fistulas and insisted that they should be opened before they rupture in the rectum. His predecessors like

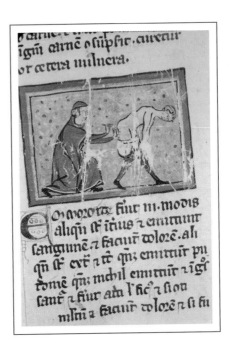

Figure 1.1 Arderne's proctological procedures.

Albucasis (d. 1106), was of the opinion that fistulae were incurable and all operations and applications of ointments were but labour in vain. William de Salicet (fl. 1245), considered to be the most skilful surgeon of his age, wrote 'when the fistula is complete, it is assuredly so difficult to cure that it is better and more honourable for the surgeon to leave the case at once'. Again, Lanfranc (d. 1315) contented himself with saying that fistulae were incurable while de Mondeville merely enlarged the opening of the fistula with a tent and condemned those who would operate and afterwards apply a corrosive.

In contrast to all these, Arderne laid the fistula open with a knife and was confident of success. He had a long list of patients—knights and priests, merchants and friars—whom he had cured of the disease. His post-operative treatment was also unique. Starting from simple applications like the yolk of a raw egg, ordinary oil, or oil of roses for the early post-operative period, he used his powder 'pulvis sine pare' after eight or nine days. Simple enemata, administered through a clyster-pipe that he described, were used after 48 hours to empty the bowel, and instructions were given as to the cleansing and drying of the wound after motion.

Thus, we are given a fascinating account of this fourteenth-century surgeon's operating methods. From Arderne's descriptions, there is no doubt that he dealt with severe and complicated cases, probably much more serious than we are accustomed to seeing today. There is little doubt that he achieved considerable success in those difficult cases by using a method of operating and, what was equally important, a routine of after-care, which was far advanced than those of his contemporaries and remarkably approximated our present-day methods.

Though Arderne's central theme was fistula-in-ano, he also dealt sufficiently with most of the other anorectal conditions that we have to treat today. He had a long dissertation on haemorrhoids, an excellent description of cancer of the rectum, and shorter sections on proctitis and ulceration of the rectum, prolapse of the rectum, pruritus ani, and tenesmus.

Arderne indulged in the use of, and was an expert in the preparation of, concoctions like ointments, plasters, pills, confections, and valences for both internal and external applications so much so that his reputation as a pharmacist excelled his reputation as a surgeon. John Arderne learnt by experimentation rather than by authority. He preferred personal experience to the teaching of the schools, which was often divorced from experience, and with a characteristic frankness, he related his failures as well as his successes. For some hundreds of years after him, surgeons continued to use tents, escharotics, and the cautery and to fret the fistula with threads. These methods remained the standard practice till Percival Pott, in his monograph on fistula written in 1765, once again strongly advocated laying open the fistulous tract by simple incision, and condemned the other methods of treatment as well as the operation of excision of the fistulous tract and the overlying tissues, which was then being practised.

Rectal prolapse had also received a large amount of attention in the medical literature dating back to Hippocrates and comprised fomentations and reductions and then gradually with more sophisticated attempts with haemorrhoidectomy, incision, cauterisation, and excision.

The seventeenth century produced a notable event in the form of Louis XIV's operation for fistula, which was performed by Charles Francois Felix, a surgeon who performed this surgery at Versailles, which proved a complete success. For this, he received 300,000 livres and was made a nobleman, and the year 1686 came to be known as 'l'anee de la fistule.

After Arderne, there is little to note until the early eighteenth century, when Heister of Helmstadt published an outstanding work in German on surgery, which was translated into English in 1743. Heister gives an excellent account of the varieties of fistula. He advises injecting 'milk, if it is so crooked that a probe cannot follow it', thus anticipating our more advanced method of injection with methylene blue or lipiodol. He is in favour of using a falciform knife with an obtuse point, such as was employed by Felix on Louis XIV for the cure of fistula in 1686, and was afterwards called the 'Bistouri Royal'.

In the eighteenth century, Morgagni described the crypts and columns that still bear his name. He was the first to propose an operation for the cancer of the rectum. Before the war of American independence, American medicine was the alter ego of British medicine. That war, however, allowed French medicine to exert some influence in the United States of America (USA). In 1812, the young republic waged its first foreign war with the motherland against whom her war of independence had also been fought. For Americans, this war promoted more bitterness than for the British. The resulting deteriorations of Anglo-American relations enabled French medicine to further increase its influence in the young republic.

However, the British influence remained strong in American medicine, especially American proctology. In 1813, the year Wellington's army entered France, John Syng Dorsey produced his two-volume work *Elements of Surgery*, the first textbook on surgery published in the USA.

Dorsey's work received worldwide recognition; it was reprinted in Edinburgh and used as a textbook at the University of Edinburgh. Concerning haemorrhoids, Dorsey quoted Abernethy's recommendation of a knife since the operation was safe and less painful. Dorsey mentioned that accidents from wounds of the haemorrhoidal veins caused him to prefer the ligature treatment because it was 'safe and sure', even though it was more painful. Describing the technique, Dorsey wrote about 'affixing a strong ligature upon the protruded tumours while the patient strains as if passing stool to propel them as much as possible'.

Writing on fistula-in-ano, Dorsey termed the use of leeches by British surgeons 'ridiculous'. Twenty to sixty leeches were employed to obtain 8–15 ounces of blood. It should be recalled that the French also used leeches. Napoleon's letter dated 26 May 1807 to his youngest brother Jerome stated, 'I hear you have haemorrhoids. The simplest way to get rid of them is to apply three or four leeches. Since I first employed this remedy, ten years ago, I have been no more troubled'. During the Battle of Waterloo, Napoleon had an attack of inflamed prolapsed haemorrhoids, which was a well-kept military secret for many years.

Dorsey's book had a diagram of the bistoury and cited the French surgeons Pierre-Joseph Desault and Marie François Xavier Bichat. In the first three decades of the nineteenth century, there appeared in England many small volumes dealing with anorectal diseases written by George Calvert, Thomas Copeland, William White, Frederick Salmon, John Howship, Herbert Mayo, and John Kirby—all British physicians. These publications, many going into more than one edition, testify to the considerable interest in the study of anorectal diseases in England. However, in the USA, it was not until 1837 that the first book on anorectal diseases was published by George McCartney Bushe, who came from Ireland, died of pulmonary tuberculosis at the age of 39 on 18 May 1837, the same year that his *Treatise on the Malformations, Injuries, and Diseases of the Rectum* was published in two volumes. Bushe's *Treatise* reflected his experiences as well as knowledge from his vast library of books. Bushe's reference to a large number of outstanding physicians is in contrast to books on proctology by other physicians of the nineteenth century. Herbert Mayo (1833) in his chapter on piles cited only a case report by Sir Benjamin Collins Brodie. What doctors of the past wrote about haemorrhoids is always fascinating. Of particular interest, Bushe thought that haemorrhoidal disease was seasonal, most likely to occur in spring. He wrote 'the spring is the period most favourable to the development of haemorrhoids; first, because the volume of the blood is increased as the secretions having been diminished during the winter; second, because the absorption of caloric expands the blood; and third, because the phenomena of life are more active at this season'. Some authors have noticed that the haemorrhoidal flux is most likely to occur when the winds are northerly, and others say that it is apt to take place during the solstices and equinoxes.

Bushe's work was widely acclaimed. Howard Kelly of the Johns Hopkins Medical School wrote that Bushe's *Treatise* was 'long considered the ablest work on the subject in any language'. In England, T.B. Curling (1863), W. Allingham (1896), T.J. Ashton (1857), and F.J. Gant (1878) cited Bushe. Bushe's *Treatise* was cited for six decades. At a time when no American physician specialised, Bushe recognised the need for the greater dissemination of knowledge of anorectal diseases, and significantly promoted American proctology by his *Treatise*. In the first half of the nineteenth century, although Bushe's *Treatise* was devoted only to anorectal diseases, there were works on general surgery, which included the treatment of anorectal diseases.

The middle of the nineteenth century was the 'dawn of anaesthesia'. Nitrous oxide gas was first used as an aesthetic by Horace Wells, John M. Riggs, and Gardner Q. Colton in 1844, although discovered by Joseph Priestly in 1772; ether by William Thomas Green Morton in 1844; and chloroform by James Young Simpson in 1847. In 1867, Joseph Lister published his article on 'The Antiseptic Principle in the Practice of Surgery'.

The Institutes and Practice of Surgery by William Gibson (1788–1868) went through eight editions and was a famous text in many medical schools. Although Gibson did not produce a particular monograph on proctology, Benjamin Collins Brodie's (1783–1862) writings on anorectal diseases had a considerable influence on both sides of the Atlantic Ocean. In fact, up to a few years ago, American books on proctology identified the sentinel pile of an anal fissure as Brodie's pile. Even though he did not receive a doctorate of medicine, James Syme, the outstanding professor of surgery belonging to the University of Edinburgh and Joseph Lister's father-in-law, influenced surgery and proctology in the British Isles, on the Continent, and in the USA. He wrote texts on general surgery, as well as a treatise on anorectal diseases that went into three editions.

Further interest in proctology was shown by the publication of several books on anorectal diseases by George Calvert, Thomas Copeland, William White, Frederick Salomon, John Hawship, and John Kirby.

In 1868, M. Demarquay strongly advised the red-hot cautery as a cure for internal piles. William Allingham, in the fifth edition of his book *The Diseases of the Rectum* (1888), gives an exhaustive account of almost all the operations and methods of treating piles that have been tried. He mentions no less than 13, most of which are now obsolete. The list includes injection treatment; clamp and cautery; Whitehead's operation; Allingham, Jr.'s, modified Whitehead's operation, and so on. After having tried many methods, Allingham pronounces himself in the favour of the ligature method.

Frederick Salmon (1796–1868) influenced American proctology not so much by his writings but by the establishment of St. Mark's Hospital, London, for the treatment of rectal diseases. In 1835, he founded a seven-bed infirmary known as 'The Infirmary for the Relief of the Poor suffering with Fistula and Other Diseases of the Rectum'. In 1854, this became St. Mark's Hospital with 25 beds and St. Mark's, in turn, became the fountainhead for the education of rectal surgeons in England and for most of the world.

This hospital significantly influenced American proctology in the nineteenth century, a force that continues today. Joseph M. Mathews, who is considered as the first ethically educated proctologist of America, also trained at St. Mark's Hospital. In 1864, he published *A Treatise on Diseases of the Rectum, Anus, and Sigmoid Flexure*, which was the first credible book on this subject in the USA. He, along with J. Rawson Pennington, Samuel G. Gant, and James P. Tuttle, took many efforts to establish the American Proctologic Society and became its first president.

The American Proctologic Society continues as a major force in American medicine. The editors selected William Allingham, a surgeon at St. Mark's Hospital, to write about diseases of the rectum and colon in the six-volume *International Encyclopaedia of Surgery*, published in 1886 in New York.

Even today, the value associated with a St. Mark's Hospital surgeon is not forgotten. For the section on rectal diseases in the latest edition of *Christopher's Surgery*, a traditional American surgical textbook, the editor selected a St. Mark's surgeon, Alan Parks as the author.

During the nineteenth century, various surgical treatments for rectal cancer were introduced. Richard von Volkmann reported on the excision of the rectum and M. Verneuil suggested removal of the coccyx to improve exposure. Kocher began closing the anus with a purse string suture and excising a portion of the sacrum and the coccyx that allowed for more radical excision. During this time, there was an increase in the knowledge of the anatomy of the colon and rectum, most of which was contributed by the extensive work from John Hilton, William E. Horner, and D. Girota.

Thomas Blizard Curling, in his book *Diseases of the Rectum*, made some mention of the surgical instruments suitable for proctological work. The book describes the pathology, clinical features, and treatment of most of the anorectal disorders with which we are familiar at present. The description of these common anorectal conditions will give the reader a glimpse into the similarities and differences of proctology 100 years ago. In some respects, times have changed a little, as can be seen both from the extensive list of preparations recommended for pruritus ani and Curling's comment that 'the complaint is often very obstinate, and much perseverance is required on the part of the practitioner and also of the patient to effect a cure'.

The first decade of the twentieth century brought forth two of the standardised operations for colon and rectal carcinoma. It was J. von Miculicz for the cancer of the colon and W.E. Miles for the carcinoma of the rectum.

With modern methods, the treatment of anorectal diseases by surgery meets all of the three ancient admonitions to carry out operation; that it should be done *tuto* (safely), *cito* (quickly), and *jucunde* (pleasantly). The progress from the days of John of Arderne to the present-day status of the colorectal surgeon being a well-trained abdominal surgeon as well as a specialist in anal problems has been significant. Improved results in the therapy of diseases of rectum and anus will rest on the continued development of fully trained surgeons who have continuing interests in these problems.

Coloproctology or the disease of the colon, rectum, and anus has been receiving well-merited attention from not only British and American universities, but also those bodies of specialists constituted to license specialities. Many universities today have departments for this speciality with a professor and other staff.

In this study of medical history, one fact stands out—people will seek the doctor who excels in the treatment of anorectal disease. The quest for knowledge of this transcends national boundaries.

CLINICAL PEARLS

- Proctology is an integral part of the surgery, and its developmental path was inseparable from the historical development of operational medicine.
- In the ancient Egypt, proctology was an important branch of medicine.
- Of the so far known medical papyri in the history of proctology, the most important one is *Beatty papyrus*, which is a short monograph on diseases of the anus and their treatment.
- Operative proctology reached the highest level in the time of Hippocrates. He wrote in detail about the operative procedures for perianal fistula and haemorrhoids.
- The most famous Roman medical writer Celsus described the surgery of haemorrhoids by their ligature and the surgery of anorectal fistula in two ways— ligation of the fistula channel by a string of raw flax and fistula incision through the probe placed through the fistula channel.
- Surgeons of eighteenth and the nineteenth centuries introduced more complicated surgical procedures for the treatment of anorectal diseases.

(Cont'd)

- The French surgeons were the leaders. M. Littré performed, for the first time, anus praeter naturalis and Jacques Lisfranc pioneered the method of perineal resection of the rectum for cancer.
- The first rectoscope was constructed in 1895, and in 1903 Kelly introduced it into practice.
- A swift progress in the diagnosis and treatment of anorectal diseases occurred after the World War II, and the trend has continued to this day.

SUGGESTED READINGS

Ashrafian H. Arius of Alexandria (256–336 AD): the first reported mortality from rectal prolapse. *Int J Colorectal Dis*. 2014;29(4):539.

Banov L, Jr. An historical sketch of proctology from ancient Egypt to modern South Carolina. *J S C Med Assoc*. 1985;81(7):359–60.

Bonello JC, Cohen H, Gorlin RJ. Of heliotropes and haemorrhoids: St. Fiacre patron saint of gardeners and haemorrhoid sufferers. *Dis Colon Rectum*. 1985;28:702–4.

Ellesmore W, Charles MV. Surgical History of Haemorrhoids. In: *Surgical Treatment of Haemorrhoids*. London: Springer; 2002;1–4.

Glaser S. Hippocrates and proctology. *Proc R Soc Med*. 1969;62(4):380–1.

Guardasole A. A look at the Hippocratic Treatise on haemorrhoids in the Byzantine era. *Stud Anc Med*. 2005;31:457–63.

Vieni S, Latteri F, Grassi N. Historical aspects of a frequent anal disease: haemorrhoids. *Chir Ital*. 2004;56:745–8.

Viso L, Uriach J. The 'guardians of the anus' and their practice. *Int J Colorectal Dis*. 1995;10(4):229–31.

Viso Pons L. The analysis of a basic legacy. Hippocrates and proctology. *Rev Esp Enferm Dig*. 1991;80(5):348–51.

Wake WC. Who Was Hippocrates? *The Listener*. 1966:968.

Welling DR, Wolff BG, Dozois RR. Piles of defeat: Napoleon at Waterloo. *Dis Colon Rectum*. 1988;31:303–5.

Chapter 2

The rectum and the anal canal

Developmentally, the anorectal region is composite in structure, comprising two tube-like components, one within the other. The inner visceral part comprises the termination of the alimentary tract and contains only smooth muscle innervated by the autonomic nervous system. The outer (somatic) component comprises skeletal muscle which forms the external sphincter. The muscle is mainly under reflex control but is also influenced by conscious motivation. This component not only has a sphincteric action, but its upper part is continuous with the levator ani muscles which fan out to close the pelvic hiatus.

The rectum begins as an ill-defined anatomical location; however, surgically, the rectosigmoid junction lies in opposition to the sacral promontory. The rectum usually follows the curve of the sacrum to end at the anorectal junction. Over this intersection, the puborectalis muscle encircles the posterior and lateral aspects of the junction, creating the anorectal angle (usually 120°). The outer layer of the rectum, unlike the colon, is covered circumferentially by longitudinal muscle; the colon is covered by the three taeniae bands. When the rectum collapses, it appears as a nearly straight tube following the curve of the sacrum; however, during distension, it becomes distinctly sacculated. The part of the rectum that lies below the middle valve is much wider in diameter than the upper one-third and is better known as the ampulla of the rectum. These valves are chiefly made up of connective tissues and circular muscular fibres overlapped with mucous membrane.

The adult rectum is about 18–20 cm in length and is divided into three equal parts. The upper one-third is mobile and has a peritoneal coat except near to the middle one-third where only the anterior and part of the lateral surfaces are covered with the peritoneum. The middle one-third is the widest part of the rectum and is conned within the diameter of the bony pelvis. Moreover, the lowest one-third lies within the muscular floor of the pelvis and has significant relations to fascial layers (Figure 2.1).

A fascial condensation (Denonvilliers' fascia) separates the lowest part of the rectum in front from the prostate and the Waldeyer's fascia from last two sacral vertebrae and the coccyx separates it from behind. These fascial layers act as a barrier to malignant penetration, have significant surgical importance, and are valuable guides during surgery.

The lowest part of the rectum is covered with endopelvic fascia and is free of peritoneum. The fascia is quite strong to cover the entire anterior surface of the sacrum and the underlying vessels and nerves. The presacral fascia runs forward and downward at around the level

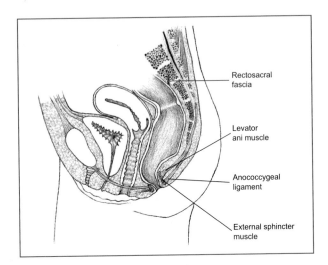

Figure 2.1 Anatomy of the rectum.

Illustration: James Oinam.

of S-4, and attaches to the rectum. This part or space is referred to as the recto sacral fascia. The lateral endopelvic fascia, which is thicker, is referred to as the lateral rectal stalks.

The peritoneum covers the upper two-thirds and upper one-third of the rectum anteriorly and laterally. The anterior peritoneal reflection ends at about 6–8 cm from the anal verge.

ANAL CANAL

The anal canal runs from the level of the levator ani to the anal margin. In an adult, it is about 4 cm long and is wrapped by muscular sphincters. The arrangement of these muscles, the character of the epithelial lining, and the nature of the subepithelial tissues are all relevant to anal and perianal disorders (Figure 2.2). The visceral component of the anal canal has a longitudinal layer of muscle, a circular layer (the internal sphincter), submucosa, and mucosa. The internal sphincter is a relatively large muscle mass that superficially resembles the thickened segment of the circular muscle of the lower rectum. There are, however, profound functional and anatomical differences between them.

The upper half of the anal canal is lined by columnar, mucous-secreting epithelium identical to that of the rectum. In the course of development, ectoderm migrates into the lower half of the anal canal which, as a result, is lined by squamous epithelium. The importance of this is that it is dry and does not secrete mucous; it is also richly innervated by the pudendal nerve and plays an important part in the maintenance of continence. The mucocutaneous junction, about half way along the anal canal, is fixed to the underlying internal sphincter so that columnar epithelium cannot prolapse externally. The somatic or

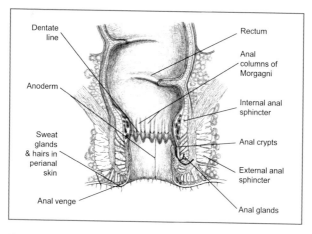

Figure 2.2   Anal canal.

Illustration: James Oinam.

skeletal muscle component of the pelvic floor comprises the external sphincter, the puborectalis, and the levator ani muscles (pubococcygeus and iliococcygeus). The external sphincter is usually divided into three parts, but functionally it is a unit. The innervation is derived from the inferior haemorrhoidal nerve.

The muscular wall of the anal canal continues from the circular muscular layer of the rectum, is thickened, and is termed as the internal sphincter. The internal sphincter continues down the anal canal for a distance of about 2.5 cm and ends at the skin margin, and it has been called as the 'white line of Hilton'. The anal canal is encircled by two muscles, the external sphincter and the puborectalis, which form three U-shaped loops.

The puborectal muscle which originates from the pubis forms the first loop. The intermediate loop originates at the tip of the coccyx and is known as the anococcygeal ligament. It comprises the superficial external sphincter. The basal loop is made of a subcutaneous portion of the external sphincter muscle (Figure 2.3). The cephalad end of the anal canal, where the internal sphincter muscle is thickened and is wrapped by the puborectal muscle, is called the anorectal ring. Though one can see it on proctoscopic examination, one cannot palpate it.

From the level of the anorectal ring caudally and between the internal and external sphincter muscles, fibres of the puborectal and levator ani muscles merge with the longitudinal muscle coat of the rectum to form the conjoined longitudinal muscle. These muscle fibres traverse the lower portion of the distal external sphincter to be inserted in the perianal skin that causes wrinkling of the anal verge and is called as the corrugator cutis ani.

At about the centre of the anal canal, about 2 cm from the anal verge, is a surging demarcation called the dentate or pectinate line.

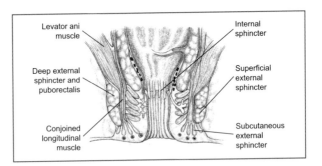

Figure 2.3 The musculature of the anal canal.

Illustration: James Oinam.

The dentate line is nothing but a remnant of the embryonic procto-deal membrane, that is, the juncture of the endoderm and ectoderm. While distal to the dentate line, the anal epithelium looks like the skin except that it is non-keratinised and is devoid of hair or glandular structures. This part is also called as the anoderm. This lining becomes that of true keratinised skin with hair, sebaceous glands, and sweat glands.

Between the anal margin and the lower border of the internal sphincter, the anal canal is lined with skin containing hairs, sebaceous and sweat glands, and large apocrine glands, the so-called circumanal glands of Gay. The next 10–15 mm of the canal, originally called the 'pecten', is lined by stratified squamous epithelium. This is devoid of hairs and glands but has a thin horny layer. At or below the anal valves, the epithelium becomes stratified columnar or thinner stratified squamous epithelium with surface cells more cuboidal than in the pecten. The boundary between epithelial types is very ragged, and longitudinal sections of the same anal canal can show differing epithelial relationships. It is not unusual to find islands of columnar epithelium amid stratified squamous epithelium. These occur more commonly between anal columns, while the columns themselves are usually covered with stratified squamous or cuboidal epithelium.

The zone of stratified squamous, cuboidal, or columnar epithelium extends proximally from the anal valves for a variable distance of 5–10 mm, to its sinuous, but somewhat abrupt, junction with rectal-type mucosa. Rectal-type mucosa, with tubular intestinal glands, lines the canal up to its proximal termination at the level of the levator ani. Although the anal valves and columns are not always apparent, they provide the only unambiguous macroscopic landmark. Because of the possibilities of confusion, terms such as 'ano-cutaneous' or 'mucocutaneous' are best avoided in descriptions of operative procedures.

The lining of the anal canal proximal to the pectinate line is thrown into pleats or columns due to the reducing size of the canal as it moves distally. The columns, 5–15 in number, are termed the columns of Morgagni. These columns end as small hollows, which are called as the crypts of Morgagni, and the free edges of the mucous membrane that guard the crypts are the anal valves. At the lower end of each column, and between each column, is a small pocket named the anal crypts that are connected to the anal glands.

Anal glands begin at the crypt and extend behind and outwards. The passage of the anal glands is bordered by squamous epithelium. This epithelium transits into a columnar epithelium deep in the gland. Interspersed along the length of this epithelium lies the mucous-secreting cells or goblet cells. They secrete into the anal canal via anal ducts that open into the anal crypts along the level of the dentate line. The glands are usually located at varying depths in the anal canal wall, some of them being between the layers of the internal and external sphincter (the inter-sphincteric plane). The cryptoglandular theory is based on the obstruction of these ducts due to an accumulation of foreign material in the crypts, to lead to perianal suppurations and abscess and fistula formation.

All but the most distal part of the anal canal is surrounded by a double sleeve of muscle. The outer layer is striated and comprises the external sphincter and the puborectalis portion of the levator ani. The inner layer is made up of circularly arranged smooth muscle fibres. The layers are separated by a tissue space containing longitudinally arranged muscle fibres continuous with the longitudinal muscle layer of the rectum. This inter-sphincteric space has a strategic role as it often contains the anal glands, structures which are thought to be implicated in the pathogenesis of anal abscess and fistula. There are eight to twelve of these glands and their ducts pass through the internal sphincter and drain into the anal canal at the bases of the anal crypts. The 'inter-sphincteric space' is important surgically for it is a plane for excision of the rectum and anal canal in inflammatory bowel disease.

It is usual to divide the external sphincter into subcutaneous, superficial, and deep parts. There is, however, little distinction between the three sections and from the surgeon's point of view the external sphincter, together with the levator ani, forms a continuous muscle sheet. The deep part of the external sphincter and the puborectalis in conjunction with the internal sphincter forms the palpable inter-sphincteric groove. The longitudinal muscle that lies between the two sphincters ends by fanning out into numerous fascicles which traverse the subcutaneous part of the external sphincter and attach to the overlying epithelium. It is agreed that they provide pathways for the spread of perianal infections and that the intense pain of perianal lesions is due to the way they divide the subepithelial tissue into tight compartments.

The levator ani, a broad, slim muscle, and the iliococcygeal muscle make the pelvic floor. It is innervated by the fourth sacral nerve. The levator ani muscle has been traditionally considered to consist of three muscles—iliococcygeal, pubococcygeal, and puborectal (Figure 2.4). The puborectal and levator ani muscles have corresponding actions; as one contracts, the other relaxes. During defecation, puborectal relaxation is accompanied by levator ani contraction, which widens the hiatus and elevates the lower rectum and anal

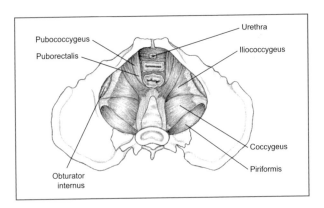

Figure 2.4 Pelvic floor musculature.

Illustration: James Oinam.

canal. When a person is in standing position, the levator ani muscle supports the viscera.

The puborectalis muscle, probably the most powerful, arises from the pubic ramus near the midline anteriorly and passes behind the upper anal canal as a sling. It, therefore, has a sphincteric action on all the viscera of the pelvic hiatus and at the same time has the important task of maintaining the angulation between the lower rectum and the anal canal. The levator ani muscles have no sphincteric activity but have an antigravity function, that is, preventing herniation of the viscera through the pelvis. Innervation of the levator ani muscles, and probably the puborectalis, comes from the branch of S4 which descends on their internal surface. On the other hand, the vessels of the skeletal muscles of the pelvic floor enter via their external aspect.

In between the two components of the pelvic floor, there is an embryonic plane of fusion. In the normal person, very few blood vessels cross this plane and practically no nervous structures. It is of practical importance in as much as fistula tracts tend to spread within it. In addition, it is a useful plane of dissection for certain operative procedures, as no important structures are encountered.

There are some areolar tissue filled clinically significant potential spaces surrounding the anorectal region as they are sites where abscesses can form (Figure 2.5). The perianal area encloses the anus. The perianal area is laterally in continuity with the subcutaneous fat of the gluteal region and medially bounded by the anoderm to the level of the dentate line. The ischioanal space is like a triangle lying below the levator ani muscle that is bounded medially by the external sphincter complex, laterally by the ischial bone, and inferiorly by the transverse septum of the ischiorectal fossa. The ischioanal space on both sides is occupied by fat and contains the inferior rectal vessels and lymphatics. The deep postanal space attaches the ischioanal space on each side posteriorly and lies in the middle of the levator ani muscle above and the anococcygeal ligament below. The deep postanal

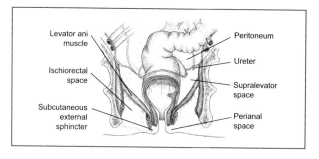

Figure 2.5 Spaces around the rectum and anal canal.

Illustration: James Oinam.

space is an essential pathway in the formation of abscess; it is spread from one ischiorectal fossa to the other, resulting in a so-called horse-shoe abscess. The inter-sphincteric space lies amongst the internal and external sphincter muscles. It is constant with the perianal space below and extends above into the wall of the rectum. The supra levator spaces are situated on each side of the rectum above the levator ani. The supra levator spaces communicate posteriorly and may allow a spread of infection cephalad into the retroperitoneum.

ISCHIORECTAL FOSSE

The ischiorectal fossae are fascia-lined wedge-shaped spaces that are found on the sides of the anal canal and rectum. They are the spaces that lie above the skin of the anal canal and under the roof of the perineum that is formed by the levator ani muscles. These two fossae communicate posteriorly, behind the anal canal via the retro anal space of Courtney. These fossae act as distensible space fillers while also giving support to the anal canal. The ischiorectal fossae are filled with adipose tissue that is infiltrated with numerous fibrous bands and few septa, part of which are derived from the longitudinal muscle of the anal canal, and this adipose tissue is notable for its tough and stringy nature.

The ischiorectal fossae help in distension of rectum and the anal canal during the passage of faeces. Both the perianal and ischiorectal spaces are the usual site of abscess formation. As the blood supply is poor and coarse, the lobulated fat predisposes it to infection. The ischiorectal abscess is the result of a spread of infection from the nearby area as the skin, the lumen of the bowel, or perirectal tissue above the levator ani, or through blood or lymphatics. They can be drained liberally because of the poor vascularity of the fossa, but it should be done gently to avoid injury to inferior rectal neuromuscular bundle and prevent paralysis of the external sphincter.

Blood Supply

The superior rectal artery is a branch of the inferior mesenteric artery and is the primary arterial supply of the rectum. In front of the third

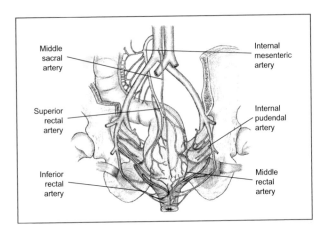

Figure 2.6 Blood supply to the rectum and the anal canal.

Illustration: James Oinam.

sacral vertebra, the artery divides behind the lower one-third of the rectum into two branches—one anterior and another posterior. The arteries and their associated lymphatics are kept embedded at the back of the rectum by the mesorectum or 'rectal fascia', which is a dense connective tissue.

The middle rectal artery arises on each side from the internal iliac artery (Figure 2.6) and passes to the rectum in the lateral ligaments. It is usually tiny and breaks up into several terminal branches. However, the middle rectal arteries are inconsistent and cannot be relied on after ligation of the superior rectal artery.

The inferior rectal artery is a branch of the internal pudendal artery that enters the Alcock's canal. It joins the inferior surface of the levator ani muscle while crossing the roof of the ischiorectal fossa to get into the anal muscles.

Although no extramural anastomoses are seen on cadaver dissection between the superior, middle, and inferior rectal arteries, arteriography shows quite abundant intramural anastomoses between them, notably in the lower rectum. The middle sacral artery does not supply any significant amount of blood to the rectum. It arises posteriorly, just above the bifurcation of the aorta, and ascends over the lumbar vertebrae, sacrum, and coccyx.

Venous Drainage

The tributaries of the superior and inferior haemorrhoidal veins lie in separate but poorly defined spaces in the subepithelial tissue. Their boundaries and the nature and attachment of the smooth muscle which they contain are disputed. Clinical observation suggests that there is some tethering of the epithelial lining of the canal. In the article 'Pathogenesis and treatment of fistula-in-ano', Parks suggests that this occurs at the level of the valves, the epithelium being held in place by strands of fibrous tissue that he calls the 'mucosal suspensory ligament' near the dentate line which divides the space into the 'submucous' to the space above the valves, and 'marginal' to space below. The venous drainage of the rectum and anal canal parallels the arterial supply. Therefore, blood from the rectum and upper part of the anal canal returns through the superior rectal veins into the portal system, whereas the middle and inferior rectal veins empty into the caval circulation.

Whatever the details of the distribution, there is undoubtedly more connective tissue underlying the epithelium which covers the distal part of the internal sphincter than that covering the proximal end. According to some, the smooth muscle in this region is merely the inferior extension of the muscularis mucosae of the rectum, while others consider it to consist of separate muscles; the 'corrugator cutis ani' in the anal margin, and the 'muscularis submucosae ani' within the distal part of the canal.

Lymphatics from the upper and middle parts of the rectum ascend along the superior rectal artery and subsequently drain into the inferior mesenteric lymph nodes. The bottom of the rectum drains upwards by way of the superior rectal lymphatics to the inferior mesenteric nodes, and laterally via the middle rectal lymphatics to the internal iliac nodes. Lymphatics drain cephalad through the superior rectal lymphatics into the inferior mesenteric nodes and laterally along both the middle and inferior rectal vessels through the ischioanal fossa to the internal iliac nodes from the anal canal above the dentate line. Lymphatics lying below the dentate line mostly drain to the inguinal nodes. In case of obstruction to the primary drainage it may drain to the superior rectal lymph nodes or along the inferior rectal lymphatics to the ischioanal fossa.

Sympathetic and parasympathetic nerves of the autonomic nervous system innervate the anorectum, and few branches are sent to the adjacent urogenital organs. Nerve trunks lie very close to the rectum that is prone to injury during mobilisation of the rectum, and specific precautions should be taken during such dissection.

Sympathetic nerve fibres to the rectum originate from the first three lumbar segments of the spinal cord. These fibres pass through ganglionated sympathetic chains before forming the preaortic plexus. Preaortic fibres extend below the bifurcation of the aorta to form the hypogastric plexus or the presacral nerve.

The plexus thus formed is divided into left and right branches on each side of the pelvis and is joined by the parasympathetic nerves. The nervi erigentes supply the pelvic parasympathetic nerve, which originates from the second, third, and fourth sacral nerve roots. These fibres pass inward and forward to join the sympathetic nerve fibres and form the pelvic plexus.

The pelvic plexus on each side is encased in the midst of the lateral stalk, which is situated just above the levator ani muscle. From each pelvic, both types of nerve fibres are distributed to urinary and genital organs.

The pelvic plexus produces the periprostatic plexus, which is an important subdivision needed for sexual function in men. This periprostatic plexus distributes fibres to the prostate, corpora cavernosa, seminal vesicles, last part of the vas deferens, ejaculatory ducts, prostatic and membranous urethra, and bulbourethral glands. The erection is governed both by the sympathetic and parasympathetic nervous systems. Nerve impulses from the parasympathetic nerves lead to an erection and produce vasodilatation and increase blood flow in the cavernous spaces of the penis. The activity of the sympathetic system adds to vascular engorgement and sustained erection.

The importance of the squamous mucosa of the lower 2 cm of the anal canal has been mentioned. Its rich innervation gives rise to conscious sensory information. If flatus or faeces enter the anal canal, stimulation of the receptors causes immediate contraction of the external sphincter. The internal sphincter itself maintains closure of the anal canal in the resting state. The effective length of the sphincter can be observed by inserting a pressure probe into the lower rectum and drawing it down through the canal, recording the pressure changes 'en route'. The length (about 3.5 cm) is greater in men than women by about half centimetre and is unrelated to age or parity. The resting pressure is the same for men and women and diminishes with increasing age in both sexes.

The maximal pressure is found a half way along the internal sphincter; this is also observed in patients with a Cauda Equina lesion, a lesion of the sacral nerve roots and after the transaction of the spinal cord serial distension of the rectum with small volumes produces transient relaxation of internal sphincter after each increment. With each increment, the baseline pressure falls and after a rectal distension of between 150 and 200 mL, the internal sphincter completely relaxes; the balloon descends into the anal canal, and only minimal straining is required to expel it.

In patients with Hirschsprung's disease, the reflex is absent, and the internal sphincter fails to relax at all. In this condition, the intrinsic neural plexus of the rectum is abnormal, which suggests that the receptor site is in the viscus itself.

The skeletal muscles of the pelvic floor have a dual role—they combat the force of intra-abdominal pressure, thus preventing a pelvic hernia, and the external sphincter group (which includes the puborectalis muscle) plays the most important part in the maintenance of continence. Muscles which are actuated only by voluntary means would be useless for the task of maintaining continence or of combating gravitational forces, as the person's attention would need to be continually drawn to them. An automatic mechanism is essential. If an electromyographic needle is inserted into most skeletal muscle, no electrical activity at all is found at rest; it only develops as a result of the voluntary or synergistic activity.

The pelvic floor is entirely different; the muscles are constantly contracting at rest and even during sleep. However, this is not all as, using automatic reflex action, the muscles will either additionally contract or relax according to circumstance. Thus, when intra-abdominal pressure rises (for example, as a result of coughing, walking, or lifting), there is a rapid reflex reinforcement of the tonic activity of the pelvic floor muscles to resist this pressure. Voluntary contraction can be sustained for about 60 seconds but not much longer, after which activity fades.

MOTOR INNERVATION

The sympathetic and parasympathetic nerves innervate and induce inhibition of the internal anal sphincter. The external sphincter is supplied by the inferior rectal branch of the internal pudendal nerve and the perineal branch of the fourth sacral nerve. The levator ani is supplied both by the pudendal and the last three sacral nerves, where the fifth nerve is lying above the pelvic floor.

SENSORY INNERVATION

The inferior rectal nerve, a branch of the pudendal nerve, innervates the anal canal by sensory nerve endings close to the vicinity of the dentate line. Painful sensations in the anal canal are present at sites up to 1.5 cm proximal to the dentate line.

The anal canal is relatively short in women than men (3–7 cm vs 4–6 cm respectively). It has a high-pressure zone resulting from tonic contraction of the two sphincters, which is responsible for continence. Voluntary contraction may double this pressure (squeeze pressure).

Distension of the rectum by a balloon first increases the activity of the skeletal muscles. This again will protect against involuntary evacuation. When inflated to a greater size, reflex relaxation of the entire sphincter mass occurs. While this rarely occurs in normal circumstances, it is seen in cases such as the occurrence of impaction of faeces in patients with idiopathic megacolon, in the old and in some post-operative states. Here, the rectum is grossly overloaded, and the external sphincters are totally patulous. The main complaint of such a patient will be incontinence; he has no control over defecation. Liquid stool passing around the impacted mass leaks out without let or hindrance. This unusual physiological state also has clinical relevance, demanding vigilance on the part of the doctor, especially when looking after the elderly. Fortunately, it can be readily treated.

The mechanical valve effect is maintained by the tonic contraction of the external sphincter and puborectalis muscles. The lower rectum makes a double right angle just before and on entering the upper anal canal. As a result, the upper part of the canal is closed by the anterior wall of the lower rectum, which impinges upon it. Any increase in abdominal pressure will automatically force that part of the lower rectal wall even more firmly upon the closed upper anal canal and will block it, provided the anal sphincters remain active. In this way, a flap valve is formed between zones of high and low pressure. Thus, any increase in abdominal pressure will automatically seal the upper anal canal and prevent stress incontinence occurring. The angulation between the anal canal and lower rectum is maintained by the puborectalis muscle.

Assessment of any sensation, whether qualitative or quantitative, is always difficult. However, there is no doubt that in a normal person rectal distension produces a sensation of fullness in the perineum associated with a feeling of impending evacuation. Distension above the ampulla produces only intestinal abdominal colic. It was originally thought that receptors responsible for 'rectal' sensation were present in the rectal wall. Recently, however, it has been shown that the sensory mechanism remains intact even after total excision of the rectum with anastomosis of the colon to the upper anal canal. It is, therefore, apparent that the rectum itself is not the site of sensory information. The rectal ampulla lies in a cradle formed by the levator ani muscles, and it is probable that changes in volume stimulate stretch receptors in these muscles. Further evidence for this comes from patients who have had total excision of the colon and rectum for ulcerative colitis and have been given a pelvic pouch anastomosed to the anal canal. As the pouch distends, they get a sensation identical with that experienced in their previously normal state.

In summary, the internal sphincter keeps the anal canal closed and provides a pressure gradient acting against the rectum, the latter functioning as a reservoir for faeces and flatus. The tone of the levator ani and external sphincter is maintained by a reflex arc. Sensory impulses arise from receptors in the pelvic floor muscles and the squamous mucosa of the anal canal, providing information at both reflex and conscious levels. The tonic contractile activity of the pelvic floor muscles continually adjusts to changes in abdominal pressure. Contraction of the puborectalis muscle, situated at the anorectal junction, maintains the right angle between the axis of the rectal ampulla and the anal canal itself. This, in turn, establishes a flap valve mechanism, which automatically occludes the upper anal canal. The seal of the valve is usually only broken by intraluminal contents entering the lower part of the ampulla.

CLINICAL PEARLS

- The anal canal is the most terminal part of the lower gastrointestinal (GI) tract and lies between the anal verge (anal orifice, anus) in the perineum below and the rectum above.
- The pigmented, keratinised perianal skin has skin appendages like hair, sweat glands, and sebaceous glands.
- The demarcation between the rectum above and the anal canal below is the anorectal ring or anorectal flexure, where the puborectalis muscle forms a sling around the posterior aspect of the anorectal junction.
- The epithelium of the anal canal between the anal verge below and the pectinate line above is described as the anoderm; it looks like skin, is very sensitive, and is keratinised.
- The pectinate line is the site of transition of the proctodeum below and the post allantoic gut above.

(Cont'd)

- At the bottom of anal columns are anal sinuses or crypts, into which open the anal glands and anal papillae. Infection of the anal glands is likely the initial event in the causation of perianal abscess and fistula-in-ano.
- Three of these columns are prominent; they are called anal cushions and contain branches and tributaries of superior haemorrhoidal artery and vein. When prominent, veins in these cushions form the internal haemorrhoids.
- The terminal branches of the superior rectal (haemorrhoidal) artery supply the anal canal above the dentate line, which is the terminal branch of the inferior mesenteric artery. The middle rectal artery (a branch of the internal iliac artery) and the inferior rectal artery (a branch of the internal pudendal artery) supply the lower anal canal.

SUGGESTED READINGS

Cirocco WC, Reilly JC. Challenging the predictive accuracy of Goodsall's rule for anal fistulas. *Dis Colon Rectum*. 1992;35:537–42.

Dailey AR. The riddle of the sphincters, the morphophysiology of the anorectal mechanism reviewed. *Am Surg*. 1987;53:298–306.

Goligher JC. Surgical anatomy and physiology of the colon, rectum, and anus. In: *Surgery of the Anus, Rectum, and Colon* 5th ed., Goligher JC (ed.). London: Balliere-Tindall;1984.

Parks AG. Pathogenesis and treatment of fistula-in-ano. *Br Med J*. 1961;1:463–9.

Pead RK, Monsen H, Abcarian H. Surgical anatomy of the pelvic autonomic nerves, a practical approach. *Am Surg*. 1986;52:236–7.

Pearl RK. Anorectal fistula; role of the seton. In: *Current Surgical Therapy* 4th ed., Cameron JL (ed.). St. Louis:Mosby-Year Book 1992.

Prasad ML, Read DR, Abcarian H. Supralevator abscess: diagnosis and treatment. *Dis Colon Rectum*. 1981;24:456–61.

Rociu E, Stoker J, Eiijkemans MJC, Lameris JS. Normal anal sphincter anatomy and age and sex-related variations at high spatial-resolution endoanal MR imaging. *Radiology*. 2000;217:395–401.

Seow-Choen F, Ho JM. Histoanatomy of anal glands. *Dis Colon Rectum*. l994;37:1215–18.

Shafik A. A new concept of the anatomy of the anal sphincter mechanism and the physiology of defecation. The external anal sphincter: a triple-loop system. *Invest Urol*. 1975;12:412–19.

Chapter 3

Examination of the patient with proctological complaints

Perhaps in no other region of the body does one find more opportunities for effective diagnosis than in the case of the rectum. Unfortunately, ignorance of methods of analysis and arriving at a clinical diagnosis is surprisingly rampant among most of the medical practitioners who have graduated recently. The interns at hospitals come with a little idea of even the anatomy of the rectum and anus. The frequency with which rectal examination is performed in general practice is inadequate. Up to two-thirds of patients who present with anorectal symptoms do not undergo a rectal examination and are rarely referred to a specialist. It is unfortunate as a third of rectal cancers are palpable, and omission of the routine anorectal examination may lead to delays in referral for resectable malignancy. Various factors contribute to rectal examinations not being conducted. These include apathy of family physicians towards such patients; longer stay, which may get prolonged for up to two weeks, for outpatient to avail expert services from the coloproctologist for the rectal examination; male patients shying away from such an examination by a female practitioner; or cases where a patient is too ill to undergo a rectal examination.

Several factors can aid a thorough rectal examination: interpersonal skills that allow for a good doctor–patient rapport and open communication; knowledge of detailed examination required and supplemented by instructional materials explaining the examination; adopting an orderly, thorough, and gentle examination technique; and sharing complete findings and feedback with the patient.

Thus, a rectal examination should be recognised as a speciality as much as any other, and indeed should be taught more thoroughly in our medical schools by competent teachers.

An almost accurate diagnosis can be achieved with the patient history and confirmation by visual inspection, anoscopy, and rectoscopy. Bleeding per rectum, anal pruritus, irritation, and proctodynia rank among the most common symptoms of anal diseases seen in primary care practices.

OBTAINING THE HISTORY

The best practice is to listen to the patient. The discussion will give a clue to diagnosis. The patient's history with anorectal ailments, with careful and focused elaboration, should be the starting point. Patients suffering from any symptom related to the anal region often incorrectly think that their symptoms are because of haemorrhoids.

Someone has rightly said that nearly every lesion around the anus is invariably called 'piles' by the patient and at times even by his or her physician. There is a well-known saying, 'Practically, everybody experiences haemorrhoids eventually in their lives'.

When a patient has described his primary symptom, a checklist of few other symptoms must be ensured. This includes the following features.

Bleeding

The pattern of bleeding can be helpful in pointing to a diagnosis and indicating the evaluation. Is bleeding associated with a bowel movement; what is the amount of bleeding—a little soiling on the tissue or a significant amount in the toilet; does it come in a jet in different directions of the pan—the answers to these simple questions can give important clues in a diagnosis.

The type of the bleeding should also be noticed; whether the blood is fresh, purely liquid, or coming as clots. If the blood seen in the pan is pure, it is mostly because of the haemorrhoidal bleeding and is unlikely to be with fissures. Bleeding related to rectal or colonic malignancies is more often dark and mixed with not only faeces, but with flatus, and is an ominous symptom.

Occasionally, a patient feels the call to defecate and is surprised at passing the large volume of blood on one occasion only. This is almost diagnostic of diverticulosis. Rarely, women confuse rectal bleeding with either vaginal bleeding or haematuria.

Pain

The causes of anal pain may include the anal fissure, perianal abscess, levator ani syndrome, or a thrombosed external haemorrhoid. The history is diagnostic in most cases, and physical examination is only to reconfirm the cause. Any association between pain and bowel movements is important to determine the lesion. Significant pain with bowel movements that then recedes is usually an anal fissure. Anal abscesses and thrombosed haemorrhoids can be seen with exacerbation of pain during bowel movements but mostly manifest with a persistent pain that does not alter with bowel activities. Pain due to levator spasm is relieved after a bowel movement. Another information that may be obtained from the history is that thrombosed external haemorrhoids (TEH) usually start with a lump that becomes progressively more painful. Anal abscesses usually start with pain and swelling occurs later. Anal fissures usually start after a hard or strenuous passage of stool. Levator spasm begins following prolonged sitting, mostly in patients experiencing increased stress in life.

The presence of a rectal malignancy is suggested by tenesmus or a change in calibre of stool. Cutting or shearing pain with bowel movements indicates a fissure. Constant, nagging pain progressing over time may be associated with anal cancer with the invasion of the sphincter complex. A complaint of a firm or soft mass peeping out while defecation, and is either reducing on its own or with manual push, is suggestive of either advanced grades of haemorrhoids or full-thickness rectal prolapse calling for a specific investigation.

Itching

The differential diagnosis for itching includes pruritus ani, pinworms, dermatoses (for example, lichen sclerosis et atrophicus), Bowen's or Paget's disease, and anal warts. Perianal itching and burning (pruritus ani) are usually an indication of repeated irritation or trauma. The underlying cause could be any condition that produces repeated wetness onto the perianal tissues. Often, the patient himself is unwittingly causing or worsening the problem since most patients with anal discomfort clean the area with soap or by frequent scrubbing.

Prolapse

The differential diagnosis of prolapse includes internal or external haemorrhoids, rectal prolapse, and hypertrophic anal papilla. An in-depth history will clinch the diagnosis and treatment. Painless prolapse that reduces spontaneously, and is associated with bright red bleeding, is usually second-degree haemorrhoids.

Lump

History of a lump, which is prominently present at the anus, may be an anal haematoma, a skin tag, a sentinel pile, or prolapsed internal haemorrhoids or external haemorrhoids.

Lump appearing on defecation indicates internal haemorrhoids, an anal polyp, or a complete rectal or mucosal prolapse.

Discharge

A mucoid discharge may be due to carcinoma, proctocolitis, villous papilloma, or protruding internal haemorrhoids or rectal prolapse. A purulent discharge is mostly from an abscess or anal fistula.

Bowel Movements

When a patient complains of diarrhoea, it is worth enquiring carefully whether its onset followed a course of an antibiotic. Morning diarrhoea, real not spurious, and without other symptoms are unlikely to be due to organic disease.

Past History

A complete medical history is necessary, and this should include a medication review. Some drug therapy may aggravate anorectal symptoms by causing dyschezia (for example, calcium channel blockers) or frequent stools (for example, proton pump inhibitors). They may contribute to haematochezia (for example, Coumadin, nonsteroidal anti-inflammatory drugs). Patients might not be remembering procedures that have been performed in the past. One should elicit a history of anorectal surgery. Other abdominal operations, which the patient may think unimportant but may lead to gastrointestinal symptoms, should be specifically questioned. Symptoms related to such procedures, like incontinence, may also reveal the aetiology of the current complaint, as well as provide information to counsel the patient if any additional surgery is required. Any previous investigations like flexible sigmoidoscopy or colonoscopy may be significant, so is the history of polypectomy performed along with one of these procedures. Although a rare cause of rectal bleeding, anal trauma attributable to anal intercourse should also be included to complete the history.

THE ANORECTAL EXAMINATION

Most patients with anorectal disease are scared, embarrassed, uncomfortable, and nervous. A relaxed, silent, and professional approach helps in gaining the trust of the patient. To be more elaborate, few anatomic models, figures, and videos may help address a patient's queries and clarify any doubts. A separate examination room that is peaceful is quite helpful; an examination table behind flimsy curtains may not make the patient feel comfortable. It is advisable to have the patient's body as much covered as possible. An associate, for instance a member of the nursing staff, should be asked to be present during the examination. The aim to have such a person is not only to aid the examiner, but also to make the patient feel secure. Additionally, instances of alleged physical abuse are more likely during the intimate examination and this practice would help counter such situations. If there is someone accompanying the patient, they could be asked if they would like to stay during the examination, as a chaperone. It is often experienced that the patient's attitude towards such an examination is guided by previous experiences, both positive and negative, as well as by cultural or religious beliefs in some cases.

The advantages of different examination positions for determination of the causes of anal symptoms are unknown. The knee–elbow position provides a better field of view than the routinely used left lateral Sims' position, as the buttocks fall apart, and fingertips of the investigator are free for the eversion of the anal skin under a good lighting. However, the major drawback of this position is that haemorrhoids fall back in the knee–elbow position due to the sloping stature of the patient and hence they are unable to protrude. The Sims' position is relatively more comfortable, as the patients achieve it easily and quickly by themselves; saving the investigating physician's time towards manoeuvring the patient in a particular position. The hips of the patient should be at the edge of the bed or on the examining table.

The left leg is extended while the right knee is flexed, and the right thigh is drawn up to the abdomen. The left arm is brought back to the patient, which allows the patient's chest to touch the examination table. The hips are in the vertical line. The patient is instructed to take deep breaths allowing the abdominal muscles to relax. If the patient is thus placed, the bowels tend to fall away from the pelvis, as in the knee–elbow or inverted position, to facilitate the examination.

A weak, frail, and old or a semiconscious patient may be examined in a supine position with the knees and hips flexed closed to the abdomen by an assistant (modified lithotomy position). Another position for rectal examination is standing up and leaning over the examination couch. This certainly provides a better hand position to the examining doctor for prostate palpation but not necessarily for the rest of the rectal walls. Instead, you can show a picture to your patient about how to take the position, rather than giving many instructions to make him do what you want (Figure 3.1).

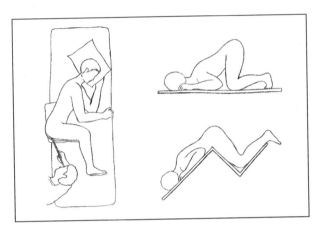

Figure 3.1 Positions for anorectal examination.

Illustration: James Oinam.

EXTERNAL INSPECTION

The external examination should be the first step in evaluation. Much information can be obtained by careful inspection of the entire area. An insightful external examination can give much information and gives enough time for the patient to become mentally prepared to allow for the internal examination. However, do not rush inspection. Spreading the buttocks with gentleness will help visualisation of the entire skin-covered portion of the anal canal possible. At the same time, the patient should also be asked to strain as if he is passing stool. Valsalva manoeuvre may further aid in the examination of a long anal canal or a funnel-shaped anus. If the patient is in the Sims' position, separate the buttocks by using your left hand to lift up the right buttock. Another way is to press on both buttocks with both hands. You should now have a clear view of the sacrococcygeal, peri-anal, and anal area. The sacrococcygeal area can be the site of various sinuses or even a high anal fistula. The presence of a pilonidal sinus is suggested by swelling or mass, scars, oedema, sinus openings, and abundance of hair around. It is usually sited some distance from the anus, in the midline of the natal cleft.

The perianal area often has abnormalities of the skin. Hutchinson describes the variation from mild erythema to red, raw dermatitis. These dermal afflictions can be the result of excoriation from diarrhoea and, which when becomes chronic develops in a thickened white skin leading to exaggerate the anal skin folds, forming anal skin tags.

Skin tags can be due to many causes:

- Chronic inflammation and irritation in cases of pruritus ani
- Chronic haemorrhoids
- Sentinel pile from a chronic anal fissure
- Crohn's disease

Skin tags may be confused with anal warts (condylomata acuminata), but warts are usually pedunculated with a white surface and a red base. To be able to view conditions in the perianal area, stretch the anal orifice by exerting tension on the skin on each side of the anus to evert it. Instead of simply the hand on the butt cheek, this strategy recommends that pressing with both thumbs (or thumb and index finger) nearer to the anus will prompt an enhanced diagnostic precision. Rectal prolapse appears as varying degrees of rectal mucosa protruding from the anus. Perianal haematoma or thrombosed external haemorrhoid is seen as a 'tense bluish swelling' and is covered by anal skin while internal haemorrhoids are covered by rectal mucosa and are not visible unless they prolapse when they appear as deep-red or purple masses.

Suspicion should arise if the patient gives a history of intense pain on passing stool and a breach in the anal mucosa either in the posterior or, less commonly, on the anterior midline. With a chronic anal fissure, a skin tag may be seen. Any opening within about 4 cm of the anus may also be viewed as a 'bead of pus'; similarly, opening with surrounding granulation tissue may represent the opening of an anal fistula. It is an inflammatory tract, which runs from the anus or rectum to the perianal skin, usually because of perianal or perirectal abscess draining.

There would be a distinct area of tenderness in the perianal area on palpation, alerting and indicating towards the presence of a fistula, fissure, or a perianal abscess, which may also be felt as a lump. A zone of swelling, deforming the outline of the anus may be seen. Rectal polyps may protrude through the anus and carcinoma of the anus may be considered as a 'fungating mass at the anal verge'. Ask the patient to strain. See for rectal prolapse upon straining, haemorrhoid prolapse, or incontinence. Ask whether this straining is painful.

A digital rectal examination in conditions like an abscess or a fissure-in-ano is painful and serves no purpose other than making the patient miserable. It should best be avoided.

If you are suspecting a rectal or haemorrhoid prolapse, take the patient to the toilet and ask him to strain as if he is passing stool. The anal area may then be inspected with a hand mirror. If the patient has difficulty doing so and yet there is a strong suspicion, administration of a suppository or enema may help to detect the prolapse.

Many conditions can be diagnosed merely with an external inspect. Prolapsed polyps or tags, incarcerated haemorrhoids, fistula opening, abscess, external thromboses, fissures, rhagades, ulcerations, or sentinel tags may be immediately apparent. The typical Crohn's anus may also be evident and cautious note should be made of the waxy or oedematous tags with multiple deep fissures or fistula openings. An advanced anal cancer protruding beyond the anal canal may sometimes be visible on the anal verge.

Various dermatologic conditions of the perianal region can also be identified during this part of the anorectal examination. Perianal excoriation of the skin may at times be so severe as to bleed, and this may be defined by the patient as pain and blood on the tissue. Malignant lesions of the perianal skin can manifest in the form of bleeding in the advanced stage.

To summarise the findings of inspection, the following points are to be considered:

- Soiling due to incontinence, faecal impaction, or lack of fastidiousness.
- Discharge or seepage.
- Dermatitis or evidence of pruritus, such as excoriations.
- External invaders like lice and worms.
- The multiple wart-like growths of condylomata accuminata. (Condylomata lata, due to syphilis, differs in appearance and is far less common.)
- Skin tags, including a 'sentinel pile' below an anal fissure.
- The bulge of external haemorrhoids.
- The tense swelling of a perianal haematoma.
- The bulging and redness of an abscess of the perianum or ischio-rectal space.
- The multiple superficial abscesses and sinuses of hidradenitis suppurativa.
- The external opening of an anal fistula.
- Exposed mucosa (may be due to prolapsing haemorrhoids, to mucosal prolapse, or to eversion caused by the previous operation).
- Scars of the previous operation.
- Squamous carcinoma, which may occur in the perianal area or the anal canal; any suspicious or bizarre lesion should be biopsied.
- Dermatologic lesions. Any tumour or other diseases of the skin may also affect this area.

PERFORMING A RECTAL EXAMINATION

For the rectal examination, lubrication is necessary, and it should preferably be water soluble like K-Y jelly. If necessary, a mild topical anaesthetic, such as plain viscous lidocaine, may be applied externally. The patient should be informed and assured just before putting in the finger. Draw the patient's right buttock up with the left hand and place the right index finger against the anus, with the finger pointing in the direction of the patient's front (Figure 3.2). At this point, the patient may feel the need to pass a bowel but reassure the patient that it is not required.

Sometimes insertion is difficult because of a tight sphincter. If you continue to proceed when the sphincter is tightly closed, you will cause the patient much pain—so avoid doing so. The tight sphincter is telling you relevant information. It may simply be due to apprehension. If that is the case, when you feel resistance on advancing your finger, stop moving forward, hold your finger in place and wait, with the patient breathing slowly, until the sphincter is adequately relaxed, and then advance. If the patient has an anal fissure, the anal sphincter goes into spasm, which cannot be overcome by relaxation, patience, or gentleness. So, if resistance and severe pain are encountered, do not try to perform the digital examination. Search the anal area for a tear. A complete digital examination can sometimes only be performed under a general anaesthetic. Other causes of tight sphincter include anal stricture, fibrosis of anal muscles, and

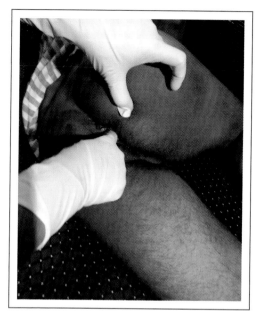

Figure 3.2 Digital rectal examination.

Courtesy: Pravin Jaiprakash Gupta.

anal carcinoma. The normal muscle tone of the anal sphincter should 'grip the finger firmly'. The relaxed (or weakened) anal sphincter may be due to torn or lacerated anal muscles or atony of the muscles from neurological lesions.

The external sphincter is derived from skeletal muscle and is under voluntary control while the internal sphincter consists of smooth muscle and is under involuntary control. On entering the anus when the patient is relaxed, you can appreciate the tone of the internal sphincter (resting tone). Later, when you ask the patient to squeeze, you are assessing the external sphincter tone.

The best manoeuvre is to press on the anus until the anal sphincter opens up and then slowly insert the finger into the rectum, pointing the finger in the direction of the patient's head. Examine the walls of the rectum in an orderly fashion, sweeping the finger clockwise passing through each quadrant. You may need to kneel down to have your arm in the most comfortable position for your finger to examine the prostate in the male or the cervix in the female. Make the patient bear down by which sweeping the examining finger will yield an extra centimetre of the rectal walls. You can stand up while performing this 360° sweep or upon completion. The patient should be completely relaxed. Ask the patient to squeeze to assess external sphincter tone. Gently remove the finger, checking the colour of faeces and for any presence of blood on your glove. You can ask the patient if he would like you to wipe the anal area for him, or still better, get it cleaned by the chaperone or the nurse.

Haemorrhoids are not palpable unless they are very large or thrombosed. An anal papilla can easily be differentiated from an anal mass. In males, the prostate should be examined for texture, any tenderness, size, and any masses. The overlying mucosa should be able to slide over the prostate. In the females, the cervix can often be palpated along the wall of the rectum, and should not be confused with a rectal mass. Make no confusion with the presence of foreign bodies, such as a pessary or a tampon in the vagina, which can also be felt on rectal exam.

Simple anorectal inspection and palpation are usually all that is required to confirm the diagnosis in a patient with anorectal pain. A thrombosed external haemorrhoid is a prominent, tender, discrete, hard, and bluish swelling. A perianal abscess can be identified as an indurated, erythematous, and diffusely tender mass and it may often be found at the base of a draining fistula opening. A deep abscess may only be palpable on a deep digital rectal examination. An anal fissure is often related to a contracted 'tiny looking' anus that is in spasm. One may notice a sentinel skin tag guarding the distal part of the fissure.

Anal fissures can easily be located by a gentle spreading of the perianal skin in the anterior and posterior midline. Associated sentinel skin tags are caused by chronic inflammation and should easily be differentiated from haemorrhoids since they are usually in the anterior or posterior midline; whereas, haemorrhoids are typically found more laterally in the classic left lateral, right anterior, and right posterior quadrants. The anus will look altogether normal in a patient having levator spasm, and the diagnosis is made when a tender, tight levator muscle is noticed on digital rectal examination.

The pain of a perianal abscess is constant, and unaffected by the bowel movement. Before localisation, a perianal abscess is not evident upon external inspection or external palpation. An important diagnostic procedure is bi-digital palpation of the perianal tissues, with the index finger inserted into the rectum and flexed to oppose the thumb outside the canal. Palpation of a deep area of tender induration by this means is an indication for prompt incision and drainage. Pain related to a fistula-in-ano is evidence of inadequate drainage of an area of acute infection somewhere in the course of the fistulous tract.

Rectal cancer can be diagnosed by a digital exam as a firm mass, with a rough or ulcerated surface, and not freely mobile. On occasions, a thrombosis within the anal canal may be misinterpreted as a polyp or cancer; that is why the visual assessment of the anal canal and rectum is necessary. There is also an opportunity to reduce the prolapsed haemorrhoids or a full-thickness prolapse gently.

In the assessment of rectal bleeding, testing for occult blood in the stool essentially has no role—when blood has been visualised, tests that are more specific are needed to identify an apparent source.

The perianum is palpated for areas of tenderness, induration, or heat if an abscess is suspected. Scars are palpated, and their induration or pliability noted.

A fistula tract may be palpated as a cord-like structure when traction is placed on it, and pressure may result in the release of a bead of pus from its external opening.

The bi-digital examination may reveal a small lesion such as a perianal abscess, which is otherwise not apparent. It is performed in a clockwise fashion, palpating the tissues between the examining finger in the anal canal and the externally placed thumb of the same hand, the suspicious area being compared with adjacent tissues and with the corresponding tissues on the other side.

While examining a female patient, one should be cautious enough that finger should not slip into the vagina. It can happen at times because an anxious patient with a tight anus has a lax vagina. The patient may not excuse you for this mistake. Better to put one finger on the coccyx to avoid this complication.

CLINICAL PEARLS

- Anorectal disorders are commonly encountered in day-to-day practice. Most of the organic lesions are discovered while performing a routine examination or assessment of symptoms.
- Haemorrhoids are the most prevalent anorectal disorders and are the most common cause of haematochezia.
- Anal fissures are the number one cause of anorectal pain. Though most of them are idiopathic, some may be due to a particular pathology and majority of them are located in the posterior midline.
- Anorectal abscesses are categorised into four types. Most are secondary to cryptoglandular infection containing mixed organisms.
- The abscess turning into fistula varies from 25% to 50% and is much more common with gut-derived organisms like *Escherichia coli*.
- Anal carcinomas are not very common, and the majority of them are a squamous cell or epidermoid carcinomas.
- The most common presenting complaint of anal tumours is rectal bleeding.
- Rectal injuries can occur following a penetrating or blunt trauma, iatrogenic injuries, or from foreign bodies.
- A detailed physical examination is essential to detect and evaluate all anorectal lesions. This must include abdominal examination, visual inspection of the anal and perineal areas, digital rectal palpation, and anoscopic visualisation, preferably using an Ive's slotted anoscope.
- Advanced diagnostic tools like sigmoidoscopy or colonoscopy are indicated in few of the patients. Although all four anal disorders cause some anal discomfort or pain, other symptoms vary, depending on the particular anal problem.

SUGGESTED READINGS

Barber MD, Lambers A, Visco AG, Bump RC. Effect of patient position on clinical evaluation of pelvic organ prolapse. *Obstet Gynecol*. 2000;96:18–22.

Beer-Gabel M, Carter D, Venturero M, Zmora O, Zbar AP. Ultrasonographic assessment of patients referred with chronic anal pain to a tertiary referral centre. *Tech Coloproctol*. 2010;14:107–12.

Jeppson PC, Paraiso MF, Jelovsek JE, Barber MD. Accuracy of the digital anal examination in women with fecal incontinence. *Int Urogynecol J*. 2012;23:765–8.

Nicholls RJ, Dube S. The extent of examination by rigid sigmoidoscopy. *Br J Surg*. 1982;69:438.

Perry WB. History and physical examination. In: *Handbook of Colorectal Surgery*. Beck DE (ed.). St. Louis: Quality Medical Publishing;1997; 30–8.

Roberts PL. Patient evaluation. In: *Fundamentals of Anorectal Surgery* 2nd ed. Beck DE, Wexner SD (eds). London: WB Saunders Co Ltd;1992;25–36.

Salazar M, Jackson RJ. Reasons for incomplete proctoscopy. *Dis Colon Rectum*. 1969;12:19–21.

Toomey P, Asimakopoulos G, Zbar A, Kmiot WA. 'One-stop' rectal bleeding clinics without routine flexible sigmoidoscopy are unsafe. *Ann R Coll Surg Engl*. 1998;80:131–3.

Chapter 4

Investigating a patient of anorectal complaints

Anoscopy, proctoscopy, and proctosigmoidoscopy are few of the simplest, most rewarding, but most neglected diagnostic manoeuvres available to a physician. About 70% of all the diseases that involve the anal canal and the rectum can be diagnosed with the help of proctoscopy (Figure 4.1). Mostly, this is an office procedure, and usually it does not require anaesthesia.

The majority of anorectal disorders are present immediately above and below the anorectal or pectinate line, but due to lack of adequate illumination and the use of the ordinary conical speculums, a thorough examination is often challenging and mostly unsatisfactory. However, proper illumination and inspection of the diseased area are essential for making the correct diagnosis.

ANOSCOPIC EXAMINATION

Mere palpation without visual inspection is inadequate to evaluate the anus and rectum adequately, and unfortunately there is no single instrument that can fully evaluate both. A careful examination of the anus can be carried out with an anoscope, which is available in small, medium, and large sizes depending on the calibre. The size of the anoscope selected depends on whether or not there is anal narrowing, anal spasm, or inability of the patient to cooperate.

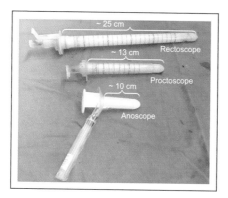

Figure 4.1 Various scopes to visualise the anal canal and the rectum.
Courtesy: Pravin Jaiprakash Gupta.

Although some endoscopists can examine the distal rectum by retroflexion of a flexible scope, this will not help them to visualise internal haemorrhoids as efficiently as with an anoscope, and the procedure itself is quite uncomfortable in a conscious patient. Therefore, an adequately equipped proctologic setup should have a selection of anoscopes available.

Anoscopy is a critical visual evaluation, after digital examination, to assess the several distal centimetres of the anal canal. There are some different instruments available, and decision-making needs to be made in setting up the ambulatory proctology clinic regarding the use of disposable or non-disposable equipment. This decision influences the lighting source to be utilised; hence, a fibreoptic system is the preferred choice for examination.

These systems need almost no maintenance and last for years, although they have portability problems. The simple torchlight systems that go into the plastic side channels of disposable systems are an ingenious idea. However, the lighting is suboptimal. The bevelled anoscopes that are non-disposable and permit single entry into the anal canal and rotation of the instrument without the need for reinsertion and examples include the Hirschman or Buie anoscope, which suits this purpose adequately. This assessment can define haemorrhoidal grade on straining as well as location and the separation of typical haemorrhoidal position from circumferential haemorrhoids or from circumferential mucosal prolapse that itself can be graded. Pressure on the perineum or an external fistulous opening can show purulent emanation from the potential site of an internal opening, notably predicted by Goodsall's rule if this is anatomically followed. A small Lockhart–Mummery type probe may be passed through the external opening defining its internal entry point by rotating the anoscope. The various types of anoscopes available are Plastic, Clear, Opaque, Metal, Bevelled, Graduated, Lighted, and Slotted (Figure 4.2).

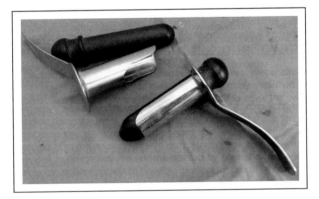

Figure 4.2 A slotted anoscope.

Courtesy: Pravin Jaiprakash Gupta.

In assessing the anal canal, one ought to search for the three haemorrhoidal sections, right anterior and posterior, and left lateral. In the ordinary state, where the patient is in an inclined position, these ought to be non-engorged and flat. In patients with significant haemorrhoidal disease, they will bulge into the slot on the anoscope, and in some cases would appear friable or having visible blood on the overlying mucosa.

Long-standing haemorrhoidal prolapse is often accompanied by a pale discolouration of the mucosa, which indicates squamous metaplasia. Haemorrhoids can be gently grasped with an instrument, but only above the level of the dentate line, and pulled down to determine if they easily prolapse outside of the anal canal. If the patient has watery faeces or bleeds during examination or manipulation then the head-down supine position is preferred so that the fluid or blood tends to run away from the instrument.

Various conditions that may be visualised on the anoscopic examination include hypertrophied papilla, fissure, ulceration, and distal proctitis. The presence of an ulcer may be related to human immunodeficiency virus (HIV) or other sexually transmitted disease, Crohn's disease, or anal cancer. While usually painful below the dentate line, but if the ulceration extends above the dentate line, then a biopsy may be taken through the anoscope. Lesions at or below the dentate line can be biopsied under a topical or injectable anaesthetic with a flexible biopsy forceps available with a flexible sigmoidoscope. Alternatively, this procedure will need to be done in the operating room under anaesthesia.

Anoscopy provides an opportunity for the biopsy of lesions including tumours, proctitis, solitary rectal ulcers, and the like. The office may be set up to assess high-risk cases for pre-cancerous syndromes of the anal canal (the so-called anal intraepithelial neoplasia [AIN]) and this high-resolution anoscopy (HRA) may be supplemented by magnification using an expensive colposcope type setup or using a magnifying working portable lens that is readily commercially available from art and craft stores. This kind of HRA assessment may be supplemented by cytological samples, which can also be sent for polymerase chain reaction (PCR) analysis to detect high-risk human papillomavirus (HPV) subtypes as well as by acetic acid staining which can direct formal biopsy to determine the histological grade of AIN. This type of practice is applied in conjunction with office infrared photocoagulation in many cases as a definitive treatment for high-risk patient groups such as those who are HIV-positive. Similarly, HIV-negative cases of men having sex with men, women who engage in receptive anal intercourse, women with high grades of cervical and vulvar intraepithelial neoplasia, and transplant patients or those who are immunosuppressed with low CD4+ T cell counts can also undergo similar treatment.

Nonetheless, treatment of many lesions at this area are office or outpatients department (OPD) procedures, but at times when a nurse or an assistant is not available, a self-retaining device is a helpful adjunct. Keeping the patient in the left lateral or Sims' position, this procedure may be performed using the illuminated

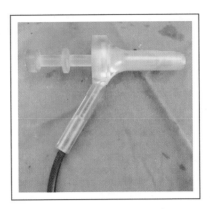

Figure 4.3   Illuminated anoscope.

Courtesy: Pravin Jaiprakash Gupta.

anoscope (Figure 4.3). The instrument is self-retaining and may be quickly introduced after the anus has been smeared with a water-soluble lubricant. The light, located in the head of the detachable handle, gives a fair illumination to perform the procedures.

Hypertrophied anal papillae, when growing to a size to prolapse, are more often the cause of pain rather than bleeding. Signs of proctitis may be visible as a circumferential area of erythema at the upper extent of visualisation in the anoscope. Further evaluation may be necessary to assess the full extent of rectal involvement.

Tips for a Better Anoscopic Examination

Before performing anoscopy, visual inspection and a digital rectal examination should be conducted to investigate for bleeding or a lump. A digital rectal examination will also help to recognise if there is a pain to defer the anoscopic examination. It is also beneficial to evacuate the rectum before such examinations. An enema may be needed to clear the rectal vault before the procedure.

At the point when utilising an anoscope with an obturator, guarantee that the obturator of the anoscope is totally embedded. Liberally grease up the anoscope with standard greasing-up jelly or lidocaine cream. Insert the anoscope tenderly and advance it gradually with a slight side-to-side curving movement while the patient bears down. In the event that resistance because of constriction of the external sphincter is huge, a steady pressure on the anoscope will exhaust the muscles and allow insertion. Keep up pressing over the obturator with the thumb amid insertion to keep the obturator from slipping out. To abstain from squeezing the anal mucosa, take out the anoscope and reinsert it if the obturator slips or drops out amid insertion. Once the anoscope is totally embedded, take the obturator out. As the anoscope is gradually pulled back, the anal canal mucosa can be viewed over the whole circumference of the canal. Any trash or blood can be swabbed for investigation, if required. As the instrument is pulled back at the anal edge, spasm of the external sphincter may prompt quick ejection. Firm counter-pressure prevents ejection.

A repeat insertion may be required for adequate visualisation of the anal verge. A common complication is minor irritation of the local mucosa, leading to discomfort and some bleeding. To avoid contamination, dispose of single-use devices after use.

PROCTOSCOPIC EXAMINATION

Proctoscopy is performed if there is no evidence of a source for the bleeding with the initial inspection, digital rectal exam, and anoscopy. The next step should be a detailed visualisation of the rectum and sigmoid. Both the rigid and the flexible proctosigmoidoscopes can be used for the evaluation of rectal bleeding, and both should be available for a proper assessment as may be required. A rigid proctoscope is handy in examining and taking a biopsy of the entire rectum, and even from the terminal part of the sigmoid colon.

Significantly, tumours that lie within the rectum above the reach of the index finger but below the peritoneal reflection can be identified. This portion can be missed by a radiographic study as the tumour is obscured either by the balloon on a barium enema or due to the bony structures of the pelvis. Similarly, to plan further treatment, the rigid scope is a standard device for measuring the distance of a rectal mass from the dentate line or anal verge, because the flexible scope may give an inaccurately high measurement. Moreover, when there is active bleeding, the proctoscope may allow for the distinction between blood originating from above the peritoneal reflection and that originating below. If the distal sigmoid colon can be visualised, the diagnosis of diverticulosis may also be made.

INDICATIONS

Diagnostic

- Bleeding per rectum
- Haemorrhoids
- Anal polyps
- Rectal polyps
- Familial polyposis coli
- Carcinoma of the anal canal
- Carcinoma of rectum
- Anal canal and rectal injuries
- Fistula-in-ano
- Follow up in cases after anterior resection
- Follow up in cases of ulcerative colitis
- Rectal endosonography
- Biopsy under vision

Therapeutic

- Injection sclerotherapy of haemorrhoids
- Band ligation of haemorrhoids
- Polypectomy

- Laser and infrared coagulation of haemorrhoids
- Transanal resection of tumours
- Transanal micros surgery

Contraindications

None. The procedure should be performed using anaesthesia in painful conditions of the anal canal.

INSTRUMENT FEATURES

Proctoscope is a rigid instrument, which has a sheath and an obturator (Figure 4.4). It is made up of either metal or plastic. It comes with a cold fibre optic light or direct light from the external source. The plastic proctoscopes are available to be used for the coagulation therapy of haemorrhoids or polyps.

PREPARATION

The exact procedure must be explained to the patient very clearly. No laxatives should be used before the examination, as they may lead to the liquefaction of faeces, which soil the anal canal and obscure the view. Inspection of the perianal area and digital examination of the rectum and anal canal must always be performed before proctoscopy.

POSITION

The anorectal examination is partly related to training where different positions can be utilised including the left lateral (the Sims' position), the prone-jack knife, or the knee–chest position. In some cases,

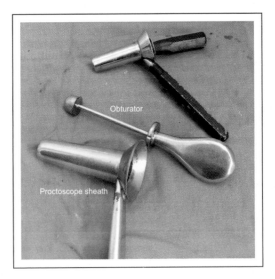

Figure 4.4 The proctoscope.
Courtesy: Pravin Jaiprakash Gupta.

assessment of the patient after a period of straining may be valuable for the diagnosis of rectal prolapse. The examination should always be done in privacy, and a female attendant must be present in a case of a female patient.

PROCEDURE

The key focuses for proctoscopic examination are as follows:

- A well-understanding and cooperative patient
- Private surroundings
- An agreeable position of the patient
- Gentle manoeuvre
- Liberal and smooth lubrication
- Gradual push on the instrument
- Knowledge of the direction of the anal canal

After the digital rectal examination has been outfitted, the greased-up proctoscope is slowly and gently negotiated into the anal canal. One ought to never attempt to push the proctoscope without its obturator present in it. No pressure is utilised to push the procto-scope. In the event the procedure of proctoscopy is uncomfortable, either the examination might be deserted, or it might be done under anaesthesia. When the proctoscope has been fully introduced, the obturator is removed. The surgeon can easily see through the scope. The colour and character of the rectal and anal canal mucosa are noticed. The condition of mucosa is noticed and written down. It may be inflamed and may bleed even on a gentle touch of the procto-scope. In the case of abnormal findings such as ulcer, new growth, papillomatous lesion, polyp, or haemorrhoids, etc., their size, site, and degree should be noted and recorded on the diagram. If a biopsy of the lesion is required, it is taken and sent for histopathological examination. Injection sclerotherapy, infrared photocoagulation, and electric or laser haemorrhoid therapy may be performed, if required. The visualisation of the rest of the anal canal is done while the proctoscope is being gently withdrawn. In case reintroduction of proctoscope is required, it must be performed again with the obturator in place.

Endorectal or transrectal sonography can also be performed with the help of the proctoscope for an early detection of cancer of the rectum. It is a very sensitive and accurate method for the pre-operative staging of cancer. Transanal resection through the proc-toscope is a minimally invasive surgical procedure. It is used as a palliative procedure for the treatment of rectal obstruction. It can also be used for villous adenomas. Proctoscopy can be used for transanal decompression procedure in acute pseudo-obstruction of the colon. However, it should not be used if the colonic perforation is suspected.

A routine bowel preparation is not necessary for proctoscopy. In some cases, if the patient has a complete and satisfactory evacua-tion in the morning and the rectum is empty, the examination can be performed with almost no preparation at all. This is quite helpful if a diagnosis of ulcerative colitis or Crohn's disease is being considered, as the mucosa is very friable and can be easily injured. In other situations, the rectum and distal sigmoid may be cleaned out with a single phosphate enema.

It is important to maintain a systematic approach to this entire examination, and to ensure that these examinations are consistent across patients. This will make it easy and quick to remember and for documentation of the findings. The examiner should also be prepared with biopsy forceps and have an assistant available, in case significant pathology resulting in sampling is encountered. Routine biopsies can be safely undertaken without any bowel preparation, but there is a slightly greater risk of igniting combustible gases that can cause a perforation of the colon when using snare and cautery in an unprepared colon. In the case where rectal cancer or polyp is identified, the rigid proctoscope is the ideal instrument for measuring the distance of the lesion from the dentate line. A polypectomy is better deferred until full bowel preparation is made and/or better can be done after colonoscopy, as the remainder of the colon will need to be evaluated to rule out the presence of synchronous lesions.

PROCTOSCOPY IN THE CHILDREN

Visual examination of the anal canal and rectum is preferably omitted by the paediatrician because the study is thought to be dangerous, difficult, time-consuming, or unrewarding. However, one should understand that there are many definite indications for this examination in prolonged or unexplained diarrhoea, the passage of tarry stools, blood, pus, or mucous, abdominal pain of unknown aetiology, unexplained protracted fever, and local conditions such as anal fistulae and abscesses. It is also suggested in any unexplained vaginal discharge or recurrent cystitis in both the sexes. Nonetheless, it is quite difficult to obtain information by routine barium enema examination in this part of the gastrointestinal tract. Specimens for bacteriological and parasitological studies of rectosigmoidal lesions are easily obtained directly from the lesion through the proctoscope. The contraindications are very few, and the procedure can be performed with an ordinary auroscope in children. It is found that the largest earpiece that could be inserted into the anal canal gives the best view. K-Y jelly can be used as lubrication in most infants, but an auroscope moistened with a little water will suffice. The auroscope is inserted in the same fashion as that used in proctoscopy in older patients, with the child in the left lateral Sims' position.

SPECIALISED PROCTOLOGY EXAMINATION CHAIR

In a clinic in which a large number of patients with colitis are seen and in which a good number of haemorrhoids are treated by injection or rubber-band ligation, the comfort of the surgeon is greater if he is examining the patient at eye level. A special chair has been developed which has a kneeling platform with thigh-retaining safety straps (Figure 4.5). The rise and fall of this can be controlled by a lever-operated hydraulic jack. This enables the patient to kneel at a comfortable level and then be raised gently until he can comfortably

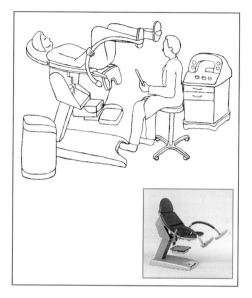

Figure 4.5 Proctological examination chair.
Courtesy: Schmitz u. Söhne GmbH & Co. KG.
Illustration: James Oinam.

bend and lie with his abdomen flat on the main table. The table can
be tilted on both sides. At the knee end, castors permit the table to be
moved easily if required.

SIGMOIDOSCOPIC EXAMINATION

Sigmoidoscopy is performed in either an outpatient or theatre setting
in association with a digital rectal examination to facilitate the diagnosis and the management of rectal and anal pathology. It is effective
as a diagnostic, case finding, and a screening tool for lesions situated
near the distal 60–65 cm of the large bowel.

It can be performed with either a rigid or a flexible sigmoidoscope. The rigid sigmoidoscope has virtually disappeared from
the ambulatory proctology clinic and has been replaced by the
flexible sigmoidoscope, the colonoscope, and, in special circumstances, the rigid video rectoscope. The disposable rigid sigmoidoscope (or more correctly, a rectoscope as it may in many cases
will not traverse into the sigmoid particularly in women because
of acute angulation) is a useful instrument to visualise some rectal
tumours and perform a biopsy, as well as to accurately determine
its height and extent from the anal verge. A rigid videorectoscopy is
done on lesions within range, particularly those which may be suitable
for transanal endoscopic microsurgery (TEMS) either using a conventional TEMS machine or the latest single-port disposable equipment

for endoanal excision (the so-called TAMIS procedure). Rigid rectoscopy can also be used to assess few patients having distal proctitis and evaluate a solitary rectal ulcer or in rare cases such as radiation proctitis and patients after prostatic brachytherapy who may have an impending rectoprostatic fistula or a post-radiation rectal ulcer.

In the case of proctitis, it has been suggested that a posterior biopsy is safer than an anterior biopsy where tamponade can be performed if there is post- or intra-procedural bleeding pushing the mucosa backwards with a long cotton-tipped swab against the sacrum. However, these are uncommon cases.

Studies have demonstrated that flexible sigmoidoscopy is two to six times as efficient as the rigid sigmoidoscope for detecting colonic polyps and cancers. Approximately, two-thirds of colorectal cancers are accessible to sigmoidoscopy, and almost half of these are situated in the rectum while the rest are in the sigmoid or descending colon. Physicians and patients are reluctant to accept rigid sigmoidoscopy because of its reduced diagnostic yield and the greater patient discomfort associated with the procedure. On the other hand, patient acceptance is significantly enhanced with the flexible sigmoidoscopy. In one study of flexible sigmoidoscopy, patients who have had a rigid sigmoidoscopic examination in the past have reported that flexible endoscope caused one-fourth the discomfort of the rigid endoscope. This finding is significant when the issue of physician and patient compliance with suggested screening and case finding protocols is examined. An appropriately performed sigmoidoscopy along with diagnostic tissue biopsies, when required, should be completed within 15 minutes and cause minimal patient discomfort.

The flexible fibreoptic sigmoidoscope (FFS) (Figure 4.6) is quite useful in diagnosing many of the common conditions, which occur in the distal 65 cm of the large bowel, and includes carcinoma, polyps,

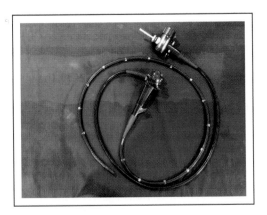

Figure 4.6 Flexible fibreoptic sigmoidoscope.
Courtesy: Pravin Jaiprakash Gupta.

ulcerative colitis, diverticular disease, Crohn's disease, colitis of various aetiologies, and haemorrhoids.

Sigmoidoscopy is a remarkably safe procedure. Few reported complications include perforation, bleeding, and transient bacteraemia. A combination of appropriate training, technique, careful patient selection, while keeping the complications in mind will minimise the incidence of perforation and bleeding. Perforation and bleeding occur in less than one in 10,000 procedures.

Indications for flexible sigmoidoscopy are a change in bowel habits, rectal bleeding, guaiac-positive stools, abdominal pain, diarrhoea, constipation, weight loss, anaemia, and high risk for colonic cancer.

Patients at increased risk of developing subacute bacterial endocarditis should be carefully identified and receive appropriate prophylactic antibiotics.

Flexible sigmoidoscopy is particularly useful for assessing bright red rectal bleeding, a common symptom in family practice. Often, no further investigations are necessary. However, a flexible fibreoptic sigmoidoscopy is not a substitute for colonoscopy. Patients with symptoms that require a complete assessment of the large bowel mucosa should undergo a full-length colonoscopy and not be subjected to an unnecessary procedure.

In most of the cases, a sigmoidoscopy too does not require a full colon preparation. A clear liquid diet a day before the examination, along with overnight fasting, is usually enough. One or two tap water enemas should be given on the morning of the examination.

The sigmoidoscope consists of a shaft, a control head, and an umbilicus (which is connected to the video processor). The control device contains the up/down and left/right buttons, a suction valve, the air or water valve, and a working channel through which biopsy forceps or other useful accessories can be guided. This circuit can also be used to hook a large syringe for pushing water inside the colon (Figure 4.7). The images from the camera can be visualised on a video monitor.

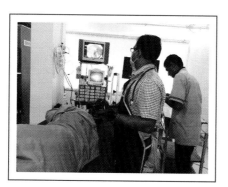

Figure 4.7   Flexible sigmoidoscopy.
Courtesy: Pravin Jaiprakash Gupta.

In most situations, no sedation is required for flexible sigmoid-oscopy. If sedation is required, then fentanyl (or meperidine) and midazolam can be given intravenously. The preferred position for the patient is the left lateral position, with the hip and knee joints partially flexed.

RIGID SIGMOIDOSCOPY

The proctoscope is for examining the anal canal and the anorectal region, that is, the lower third of the rectum and the remainder of the rectum and lower sigmoid colon are reached only by using the sigmoidoscope.

Indications for rigid sigmoidoscopy include the following:

- Symptoms suggesting anorectal pathology, including colorectal neoplasia
- To obtain a biopsy of suspected bowel condition within the reach of the instrument
- To assess the exact height (distance from anal verge) of rectal cancers
- Before anorectal procedures in a clinic or operating theatre
- In the conservative treatment of sigmoid volvulus
- During anterior resection of the rectum to gauge the lower resection margin.

Contraindications to rigid sigmoidoscopy can be either absolute or relative. Relative contraindications are further divided into surgical and medical groups.

Absolute contraindications include the following:

- Suspected or known bowel perforation
- Anal stenosis (technical consideration)

Relative surgical contraindications include the following:

- Colonic necrosis
- Fulminant colitis
- Toxic megacolon
- Acute severe diverticulitis
- Diverticular abscess
- Recent colonic surgery
- Anal fissure

Relative medical contraindications include the following:

- Severe coagulopathy
- Severe thrombocytopenia
- Acute peritonitis
- Severe neutropenia
- Extreme debilitation
- Recent bowel surgery where the risk of perforation or damage to an anastomosis is thought to be increased.

Rigid sigmoidoscopy (Figure 4.8) may also be contraindicated in patients who are highly uncooperative, agitated, or particularly anxious.

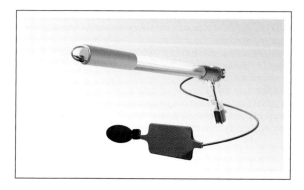

Figure 4.8 Rigid sigmoidosope.

Courtesy: Henleys Medical Supplies Ltd.

In a few cases, sigmoidoscopy after a colonic surgery is necessary for the evaluation of bleeding or obstruction. The procedure is relatively safe in stable patients, but it is wise to defer it for at least one week after the operation and reserve it for clinically significant indications.

Initially, no bowel preparation is used so that the contents of the lumen may be assessed—the consistency and colour of the stool and whether or not blood, mucous, or pus are present. If the rectum is very loaded, the patient should be given a simple 100 mL phosphate enema and re-examined.

The instrument is lubricated and gently inserted into the anal canal, passing along the rectum and hopefully into the sigmoid colon under direct vision by inflating the bowel above the scope with the aid of the double bellows. The sigmoidoscope should at least be passed to 15 cm (the rectosigmoid junction) but may be passed to its full length. It is important not to force the rigid sigmoidoscope as this will cause the patient much discomfort, not add much information, and can even perforate the bowel, whereas the flexible sigmoidoscope will easily and safely cover this area.

The normal rectal mucosa appears pale pink in colour and the intramucosal blood vessels or vascular pattern is clearly seen. The abnormalities that may be detected by sigmoidoscopy are proctitis and the presence of polyps and tumours.

The first sign of proctitis is a loss of vascular pattern and generalised reddening of the mucosa. Granularity, contact bleeding, and ulceration are the appearances which indicate increasing severity of the condition. Proctitis is a sigmoidoscopic appearance, not a pathological diagnosis. The precise diagnosis may be difficult, and a rectal mucosal biopsy for histological examination is essential.

The word 'polyp' is a clinical term to describe a tumour or elevation which projects above the surface of the surrounding flat mucous membrane. Again, histological examination is an essential investigation but should be done after total excision of the polyp, since a forceps biopsy is inadequate.

A carcinoma is usually readily diagnosed as a large, firm, indurated bleeding ulcer or tumour. The diagnosis is confirmed by forceps biopsy.

The left lateral (Sims') position is convenient, as the patient sleeps on his left side with the hips and knees flexed and parallel and allows the clinician a comfortable room to move around the entire length of the examination table. In this position, the buttocks must overhang the edge of the bed, with the patient's trunk angled obliquely across the bed, to allow for the full manoeuvrability of the scope; the more transverse across the bed, the easier the examination.

An alternate position is the prone knee–elbow or jack-knife position, in which the patient lays prone in an inverted position on a specialised table. These positions are particularly helpful to permit a considerable degree of manoeuvrability of the scope.

High-risk patients such as those with valvuloplasties need appropriate antibiotic prophylaxis.

RIGID SIGMOIDOSCOPY TECHNIQUE

The anus and surrounding areas are inspected for any abnormalities. Then a digital rectal examination is performed to assess any narrowing or painful anal pathology.

If the rectum is found to be loaded with faeces, an attempt should be made to empty the rectum with the aid of a laxative suppository or enema before performing rigid sigmoidoscopy.

With the patient in position, the rigid sigmoidoscope is inserted after applying generous amounts of a water-based lubricant to the scope.

Initial 4 cm of the scope is inserted into the anus in the direction of the patient's umbilicus. Then the scope is advanced under direct vision, using the bellows to insufflate air gently into the rectum intermittently as the scope advances. Therefore, when the scope reaches this point 4 cm from the anus, its general direction should be changed from pointing anteriorly to pointing posteriorly. Gently insufflating air into the rectum to expand the rectum in front of the scope will help in advancing the scope further. Abnormalities, if any, should be noted. A slight lateral angulation of the scope is used to manoeuvre through the rectal valves.

As the scope is withdrawn, insufflating air and changing directions while maintaining a direct vision of the lumen of the rectum will help in a quick and easy withdrawal of the scope. Small circular motions allow a complete examination and may reveal lesions missed during insertion of the scope.

COMPLICATIONS IN RIGID SIGMOIDOSCOPY

The following types of discomforts are commonly reported:

- Pain (33%)
- Discomfort from rectal preparation (13%)
- Uncomfortable desire to defecate (8%)
- Discomfort associated with patient positioning (4%)

The most likely cause of patient discomfort is while negotiating the rectosigmoid angle when the rigid sigmoidoscope is passed to a depth of 20 cm. Nonetheless, insufflation of the rectum is also responsible for the discomfort to some extent.

Torrential bleeding requiring transfusion or further procedural intervention occurs in approximately one out of 9,400 rigid sigmoidoscopies. This complication is usually related to a rectal biopsy performed during scopy. Bacteraemia occurs in 5% of patients during a rigid sigmoidoscopy, which justifies the precaution for its use in patients with neutropenia.

RECTAL BIOPSY

To take a rectal mucosal biopsy without too much trauma, a small pair of biopsy forceps is preferable. The positioning of the biopsy site is important; the rectal mucosa is usually pain-insensitive above 5 cm from the anal margin, and the posterior (sacral) aspect of the rectum is the safest site, being extraperitoneal. It is often most convenient to take the biopsy on one of the projecting rectal 'valves'. The site and distance from the anus should always be recorded to make localisation easier in the rare incidence of bleeding or perforation, which may follow rectal biopsy. For a mucosal biopsy, the jaws are partially opened, and a small bit of mucosa is taken, and the forceps then twisted 3–4 times until the biopsy separates. Twisting off, rather than cutting through the mucosa, reduces the likelihood of bleeding by traumatising the submucosal vessels. The biopsy should then be orientated flat onto a ground glass slide or a piece of filter paper so that the submucosa is on the slide and the mucosa uppermost. It is then placed in formalin for fixing; correct orientation of the specimen enables sections to be cut at right angles to the mucosal surface, which helps histological interpretation. If the specimen is placed directly in formalin, it curls up, and sections will be cut tangentially. The full thickness rectal biopsy required to make a diagnosis of Hirschsprung's disease is taken as a formal surgical excision procedure under general anaesthetic.

Polyps should be totally excised; if they are too big to fit into a pair of biopsy forceps, a more formal approach using a diathermy snare or a perianal operative technique may be required. To establish the diagnosis of carcinoma, a forceps biopsy will suffice.

During sigmoidoscopy, the samples of stool may be taken for microscopy, microbiological examination, and chemical testing for occult blood.

ANORECTAL PHYSIOLOGY TESTING

The physiology of the anorectal region is quite complex, but in the recent times, a battery of investigations has given us a better understanding of its function. The various tools that are used for the evaluation of anorectal physiology include continence tests, anorectal manometry, electromyography of the anal sphincter, defecography, and the pelvic floor, and nerve stimulation tests. These advanced tests depict a clear picture of the mechanisms of anorectal disorders and demonstrate pathophysiologic derangements in patients with disorders of the anorectal region.

Continence Disorders

One can find it difficult to define anal continence precisely, but in simple terms, it implies the ability to completely control defecation. It is important that the clinicians should agree as to what they mean when discussing incontinence, as differences in terminology can lead to confusion and sometimes wrong treatment. Incontinence can be divided into three distinct groups.

True incontinence is the passage of faeces per annum either without the patient's knowledge (that is, sensory deficit), or without adequate voluntary contraction (that is, mechanical deficit), or both. Partial incontinence is the passage of flatus or mucous per annum without either the patient's knowledge (that is, sensory deficit) or adequate voluntary contraction (that is, mechanical deficit), or both. 'Overflow' incontinence is the result of distension of the rectum, with the reflex relaxation of the anal sphincters, as occurs for instance with simple faecal impaction, when mucous and liquid faeces leak past solidly impacted faeces. In most cases, true incontinence implies an impairment of both internal and external sphincters.

Reservoir Function

The distal part of the colon functions as a type of reservoir and has a significant role to play in the continence. To add to this, lateral angulation of the sigmoid colon and the valve of Houston act as a physical wall and suppress the further advancement of faeces. Also, the compliance of the rectum is important as a reservoir.

Sphincteric Factors

The tone of the anal sphincter muscles is the most important factor in maintaining anal continence. Maximal anal resting pressure is approximately 40–80 mmHg. The internal sphincter accounts for approximately 52–85% of the resting pressure. The external sphincter is in continuous tonic activity and is active not only in the resting period, but during sleep when the other sphincter muscles are relaxed. Hence, the external sphincter muscles could be considered special muscles. During voluntary contractions, the duration of contraction is approximately 40–60 seconds.

Anal Sensory Perception

The anal canal receives several types of sensory receptors and thus rectal contents can be perceived more precisely. There are receptors for pain, contact, pressure, friction, etc., and are expressed primarily in the distal half of the anal canal. However, they may be present in the area about 5–15 mm above the dentate line.

Reflexes

When the anal area is stroked with a sharp object, the external sphincter muscle contracts and is referred to as the anal reflex.

This reflex transmits via the S1-S4 nerves and occurs through the pudendal nerve. The next is the reflex response of the anal sphincter muscles, which denotes an automatic response relaxing the internal sphincter muscles and contracting the external sphincter muscles during distension of the rectum. This reflex response of the two anal sphincters is very important for maintaining anal continence.

MECHANICAL FACTORS

Angulation between the Rectum and the Anal Canal

Angulation between the rectum and the anal canal is formed by the continuous contractile action of the puborectalis muscles, and it is the most important factor for maintaining overall anal continence. Measured by defecography, the angle formed by the anal canal and the rectum during the resting period is approximately 90°, and the angle becomes larger during defecation.

Effects of the Flutter Valve

In theory, abdominal pressure compresses the rectum from the right and the left sides of the upper anal canal; thus, the rectum forms a slit shape, which facilitates anal continence itself. According to the theory, the highest pressure point should be located in the area above the anal sphincter muscles. However, the flutter valve mechanism is controversial because the highest pressure point is located in the middle area rather the upper area.

Flap Valve Effect

When the abdominal pressure is elevated, the anterior wall of the rectum is compressed and thus flap valve blocks the faecal stream above the upper end of the anal canal. Nonetheless, this effect is also controversial. When the Valsalva manoeuvre is performed, the anal pressure is always higher than the rectal pressure; thus, anal continence is thought to be due to the reflex contraction of the external sphincter muscles rather than the flap valve effect.

Corpus Cavernosum of the Anus (Anal Cushion)

The corpus cavernosum of the anus, that is, anal cushion, consists of blood vessels, smooth muscles, and elastic connective tissues, and they allow high-quality and fine anal continence.

ANORECTAL MANOMETRY

Anorectal manometry is a test that measures the function of the anal sphincter muscles. This test can help to determine the best and appropriate treatment options for the patients with anal incontinence by evaluating the contribution levels of the nerves and the muscles involved in anal continence also detecting the site of the anal sphincter defect caused by trauma, and assess the degree of continence. It can also measure the levels of the functions of the sphincter muscles before surgery that might affect anal continence. The test can be performed in evaluating the causes of chronic constipation in children and young adults. It shows a high-pressure zone (which refers to the lengths of the anal sphincter muscles), the anorectal inhibitory reflex, the resting pressure, the squeeze pressure, and the rectal sensibility.

High-pressure Zones of the Anal Canal

The maximal resting pressure is present in the region that is about 2–3 cm above the anal canal. The measurement done by using the continuous pull-through technique is more accurate than the measurement by using the systematic pull-through technique.

The measured high-pressure zone is about 2.5–5.0 cm, and it is shorter in the females than in males. When the anal sphincter muscles contract, the anal canal becomes longer, and it becomes shorter during defecation.

Anal Resting Pressure

The internal sphincter muscles account for two-thirds of the pressure in the resting period. It is approximately 65–85 mmHg, and the maximal resting pressure is shown in the area approximately 1–1.5 cm above the anal verge.

Squeeze Pressure

Squeeze pressure is generated by a combined contraction of the external sphincter muscles and the puborectalis. It is twice that of what is in the resting period.

Anorectal Inhibitory Reflex

When the rectum is suddenly dilated, the rectal walls contract, and in the distal area of the anal canal, to begin with, the external sphincter muscles contract for a while and the resting period pressure is elevated. This is also known as the anorectal contraction reflex. Following this, in the proximal area of the anal canal, along with a decrease in the resting pressure, the internal anal sphincter muscles go into relaxation for a short period. This is referred to as the anorectal inhibitory reflex. However, in patients with colonic aganglionosis or coloanal anastomosis, the anorectal inhibitory reflex is absent.

ELECTROMYOGRAM

An electromyogram is performed to examine the presence or absence of relaxation failure of the puborectalis muscles. A surface electrode is inserted into the anus, and the electric activities of the external sphincter muscles and the puborectalis muscles during various periods are recorded.

PUDENDAL NERVE TERMINAL MOTOR LATENCY (PNTML) TEST

The most commonly conducted test is the PNTML test that along with the other motor nerve conduction tests is used for anorectal physiologic testing, and this test evaluates the nerve control of the external sphincter muscles. The method is to insert a rubber glove covered index finger having an electrode attached to it in the rectum and stimulate the pudendal nerve from the right and the left ischial spine areas to measure the latency of the external anal sphincter muscle contraction. The normal value is 1.9 ± 0.2 ms, and any value more than this implies injury of the pubic nerves. A delay in this value can be observed in anal incontinence, injury of the external anal sphincter muscles, solitary rectal ulcer syndrome, and refractory constipation patients.

DEFECOGRAPHY

Defecography is a useful test method to find functional as well as morphological abnormalities in patients with defecation disorder. It is also a very useful test method to determine appropriate surgical treatment methods. This test helps diagnose rectal intussusception, enteroceles, sigmoidoceles, paradoxical puborectalis contraction, descending perineum syndrome, and rectoceles.

ENDOANAL ULTRASONOGRAPHY

Endoanal ultrasonography is of particular help in diagnosing structural abnormalities of the anal sphincter muscles and adjacent tissues. Indications include perianal abscess, and complex and recurrent anal fistulae pre-operative staging of anal cancer, and anal incontinence.

CLINICAL APPLICATIONS OF ANAL PHYSIOLOGICAL TESTS

Anal Incontinence

Anal incontinence is diagnosed accurately by performing anorectal manometry, an electromyogram, a pudendal nerve terminal motor latency test, and anal ultrasonography; then, appropriate treatment methods are determined. For example, for patients with anal incontinence caused only by dysfunction of the anal sphincter muscles, even sphincter-saving surgery would not be of help, and in such patients, biofeedback treatments are sometimes effective.

Constipation

The estimation of colonic travel time, and in addition anorectal manometry, is of assistance to analyse extreme severe dyschezia, a megarectum, and megacolon. Biofeedback treatments are viable in a few patients.

Rectocele

Defecography is critical for analysis as well as for differential determination between an enterocele and a sigmoidocele.

Solitary Rectal Ulcer Syndrome

In an electromyogram, relaxation of the puborectal muscles may not be seen.

Descending Perineum Syndrome

In defecography, the finding of a descending anal canal 3.5 cm more than amid the resting time frame is appeared. In cases connected with anal incontinence, the anal pressure is measured to be anomalous low by anorectal manometry.

Anal Fissure

In most instances, the anal pressure is elevated during the resting period.

Injury

While planning a sphincter-saving approach, anal ultrasonography would guide and assess the presence of an appropriate volume of muscles for successful sphincter-saving surgery.

Inflammatory Bowel Diseases

The volume in the rectum is reduced in patients with inflammatory bowel diseases because of an increase in the sensitivity of the rectum and a reduction in the compliance.

BIOFEEDBACK THERAPY

Biofeedback therapy was first performed on patients with anal incontinence on an experimental basis, and now it is being performed as a routine. The idea behind this therapy is to enhance the contraction capacity of the external sphincter and make the patients learn to perceive and react during slightest dilatation of the rectum. Unfortunately, according to the Cochrane review, proofs of biofeedback therapy being effective in patients with anal incontinence were concluded not to be sufficient. Still, this therapy has the advantage in that it is non-invasive and safe. It can be recommended as the first therapeutic method to be performed for anal incontinence patients, and it is thought to be useful as an adjuvant therapy after anal sphincter repair.

CLINICAL PEARLS

- In a patient with complaints of anorectal symptoms, the assessment is initiated in the office setting. With minimally invasive diagnostic tools, one can identify the common anorectal ailment and can often treat them adequately.
- This can be achieved with a systematic approach, patience, and gentleness to get the support of the patient. This yields a patient whose anxiety has been alleviated in the course of an initial office visit.

(Cont'd)

- To obtain the best results, the patient should be positioned appropriately for the examination while maximising the patient's comfort. Therefore, a good proctologic table is an essential part of the office equipment.
- The three positions proper for the proctology examination are Sims' (changed left lateral decubitus), prone jack-knife (or knee-mid-section), or lithotomy in delicate and old patients. A colleague ought to dependably be available to help the examiner and work as a chaperone amid the examination, regardless of the sexual orientation of the patient.
- Basic palpation without visual investigation is deficient to completely assess the anus and rectum, and there is not a solitary instrument that can completely assess both.
- The lining of the anal canal is not well visualised with either a rigid proctosigmoidoscope or a flexible sigmoidoscope. An adequately equipped proctology office should have a selection of anoscopes.
- As of today, rigid proctoscopy has taken a backseat as flexible sigmoidoscopy offers greater patient compliance, ease of examination, and the ability to examine an extended portion of the colon.
- For any patient with a family history of early cancer, personal history of associated cancers or polyps, or indication based on age, it is preferable to proceed to colonoscopy rather than perform the in-office flexible sigmoidoscopy.
- Newer investigative tools include anal physiological testing, defecography, tomography, endoanal ultrasonography, and magnetic resonance imaging (MRI).

SUGGESTED READINGS

Bohlman TW, Katon RW, Lipschutz GR, McCool MF, Smith FW, Melnyk CS. Fiberoptic pansigmoidoscopy: an evaluation and comparison with rigid sigmoidoscopy. *Gastroenterology*. 1977;72:644–9.

Cirocco WC, Reilly JC. Challenging the predictive accuracy of Goodsall's rule for anal fistulas. *Dis Colon Rectum*. 1992;35:537–42.

Crespi M, Casale V, Grassi A. Flexible sigmoidoscopy. *Surg Clin N Am.* 1980;60:465–79.

Kapoor DS, Sultan AH, Thakar R, Abulafi MA, Swift RI, Ness W. Management of complex pelvic floor disorders in a multidisciplinary pelvic floor clinic. *Colorectal Dis.* 2008;10:118–23.

Liecester RJ, Hawley PR, Pollett WB, Nicholls RJ. Flexible fibreoptic sigmoidoscopy as an outpatient procedure. *Lancet*. 1982;1:34–5.

Manier JW. Fiberoptic pansigmoidoscopy: an evaluation of its use in office practice. *Gastrointestinal Endosc.* 1978;24:119–20.

Marks G, Boggs JW, Catro AF, Gathright JB, Ray JE, Salvati E. Sigmoidoscopic examinations with rigid and flexible fibreoptic sigmoidoscopes in the surgeon's office: a comparative prospective study of effectiveness in 1012 cases. *Dis Colon Rectum.* 1979;22:162–8.

Morren GL, Beets-Tan RG, Van Engelshoven JM. Anatomy of the anal canal and perianal structures as defined by phased-array magnetic resonance imaging. *B J Surg.* 2001;88:1506–12.

Nicholls RJ, Dube S. The extent of examination by rigid sigmoidoscopy. *Br J Surg.* 1982;69:438.

Pehl C, Seidl H, Scalercio N, et al. Accuracy of anorectal manometry in patients with fecal incontinence. *Digestion.* 2012;86:78–85.

Pescatori M, Quondamcarlo C. A new grading of rectal internal mucosal prolapse and its correlation with diagnosis and treatment. *Int J Colorectal Dis*. 1999;14(4–5):245–9.

Rosato O, Lumi CM. Neurophysiology in pelvic floor disorders. In: *Complex Anorectal Disorders: Investigation and Management*. Wexner SD, Zbar AP, Pescatori M (eds). London: Springer. 2005; 153–69.

Schrock TR. Complications of gastrointestinal endoscopy. In: *Gastrointestinal Disease: Pathophysiology, Diagnosis, Management*. Volume 1, 4th ed. Sleisinger MH, Fordtran JS (eds). Philadelphia: WB Saunders. 1989;216–22.

Chapter 5

Anal fissure

An anal fissure is a linear tear or split in the anodermal mucosa that traditionally extends distally from the dentate line to the anal verge. Anal fissures represent the second most common cause of a proctology specialist visit following the haemorrhoidal disease.

Anal fissure is excruciatingly painful, as it affects the multilayer squamous epithelium of the anoderm, which is richly innervated with pain fibres. During defecation, the lesion is stretched with resultant painful symptom complex. The pain can persist for a few hours and may be accompanied by bleeding. The pain can be intense enough to induce the patient to avoid defecation with consequent hardening of the faeces and exacerbation of the problem.

Anal fissures occur with equal frequency in both sexes. Additionally, anal fissures tend to occur in younger and middle-aged persons. Anal fissures are not frequent in patients older than 65 years, and in this age group must be suspected to be associated with other pathologies.

The exact aetiology of anal fissures is unknown, but the initiating factor is thought to be trauma from the passage of a particularly hard or painful bowel movement. Low-fibre diets, such as those lacking in raw fruits and vegetables, are associated with the development of anal fissures. There is no record of any particular occupation with a higher risk of developing anal fissures, whereas any previous anal surgery may be a predisposing factor. The anal canal may become more susceptible to trauma from hard stool due to stenosis and tethering caused by scarring from previous surgeries. Other risk factors include Crohn's disease and childbirth injury. Fissures are seldom seen in association with infections like tuberculosis, syphilis, human immunodeficiency virus (HIV), and herpes.

In most people, hard bowel movement often causes initial minor tears in the anal mucosa, which heal rapidly without a long-term sequel. This only accounts for acute fissures but not for the progression to chronic non-healing anal fissures even if the bowel consistency had improved. In few patients with underlying abnormalities of the internal sphincter, these injuries may progress to chronic anal fissures.

Hypertonicity and hypertrophy of the internal anal sphincter are the most commonly observed abnormalities. These may lead to elevated anal canal and sphincter resting pressures. Most patients with anal fissures have an elevated resting pressure, and this resting pressure returns to normal levels after surgical sphincterotomy. A long, high-pressure zone in the anal canal with ultra-slow waves is seen commonly in these patients.

The aetiology of fissure formation in females who have had a vaginal delivery, whether complicated or assisted, or in patients with a rectocele may be different. Scar formation may be associated with ischaemia and poor healing. However, the resting sphincter pressure is usually small.

PATHOPHYSIOLOGY OF CHRONIC ANAL FISSURE

In patients with hypertrophied internal anal sphincters, the blood supply to the posterior anal commissure is further compromised considering that it is the most poorly perfused part of the anal canal, thus rendering the posterior midline of the anal canal relatively ischaemic. This might be the reason for prolonged healing of many fissures. Pain accompanies each bowel movement as this raw area is stretched while the injured mucosa is abraded by the stool. The internal sphincter goes into spasm when the stool is passed, which has two significant effects. First, the spasm itself is painful; second, the spasm further reduces the blood flow to the posterior midline and the anal fissure, contributing to the reduced healing rate.

The internal anal sphincter hypertonia, seen in patients with an anal fissure, has long been thought to be a secondary phenomenon, occurring after local trauma to the mucosa by, for example, the passage of hard faeces. In this scenario, subsequent sphincter spasm then leads to further constipation and so a vicious cycle is created. Traditional treatment (anal dilatation and internal sphincterotomy) aims to break this cycle by disrupting the internal anal sphincter.

The blood flow to the posterior midline of the anus is potentially deficient, being supplied by end arteries, which pass through the internal anal sphincter before reaching the posterior commissure. Angiography of the vessels shows a relative deficiency of arterioles in the posterior commissure of the anal canal in 85% of individuals. This area is usually only supplied by end vessels and is thus more susceptible to ischaemia. This is the same area where the majority of chronic anal fissures tend to occur. Laser doppler flowmetry has also demonstrated that blood flow to the distal anal canal decreases with increasing anal pressure and vice versa.

As such, it has been postulated that high anal pressure and ischaemia go hand-in-hand. As the maximum resting anal pressure (MRAP) is usually greater than 90 mmHg in patients with fissures, such hypertonia will compress these end arteries and cause ischaemia of the posterior commissure. The hypertonia is not secondary to pain, as it is not relieved by the use of topical anaesthetics. The paucity of blood flow prevents healing of the anal fissure until the cycle of internal sphincter hypertonia and the decreased blood flow is broken by muscle relaxants or surgery.

In addition to the above two factors, it has been postulated that the pathogenesis of posterior anal fissures is contributed by the repeated preferential over-stretching of the posterior anal sphincter complex and perineum. This is very likely secondary to the direction of the passage of faeces due to the anorectal angle. Furthermore, there is a relative paucity of support between the coccyx and the anorectal ring.

This explains the presence of sphincter spasm, severe pain (ischaemic in nature), a predilection for the posterior midline, and poor healing in all chronic anal fissures (Figure 5.1).

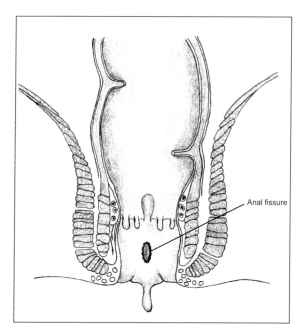

Anal fissure

Figure 5.1   An anal fissure.

Illustration: James Oinam.

CLINICAL PICTURE

Anal fissure is relatively specific in the patients who complain of severe pain during a bowel movement lasting several minutes to hours afterwards. The pain recurs with every bowel movement, and the patient commonly becomes afraid or unwilling to have a bowel movement, leading to a cycle of worsening constipation, harder stools, and more anal pain. Diagnosis can often be made based on history findings alone. There may be an intense burning pain that appears immediately or later after the evacuation of the bowels, of variable duration, described as the passing of a 'razor blade' or 'broken glass'. The pain may feel external or internal and will often last for hours after a bowel action. It may be described as sharp and often burning in nature. There may or may not be a history of chronic straining before its original onset. There is often the feeling of a perianal lump and a streak of blood after wiping on the toilet tissue.

Occasionally, a few drops may fall into the toilet bowl, but significant bleeding does not usually occur with an anal fissure. Other features include anal discharge, pruritus, constipation, dysuria, and dyspareunia.

To begin with, the fissure is just a tear in the anal mucosa and defined as an acute anal fissure. Acute anal fissures have sharply demarcated, fresh mucosal edges and granulation tissue at the base

(Figure 5.2). The majority of acute anal fissures heal spontaneously or with conservative treatment.

Some lesions do not improve even after six weeks and develop secondary changes, characteristic of chronic fissures. The skin on the distal end of the fissure becomes fibrotic and oedematous, forming a sentinel pile (Figure 5.3). The fibres of the internal anal sphincter are visible at the base of the chronic fissure, and often, an enlarged

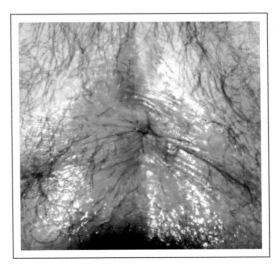

Figure 5.2   Acute anal fissure.
Courtesy: Pravin Jaiprakash Gupta.

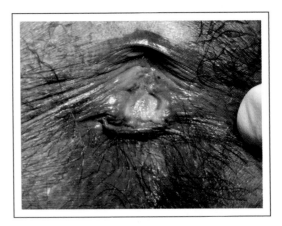

Figure 5.3   Chronic anal fissure with tag.
Courtesy: Pravin Jaiprakash Gupta.

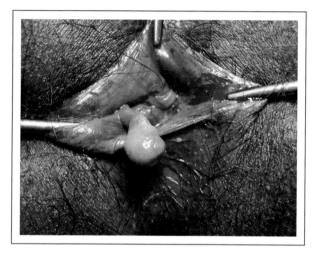

Figure 5.4   Chronic anal fissure with fibrous polyp and papilla.
Courtesy: Pravin Jaiprakash Gupta.

anal skin tag is presented distal to the fissure and hypertrophied anal papillae are present in the anal canal proximal to the fissure (Figure 5.4).

Other features of chronicity include associated haemorrhoids, induration at the edges of the fissure, suppuration in the fissure, or a bridged fissure with underlying fistula.

A chronic fissure classically occurs at the posterior midline position (6 o'clock position), with the anterior midline position occurring in 10% of females and 1% of males. Two per cent of patients have both anterior and posterior fissures. Fissures occurring off the midline should raise the possibility of other aetiologies like Crohn's disease, sexually transmitted disease, acquired immune deficiency syndrome (AIDS), or cancer.

DIAGNOSING ANAL FISSURE

If a typical anal fissure is seen located in the posterior or anterior midline, then no laboratory tests are necessary. If the fissure is off the midline (Figure 5.5), is irregular, or if an underlying illness (for example, Crohn's disease, squamous cell cancer, ulcerative colitis, AIDS) may be present, then erythrocyte sedimentation rate, stool and viral cultures, HIV testing, or biopsy of the lesion or fissure should be performed. One should also rule out other causes of perianal ulceration that includes anorectal tuberculosis, anorectal syphilis, and neoplastic disease of the anus.

A gentle perianal examination and inspection of the anal mucosa can confirm the diagnosis along with the history. A digital rectal examination is painful and may be deferred.

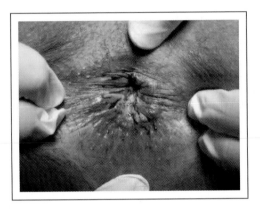

Figure 5.5 Multiple anal fissures with anal tag.
Courtesy: Pravin Jaiprakash Gupta.

Anoscopy is done occasionally only when the fissure is not easily visible, as it is not well tolerated by a patient with an acute anal fissure. Occasionally, a topical application of lidocaine facilitates the examination. A paediatric proctoscope would be an excellent tool to do the anoscopy in such cases.

Other pathologies must be excluded in patients who do not respond to appropriate therapy or those who have a recurrent anal fissure after surgical treatment. Anoscopy and rigid proctosigmoidoscopy are used for further evaluation. Patients with chronic fissures tend to have less pain and have better tolerance for either anoscopy or rigid proctosigmoidoscopy and should have this included in their evaluation.

Usually, there is no specimen available from fissure examination for pathology findings to avoid the accidental excision of internal sphincter, which usually demonstrates fibrosis. Whenever excised, the tissue typically exhibits non-specific inflammation.

MEDICAL THERAPY

Anal fissures are treated conservatively initially and more than 80% of acute anal fissures resolve without further therapy. The goals of treatment are to relieve constipation and break the cycle of hard bowel movement, associated pain, and worsening constipation.

Stool-bulking agents, such as fibre supplementation and stool softeners, are used as first-line medical therapy, laxatives are used as needed to maintain regular bowel movements, and mineral oil may be added to facilitate the passage of stool but it is not recommended for indefinite use. Sitz baths after bowel movements relieve internal sphincter muscle spasms, thus providing symptomatic relief. Use of oral analgesics is very effective in relieving pain after defecation. Recurrence may occur if the high-fibre diet is abandoned after the fissure is healed. This rate can be reduced if patients remain on a high-fibre diet. It is important to emphasise that in the case of acute anal fissures conservative treatment can provide a cure in 87% of the cases while in chronic forms, the success rate is 50%.

Similarly, application of the local anaesthetic cream, suppository or gel, ointments containing opiates, xylocaine, amethocaine, and cinchocaine to relieve pain, belladonna to alleviate sphincter spasm and silver nitrate to promote healing are also being used since long. These mixtures can be introduced on the finger or a short rectal bogie to ensure a thorough application. Although creams containing topical steroids and anaesthetics often have shown little benefit in clinical trials, many anecdotal reports support their use as a first-line treatment, with many reports of healing in approximately 50% of patients.

Sitz baths have been used to provide relief to patients with anal fissures. Shafik conducted a study on 18 healthy volunteers and 28 patients with painful anorectal diseases (18 patients with fissures and 10 with haemorrhoids). All of them used sitz baths to alleviate pain. Investigations were comprised of measuring rectal, and interstitial sphincter temperature, rectal and rectal neck pressures, and electromyographic activity of both the external and internal anal sphincters before and after the subjects sat in a warm-water bath at temperatures of 40°C, 45°C, and 50°C for 10 minutes. Pain relief was more evident and lasted longer at higher bath temperatures. There was no change in the rectal and interstitial sphincter temperatures before and after the bath in both healthy volunteers and patients. The rectal neck pressure and internal and sphincter electromyographic activity dropped significantly in the bath, but increased gradually to pretest levels 25–70 minutes after exiting the bath.

Non-surgical therapies include nitroglycerin ointment or a dermal patch (as well as analogues such as isosorbide dinitrate), botulinum toxin injection (Botox), the use of home anal dilators, calcium channel inhibitors/blockers (CCBs—delivered usually as an ointment but also in tablet form including nifedipine and diltiazem), bulk aperients (including bran and other forms of fibre), hydrocortisone or topical anaesthetic creams (principally lignocaine and clove oil with or without topical steroids), the amino acid (L-arginine), sitz baths, and additional smooth muscle relaxants that include indoramin, sildenafil, minoxidil, and trimebutine. Such therapies do not require hospitalisation. The discovery of pharmacological agents that effectively cause temporary sphincterotomy and heal most fissures has led to approximately two-thirds of patients avoiding surgery. Smooth muscle relaxation is also the first option in patients with a high risk of incontinence. Smooth muscle relaxation has been tried using a variety of agents. Some physicians use them as initial therapy in conjunction with fibre and stool softeners, and others prefer to add it to the medical regimen if fibre, analgesics, and stool softeners alone fail to heal the fissure. The effects of this medication are termed as 'chemical sphincterotomy'. Many newer drugs are being introduced in this category, but the following are mostly used.

Chemical Sphincterotomy

The mediator of the non-adrenergic, non-cholinergic pathway stimulating relaxation of the internal sphincter has been shown to be nitric oxide. Application of topical nitric oxide donors has been shown to reduce anal canal pressure. When applied topically to the anus two to three times daily, the internal sphincter is relaxed, and the fissure heals significantly better than placebo. It has been reported that blood flow at the posterior midline of anoderm is inversely related to the maximum mean anal resting pressure, and topical application of glyceryl trinitrate (GTN) ointments increases the blood flow to the posterior midline. About 375 mg of 0.4% nitroglycerin rectal ointment is prescribed twice a day, delivering 1.5 mg of nitroglycerin each time. Mean bioavailability with 0.2% nitroglycerin ointment delivering 0.75 mg nitroglycerin dose is 50%.

Such observations have generated interest in the use of nitric oxide donors as a form of chemical sphincterotomy. Temporary loss of flatus control is observed during GTN treatment, with no case of faecal incontinence. The healing rates for topical GTN ointment range from 40.4% to 68%. The majority of the patients healed within two months. However, recurrences do occur at a rate of 7.9–50%. A study investigating the effect of GTN ointment concentrations on healing rates demonstrate a better healing rate with increasing concentrations (40.4% for 0.2% vs. 54.1% for 0.4%). Its use, however, reported higher rates of side effects (a headache and temporary loss of flatus control) occurring at a rate of 5.9–56.4%. The incidence of headaches was increased with increasing concentration of GTN.

Although the application of GTN caused fissure healing and a reduction in mean resting anal pressure, there was no measurable increase in anodermal blood flow observed. This is contrary to the hypothesis that GTN heals fissures by improving blood flow to an essentially ischaemic ulcer.

A potential problem with using GTN ointment outside of a trial setting may be reduced compliance. It has been suggested that tachyphylaxis may occur when GTN is used to treat anal fissure, just as it occurs in cardiovascular disease.

Another way to use isosorbide dinitrate is in spray form in the treatment of anal fissures. Isosorbide dinitrate 1.25 or 2.5 mg (one or two sprays) applied three times a day for four weeks produced healing in 83% of patients at four months. Alternatively, GTN patches can also be applied to the buttocks in patients who have difficulty in applying the ointment. Even GTN suppositories have been tried and used successfully in patients with anal fissures.

Adverse effects of GTN often limit its use. The main negative effects are headache and dizziness; therefore, patients should be instructed to use GTN ointment for the first time in the presence of others or directly before bedtime.

The efficacy of GTN ointment has been debated, and its use is still controversial. Analogous to the use of GTN ointment, diltiazem and nifedipine ointments are also available for use in clinical trials. They are thought to have similar efficacy to GTN ointment but with fewer adverse effects.

Botulinum Toxin

Botulinum toxins (BTXs) comprise a family of neurotoxins designated as types A to G, which is produced by the anaerobic bacterium *Clostridium botulinum*. BTX-A blocks cholinergic transmission resulting in flaccid paralysis and autonomic nerve dysfunction. It is used to treat skeletal muscle disorders including blepharospasm and spasticity associated with cerebral palsy. It is also being evaluated in smooth muscle disorders including achalasia and anismus. Its use in chronic anal fissure was reported in 1993. Chronic anal fissures are caused by anal sphincter hypertonia leading to an ischaemic ulcer. BTX-A injection into the internal anal sphincter at an angle of 60° on both sides of anal fissure causes relaxation of the anal sphincters, enhances microcirculation at the fissure site, and promotes fissure healing. BTX prevents the release of acetylcholine from presynaptic axon terminals. Its action is short-lived, and full recovery of the synapse is expected within 12 weeks.

By causing temporary synaptic blockade, BTX has been shown to relax the internal anal sphincter when injected into it. By contrast, a BTX injected into the internal anal sphincter has no effect on the external anal sphincter. As the external anal sphincter is not involved in the pathogenesis of anal fissures and may be voluntarily contracted to maintain continence, it makes theoretical sense to avoid paralysing the external anal sphincter if possible. There is evidence that at least 15 units of BTX-A should be injected on either side of the anal fissure to produce a significant decrease in the resting anal pressure. The effect lasts approximately three months until the nerve endings regenerate. This three-month period may allow fissures to heal and symptoms to resolve. One study has observed that increasing the dose of Botox from 25 to 50 units increases the healing rate without a significant increase in the side effects. Initial relief of symptoms with Botox injection but recurrence after three months suggests that the patient would benefit from surgical sphincterotomy. Botox injection is a costlier therapy, but a grouping of patients on the same operating list and follow-up at the same outpatient clinic improves cost-effectiveness, as one vial can be used to treat four patients.

Gonyautoxin, a type of phytotoxin produced by dinoflagellates (shellfish), has also been tried in place of Botox. It breaks the vicious cycle of pain and spasm.

Botox has both obligatory and facultative side effects. Obligatory effects include excessive weakness of anal sphincters and injury of anal wall tissues. Transitory incontinence for flatus (18%) or faeces (5%) and perianal thrombosis or haematoma have been reported. Facultative side effects are related to Botox spreading from the target tissue to distant muscles by haematogenic diffusion.

Occasional reports of accidental injection of the toxin in the surrounding tissue resulting in a general poisoning, haematoma, and infection have been reported. As being invasive, it is uncomfortable to the patient. Many surgeons are unhappy using this technique without an anaesthetic. It can also lead to incontinence of flatus and faeces, flu-like syndrome, and acute inflammation in the surrounding area. Need for repeat injection, high cost, and slow healing are few other pitfalls in the use of Botox therapy.

Calcium Antagonists

Calcium channel blockers reduce the contractility of cardiac and smooth muscle myocytes by inhibiting the cellular influx of calcium ions. Consequently, drugs such as nifedipine and diltiazem have been used in the treatment of oesophageal dysmotility with varying degrees of success. The internal anal sphincter also has a calcium-dependent mechanism to maintain tone and receives inhibitory extrinsic cholinergic innervations. It may, therefore, be possible to lower anal sphincter pressure using calcium channel blockers and cholinergic agonists without side effects. Nifedipine is found effective in relieving the anal sphincter spasm in patients with anal fissure when 20 mg of the medicine is administered orally twice daily. Nifedipine gel (0.2%) is applied every 12 hours for three weeks. After 21 days of therapy, 95% of patients were healed according to one study. A mean reduction of 30% and 188.8% in anal pressure and squeeze pressure was observed. Side effects included mild headache, flushing, and mild ankle oedema. All side effects are seen in the first four weeks of treatment. Oral lacidipine 6 mg once daily or diltiazem 60 mg in divided doses can be used alternatively. These drugs have a short duration of action and need to be administered 2–3 times daily. Similarly, side effects like a headache, palpitations, flushing, dizziness, colicky abdominal pain, ankle oedema, reduced taste and smell, nausea, and diplopia have been reported.

Topical diltiazem shows promise as an effective therapy with relatively fewer side effects. In a randomised trial of 50 patients, topical 2% diltiazem demonstrated a more profound reduction in MRP (23% vs. 15%) and better healing (65% vs. 38%) with fewer side effects (0% vs. 33%) than oral diltiazem. Topical diltiazem appears to produce similar fissure healing with fewer side effects than GTN. It also seems to heal between 48% and 75% of fissures that have failed to improve with GTN. This agent may ultimately supersede GTN because of its better side-effect profile.

Less commonly, L-arginine ointment, potassium channel openers like topical minoxidil and nicorandil, alpha-1-adrenoceptor blockers like indoramin, phosphodiesterase-5 inhibitors like sildenafil 10% ointment, angiotensin enzyme (ACE) inhibitors like topical captopril (0.28%), and amino acid gel and cream have also been tried with some success.

Bethanechol, a cholinomimetic that promotes synthesis of nitric oxide (NO), has been shown to lower anal resting pressure in volunteers. Bethanechol as 0.1% gel applied locally three times a day for eight weeks has also been reported to give equally satisfactory results. In a small non-randomised study, bethanechol reduced fissure pain and healed 9 of 15 fissures, equivalent to topical diltiazem. No side effects were noted. No long-term follow-up data are available.

Sildenafil (Viagra®), a phosphodiesterase inhibitor, lowered anal resting pressure by 18% after a single intra-anal instillation of 0.75 mL of 10% sildenafil in patients with previously untreated fissures. One of 19 patients failed to respond.

Minoxidil is a potassium-channel opener that induces smooth muscle relaxation and vasodilatation. A small prospective randomised study using minoxidil in the treatment of anal fissure showed a healing rate of 30% or less.

In another study, six of eight fissures refractory to other treatment healed after 15 hyperbaric oxygen treatments given over three weeks. There was one relapse at three-month follow-up. Although intriguing, hyperbaric oxygen therapy has the obvious drawbacks of cost and access and is unlikely to become a widely used modality for fissure.

Surgical Therapy

Analysis of the available literature shows that by far, medical manipulation of the internal sphincter should be the first-line treatment of anal fissures. Surgical treatment is called for if the medical therapy fails, or if there is a recurrence.

Anal Dilatation

Anal dilatation was first described in 1838 and was popularised by Lord in the treatment of haemorrhoids. Lord's original eight-finger dilatation was abandoned in favour of a more gentle four-finger stretch for four minutes (Figure 5.6) and more recently a standardised dilatation procedure using a Park's retractor opened to 4.8 cm or with a 40 mm rectosigmoid balloon has been advocated in the treatment of chronic anal fissures. Although anal dilatation results in successful healing of anal fissures comparable to lateral internal sphincterotomy, there is no way to reliably standardise the procedure, and both the internal and external sphincters can be disrupted or fragmented in an irregular manner. Anal dilatation has a higher risk of incontinence than that of lateral internal sphincterotomy. Nevertheless, some authors still support a policy of gentle anal dilatation as the treatment of choice in a chronic anal fissure. The number of fingers used and the amount of time the stretch is applied varies among surgeons.

The risk of incontinence after manual dilatation has been documented by both prospective and retrospective studies. A study evaluated 12 men with faecal incontinence after manual dilatation and found that 11 had gross internal sphincter disruption (meaning 153° of the circumference), three with associated external sphincter damage.

There may be problems in standardising the interpretation and gradation of the symptoms of incontinence, but a 20–25% risk is a reasonable estimate. A study of incontinence after minor anal surgical procedures, evaluated by anal manometry and ultrasonography, found characteristic patterns of anal sphincter damage after manual dilatation in 27 incontinent patients. Incontinence grade was severe, with 17 patients complaining of incontinence to the solid stool. All 27 patients demonstrated internal sphincter injury. Ten had thinning of the posterior half of the internal sphincter, 12 had a posterior defect in the internal sphincter, and five internal sphincter fragmentation. Eight patients also had associated surgical damage to the external sphincter.

There has been a renewed interest in the technique of anal dilatation, although the current technique requires standardised dilatation to avoid excessive internal sphincter trauma. One study used cryothermal anal dilators heated to 40°C to perform anal dilatation in combination with GTN ointment application and achieved an 86.6% healing rate with a 3.3% incontinence rate. These figures are comparable with that of sphincterotomy. In contrast, in the same study GTN ointment alone achieved a 73.3% healing rate with a 13.3%

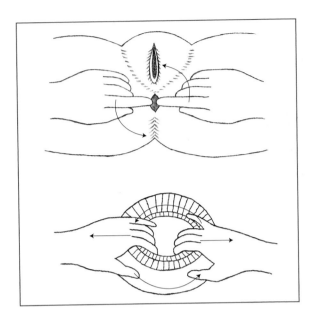

Figure 5.6   Technique of anal dilatation.

Illustration: James Oinam.

recurrence rate. A second study used intermittent anal dilatation with an adjustable anal dilator and attained a 90% healing rate with no incontinence symptoms. A further study compared pneumatic balloon anal dilatation with lateral sphincterotomy and achieved comparable healing rates (83.3% for balloon dilatation vs. 92% for sphincterotomy) but lower incontinence rates (0% for balloon dilatation vs. 16% for sphincterotomy) for balloon dilatation.

This author in his study has reported on a new technique of division of the internal sphincter, termed 'sphincterolysis'. This method involved the use of firm finger pressure over the internal sphincter fibres at 3 o'clock to produce a full-thickness division of the fibres without breaching the anal mucosa. This study achieved healing rates of 96.5% with a 3.5% temporary incontinence rate that resolved in 97% of the affected patients within one month. There were no recurrences.

Lateral Internal Sphincterotomy

Eisenhammer introduced internal sphincterotomy into surgical practice in 1951. It was initially performed posteriorly in the midline, but this often led to the so-called 'key-hole' deformity and lateral subcutaneous sphincterotomy was popularised by Notaras who first reported it in 1969. The caudal part of the internal sphincter is divided for a variable distance cephalad, usually to the dentate line. The suggested advantage of lateral sphincterotomy over manual dilatation of the anus is that it represents a surgically controlled partial internal sphincter division. Despite this, it carries a significant risk of minor but persistent disturbances in anal continence. The incidence has been poorly documented but varies between 0% and 36% for incontinence to flatus, 0% and 21% for incontinence to liquid stool, and 0% and 5% for solid stool incontinence.

Sphincterotomy can be carried out using an open or a subcutaneous technique and under local or general anaesthesia. Local anaesthesia is not always recommended but can be used in cooperative patients. The purpose of an internal sphincterotomy is to release the tension by cutting the hypertrophied internal sphincter and allowing the fissure to heal.

As per the earlier prescribed procedures sphincterotomy was performed in the posterior midline at the site of the fissure with or without a fissurectomy and this did not allow the cut to heal for the same reasons as why the fissures had a delayed healing. Currently, sphincterotomies are performed in the lateral quadrants (right or left, depending on the comfort or handedness of the surgeon). In a properly performed lateral internal sphincterotomy, only the internal sphincter is cut; the external sphincter is not cut and must not be injured.

In a closed sphincterotomy, a No. 11 blade is inserted sideways into the inter-sphincteric groove laterally and rotated medially, and drawn out to cut the internal sphincter. If the anal mucosa is cut it might result in a fistula; hence care is taken not to cut the anal mucosa. After the knife is removed, the anal mucosa overlying the sphincterotomy is palpated, and a gap in the internal sphincter can be felt through it. The sphincterotomy is extended into the anal canal for a distance equal to the length of the anal fissure.

In an open sphincterotomy, a 0.5–1 cm incision is made in the inter-sphincteric plane looping the internal sphincter on a right angle and brought up into the incision and cutting it under direct visualisation. The two ends are allowed to fall back after being cut. A gap can then be palpated in the internal sphincter through the anal mucosa, as in the closed technique. The incision can be closed or left open to heal.

A surgeon may choose to excise the fissure in conjunction with the lateral sphincterotomy in chronic anal fissures but it will be recommended to excise the hypertrophied papillae and the skin tag and leave the fissure to heal on its own instead of excising the fissure along with the sphincterotomy and worrying whether it will heal. Long-standing chronic fissures fail to heal at times even with an adequate sphincterotomy; in such cases, an advancement flap helps to cover the defect in the mucosa which the surgeon can perform at the time of sphincterotomy if the chances of the fissure to heal are less or if it is a second procedure after a failure.

Post-operative Details

Sphincterotomy is performed either in an outpatient setting or as an office procedure, and patients may return home the same day except for patients who undergo surgery under anaesthesia. They can return to normal activities the following day. Patients may witness minimal pain post-surgery and the intense pain from fissure abates immediately.

Follow-up

After surgery stool softeners and fibre supplementation are pre-scribed and indefinite use of fibre supplementation is recommended to prevent future problems with constipation. Follow-up care ensures healing of wound properly and checking whether and complaints of fissure and the spasm have resolved.

COMPLICATIONS

Infection

It is a rear complication and occurs as a small abscess in only 1–2% of patients, which can be drained out. Antibiotics are necessary only if significantly associated cellulitis occurs or if the patient is immunosuppressed.

Bleeding

Profuse bleeding which would need medical attention is rare during these surgeries; some ecchymosis may occur around the sphincter-otomy site.

Fistula Formation

Less than 1% of patients develop an anal fistula at the location of the sphincterotomy. This usually results from a breach of the mucosa at the time of the sphincterotomy. The fistula is often low and superficial and should be treated with fistulotomy.

Incontinence

Incontinence rates are much lower with an appropriately performed internal sphincterotomy than with sphincter stretch, and these rates depend on the definition of incontinence which vary dramatically amongst studies. In most patients, the minor soiling or incontinence to flatulence that may occur in the immediate post-operative period usually resolves without any long-term sequel.

Reasons for Incontinence after Sphincterotomy

Though the procedure is seemingly controlled and divides the internal sphincter only partially, with a consequently limited reduction in maximum resting pressure (MRP) of the order of 25–35%, ultraso-nographic studies have revealed that, like manual dilatation of the anus, internal sphincterotomy appears to be difficult to standardise. A study evaluated the extent of sphincterotomy with the use of anal ultrasonography. Fifteen patients underwent ultrasonography before and after the operation. Nine of 10 women and one of five men had inadvertently undergone full-length division of the internal sphincter, and three women complained of incontinence to flatus. The authors concluded that the length of internal sphincter division in women was frequently greater than anticipated, partly owing to a shorter anal sphincter, and questioned the reproducibility of the procedure. Another reason is that the sphincterotomy at times extends into the external sphincter. Overzealous or inaccurate sphincterotomy can also result in incontinence and women are particularly at risk owing to shorter anal sphincters and occult obstetric sphincter defects that may compound the effects of surgery.

Some chronic fissures are not associated with spasm, making a therapeutic reduction in resting pressure not only illogical, but also a potential threat to continence. A study performed manometry on 40 consecutive patients who presented with chronic fissure and found that 19% of men and 42% of women had low or low-normal resting pressures, placing them at potential risk of incontinence with a surgical reduction in MRP of 25%. It was also noted that surgeons were poor at identifying this at-risk group on clinical grounds.

Several surgeons have examined ways of reducing the risks associated with lateral sphincterotomy. A tailored lateral sphincterotomy has been studied in 287 patients. This procedure differs from standard internal sphincterotomy in that the division is more conservative and carried cephalad only for the length of the fissure rather than to the dentate line. This procedure appears safe and efficacious, but it has not become common practice. In an evaluation of ultrasonographically guided internal sphincterotomy, there were more complete internal sphincter divisions and a greater reduction in MRP, but healing and incontinence rates were similar when compared with standard sphincterotomy techniques.

Recurrence or Non-healing of the Fissure

The recurrence rate or non-healing rate for anal fissures after surgical treatment is 1–6%. Several studies have found that up to 50% of subjects who did not heal had underlying and undiagnosed Crohn's disease as the aetiology for their fissure.

OUTCOME AND PROGNOSIS

The recurrence rate of anal fissure after sphincterotomy is approximately 1–6%, which is higher after a sphincter stretch. Usually, any recurrent disease or an improperly or incompletely performed initial sphincterotomy may result in recurrence. The patient is given medical therapy initially but if not relieved, the surgeon must assess the original surgery by palpation during examination under anaesthesia or performing an endoanal ultrasound. If the sphincterotomy were incomplete, it could be completed on the initial side or redone on the opposite side. If the first sphincterotomy were complete, a second sphincterotomy could be completed on the opposite side.

OTHER SURGICAL APPROACHES FOR CHRONIC ANAL FISSURE

Fissurectomy

In cases where the fissure is associated with a fistula, fissurectomy with or without posterior sphincterotomy may be useful, but posterior sphincterotomy has lost favour as it may cause a 'key-hole deformity' resulting in mucous leakage in up to a third of patients. Fissurectomy includes excision of the fibrotic edge of the fissure, curettage of its base, and excision of the sentinel pile and/or anal papilla if present. When used in association with botulinum toxin in the treatment of a chemically resistant fissure, it appears to enhance healing while avoiding the risk of a sphincterotomy.

Flap Anoplasty Procedures

These are also used in the treatment of chronic anal fissures. These methods involve fashioning a local flap to cover the fissure defect. As flap procedures do not involve disruption of the internal anal sphincter, they are particularly useful in patients with normal anal pressures or in fissures secondary to obstetric trauma where there is often associated internal sphincter disruption. A study using a rotation flap achieved 81% healing rate with an 11.8% flap failure rate and 0% incontinence rate. A second study using a V-Y advancement flap produced a 98% healing rate with a flap dehiscence rate of 5.9% and 0% incontinence rate, but with a recurrence rate of 5.9% of new fissures at new locations.

In addition to the reduction of internal sphincter tone in treating chronic anal fissures, the research has been done into the reduction of trauma during defecation. One recent study looked into the use of a posterior perineal support device incorporated into a toilet seat to improve the healing rates of chronic anal fissures. This posterior perineal support device is likely to reverse the preferential over-stretching of the posterior anal sphincter complex and mucosa and thus facilitating defecation with fewer traumas. The improvement in pain, bleeding, constipation, and abdominal discomfort was statistically significant. The improvement in pain was also manifested in a decrease in pain score from five (before treatment) to zero (at three months).

Another pilot study reported on the reduction of post-lateral sphincterotomy pain, where methylene blue dye was injected into the perianal skin and inter-sphincteric space just before sphincterotomy was carried out. The median pain score of the patients decreased from 2.5 on a post-operative day one to zero on day five. Nine out of 24 patients had no pain at all post-operatively. The improvement in pain, in turn, helped in fissure healing.

ANAL FISSURE IN CHILDREN

Mechanical tears may cause fissures in children aged between 6 and 24 months. Patient history and examination can confirm diagnosis. In children stool negativism, that is, the deliberate reluctance to defecate, is not uncommon and it is important to palpate the abdomen for signs of faecal loading. Conservative treatment is recommended initially; in case of failure, local GTN or calcium channel blockers should be tried. GTN 0.2% topically twice daily has been shown to be effective in treating fissures in children. There is little information on diltiazem or BTX treatment in children. Lateral sphincterotomy or fissurectomy should be reserved for those failing to heal with medical treatment. Conservative management must heal acute fissures in 10–14 days including dietary modification and osmotic laxatives. If the fissure persists for 6–8 weeks, chemical sphincterotomy should be considered. Underlying pathologies have to be ruled out in case of chronic fissures just like in adults. Anal dilatation in the management of constipation and faecal soiling has not been found to be beneficial and is associated with a high rate of recurrence. For an indolent fissure resistant to healing, fissurectomy and lateral sphincterotomy have been found to be beneficial. The surgical technique is the same as for adults.

ANAL FISSURES DURING ANTE- AND THE POSTPARTUM PERIOD

One-third of females suffer from few symptoms of anal fissures in the ante-partum and postpartum period. The most important risk factor is dyschezia. The appearance of anal fissures can be caused by precipitated labour, large foetus, and episio- and perineotomy. The conservative treatment of anal fissures can begin with local treatment by different means, which include the arrest of the pain syndrome by analgesics, local anaesthetic, or GTN ointment, dietary regulation, and prevention of constipation. Long-term results are good. Anal sphincter hypertonia is commonly thought to underlie the development of anal fissure, yet anal fissure is particularly common after childbirth, a time when anal canal pressure may be reduced. This paradox is not understood. Postpartum anal fissure is associated with reduced anal canal pressures, and surgical interference with the anal sphincter mechanism should be avoided.

A suspicion of underlying HIV-related disease may be considered in patients with risk factors who also have deeper, broad-based, or cavitating lesions where formal fissure surgery should be avoided more often than not, particularly where there is an active proctitis, poorly controlled or advanced disease, neutropenia or a low CD4+ count, and where there is an inherently weak sphincter tone. These disorders may also be accompanied by anal intraepithelial neoplasia, where suspicious lesions merit biopsy. The pattern of anal lesions in HIV-positive patients appears not to have been affected by the introduction of highly active anti-retroviral therapy (HAART).

COMPLICATIONS ASSOCIATED WITH CHRONIC ANAL FISSURE

In a chronic or neglected anal fissure, infective organisms may invade the fissure area to lead to complications. These organisms lead to a purulent infection in and around the anal fissure leading to paraproctitis, abscess, or anal fistula (Figure 5.7).

Even a small abscess in the inter-sphincteric space at the middle of the anal canal may cause pain very similar to that of the fissure, and diagnosis may be delayed because very few physical signs are present.

A superficial fistula can occur in association with a chronic anal fissure and if present, runs subcutaneously or under a sentinel tag (Figure 5.8).

An organised abscess at the base of fissure usually follows an inadequate or delayed drainage of the anal abscess, which assumes chronicity. The abscess is treated with antibiotics to result in being walled off with fibrotic tissue and forming an antibiotic granuloma (antibioma or a sterile abscess).

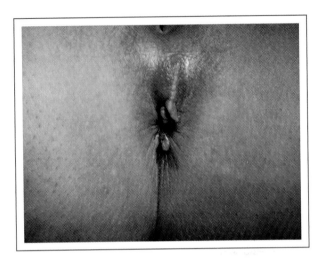

Figure 5.7 Anal fissure with abscess anteriorly.

Courtesy: Pravin Jaiprakash Gupta.

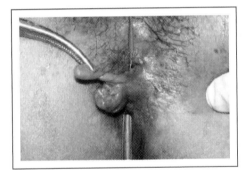

Figure 5.8 Anal fissure, sentinel pile, and fistula.

Courtesy: Pravin Jaiprakash Gupta.

Another lesion complicating a chronic anal fissure is a pyogenic granuloma, which is an acquired benign vascular lesion of skin and mucous membrane, which may occasionally present intravascularly or subcutaneously. Near the chronic anal fissure, it appears as a sessile or pedunculated, red-wine, soft little tumour of the size of millet or barley grain (Figure 5.9).

Most of the purulent pathologies are due to diseases of the anal glands. Some are probably the result of an infection in the lymphoid tissues found around the anal glands. The chronic anal fissure may act as a pathogenic factor in the development of sepsis, especially in the posterior part of the anal canal with reduced vascularity.

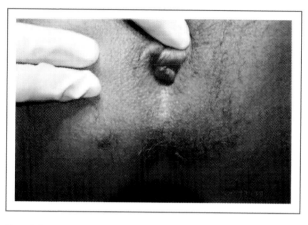

Figure 5.9 Post-fissure granuloma.
Courtesy: Pravin Jaiprakash Gupta.

These perianal infections could at times be an effect of the treatment of the fissure itself. Surgical procedures like sphincterotomy, fissurectomy, or injection of BTX are fraught with complications like ano rectal sepsis, causing abscess and fistula.

Infective pathologies associated with chronic anal fissure need a more aggressive approach. Complete extirpation of the offending tissue helps in faster and smoother recovery with reduced chances of recurrence. A careful search of such lesions can avert complex situations.

Atypical anal fissures associated with Crohn's disease or HIV should be approached cautiously. Surgical management of patients with Crohn's disease and anal fissure has been feared due to presumed risks of incontinence in a population prone to diarrhoea as well as poor wound healing, infections, and fistula formation. However, recent studies show that healing was achieved in 88% of patients after fissurectomy, closed lateral internal sphincterotomy, or a combination of both.

Anal fissure remains a difficult problem in the management of HIV-patients and should be approached cautiously, especially in a setting of advanced disease or baseline incontinence. However, recent data suggests that lateral internal sphincterotomy may be tolerated well in these patients when conservative management fails.

The following points sum up the treatment approach to anal fissure:

- Most acute fissures can be managed by general measures.
- Bulking agents are better than other laxatives and purgatives.
- Efforts should concentrate on developing a nonsurgical treatment.
- Pharmacological manipulations should be considered for both ethical and economic reasons.
- Almost two-thirds of patients can be treated without surgery.
- Combinations of modalities work better.

- Medical therapy should be extended to at least six weeks before it is considered to have failed.
- Medications chosen should have minimum side effects.
- Oral preparations should be the best choice to address compliance issues.
- However, no oral therapy comes close to the efficacy of surgical sphincterotomy.
- Surgery should be reserved for those failing pharmacological treatment. Internal sphincterotomy should be the choice of surgery.

CLINICAL PEARLS

- Anal fissures are linear splits in the anal mucosa. Acute fissures typically resolve within a few weeks; chronic fissures persist longer than 8–12 weeks.
- Most fissures are in the midline and related to constipation or anal trauma. Fissures located off-midline indicates an atypical aetiology, such as Crohn's disease, tuberculosis, leukaemia, or human immunodeficiency virus.
- Painful defecation and rectal bleeding are common symptoms. Pathophysiology is linked to high resting sphincter tone plus relative ischaemia in the posterior midline; so, therapies to relax the internal anal sphincter are useful.
- The diagnosis typically is clinical. High-fibre diet, stool softeners, and medicated ointments relieve symptoms and speed up healing of acute fissures but offer limited benefit in chronic fissures.
- Drug therapy in chronic anal fissure includes oral nifedipine, diltiazem, lacidipine, bethanechol, salbutamol, and indoramin.
- Local applications include 2% GTN ointment, diltiazem, and L-arginine gel. However, increasing incidences of adverse effects and decreasing efficacy in the long term have been the major drawbacks of these medications.
- Chemical cauterisations, use of the direct current probe, anal dilatation using anoscope or rectosigmoid balloon are few other options proposed. However, they are not substantiated with benefits on long-term follow-up and thus are not found being employed in most of the world.
- Both open and closed methods of sphincterotomy are equally effective. Surgery is highly efficacious and successful in curing the fissure in more than 90% of patients. A systematic review of randomised surgical trials shows that the overall risk of incontinence is about 10%.
- Efforts should concentrate on developing a non-surgical treatment.
- Almost two-thirds of patients can be treated without surgery.
- Medications chosen should have minimum side effects.
- Oral preparations should be the best choice to address compliance issues. Surgery should be reserved for those failing non-surgical treatment. Internal sphincterotomy should be the choice of surgery.

SUGGESTED READINGS

Altomare DF, Binda GA, Canuti S, Landolfi V, Trompetto M, Villani RD. The management of patients with primary chronic anal fissure: a position paper. *Tech Coloproctol*. 2011;15:135–41.

Arthur JD, Makin CA, El-Sayed TY, Walsh CJ. A pilot comparative study of fissurectomy/diltiazem and fissurectomy/botulinum toxin in the treatment of chronic anal fissure. *Tech Coloproctol*. 2008;12:331–6.

Cross KL, Massey EJDA, Fowler AL, Monson JRT. The management of anal fissure: ACPGBI position statement. *Colorectal Dis*. 2008; 10(Suppl 3):1–7.

Garg P, Garg M, Menon GR. Long-term continence disturbance after lateral internal sphincterotomy for chronic anal fissure: a systematic review and meta-analysis. *Colorectal Dis*. 2013;15:e104–e117.

Griffin N, Acheson AG, Tung P, Sheard C, Glazebrook C, Scholefield JH. Quality of life in patients with chronic anal fissure. *Colorectal Dis*. 2004; 6:39–44.

Hananel N, Gordon PH. Re-examination of clinical manifestation and response to therapy of fissure-in-ano. *Dis Colon Rectum*. 1997; 40:229–33.

Jensen SL. Treatment of first episodes of acute anal fissure: prospective randomized study of lignocaine ointment versus hydrocortisone ointment or warm sitz baths plus bran. *Br Med J* (Clin Res Ed). 1986; 292:1167–9.

Kenefick NJ, Gee AS, Durdey P. Treatment of resistant anal fissure with advancement anoplasty. *Colorectal Dis*. 2002;4:463–6.

Khubchandani IT, Reed JF. Sequelae of internal sphincterotomy for chronic fissure in ano. *Br J Surg*. 1989;76:431–4.

Lock MR, Thompson JPS. Fissure-in-ano: the initial management and prognosis. *Br J Surg*. 1977;84:86–8.

Lund JN, Binch C, McGrath J, Sparrow RA, Scholefield JH. Topographical distribution of blood supply to the anal canal. *Br J Surg*. 1999;86:496–8.

Lund JN, Scholefield JH. Aetiology and treatment of anal fissure. *Br J Surg*. 1996;83:1335–44.

Nelson R. A systematic review of medical therapy for anal fissure. *Dis Colon Rectum*. 2004;47:422–31.

Nicholls RJ. Anal Fissure; surgery is the most effective treatment. *Colorectal Dis*. 2008;10:529–30.

Schornagel IL, Witvliet M, Engel AF. Five-year results of fissurectomy for chronic anal fissure: low recurrence rate and minimal effect on continence. *Colorectal Dis*. 2012;14:997–1000.

Schouten WR, Briel JW, Auwerda JJ, De Graaf EJ. Ischaemic nature of anal fissure. *Br J Surg*. 1996;83:63–5.

Shub HA, Salvati EP, Rubin RJ. Conservative treatment of anal fissure: an unselected, retrospective and continuous study. *Dis Colon Rectum*. 1978;21:582–3.

Chapter 6

Haemorrhoids

References to haemorrhoidal disease have been found dating from the pre-Christian Era with the service of proctology thriving in ancient Egypt. Similarly, other cultures have devoted time to haemorrhoidal management with the Japanese establishing a temple in the city of Kanazawa entirely dedicated to it. Throughout history, prelates, presidents, and kings have all suffered from haemorrhoids. Both Henry VI and James I of England along with Louis XI of France, Frederick the Great of Prussia, and President Thomas Jefferson were described as suffering from bleeding piles with the Holy Roman Emperor Otto II apparently dying from haemorrhoidal blood loss. Martin Luther elaborated at length on his bleeding haemorrhoids with Cardinal Richelieu rather laconically recording details of his anal fissure, haemorrhoids, and ultimately his difficulties with rectal prolapse.

The list goes on and on, with sufferers including Nicolaeus Copernicus and composer Meyerbeer, with notorious Casanova suffering from 'severe haemorrhoids' while incarcerated in Venice's Piombi prison on the charge of performing magic in public. Austrian Don John, the victor over the Turkish fleet at the battle of Lepanto, died several hours after excision of a haemorrhoidal 'mass' with a more modern fraternity of sufferers including Ernest Hemingway and President Jimmy Carter. Perhaps, the most famous haemorrhoidal sufferer was Napoleon Bonaparte, who lamented along with his brother Jerome on their mutual ailment, lauding the value of locally applied leeches. Before the battle of Waterloo, Bonaparte had an attack of thrombosed prolapsed haemorrhoids and was confined for parts of the battle to his sickbed, unable to command or ride, with some historians attributing his defeat to his 'crisis haemorrhoidale'. In its wisdom, the Catholic Church has assigned curative powers to St. Goncalo. In this regard, sufferers flocked to the basilica of Murtosa in Portugal, where he was born, to expose their bare behinds to a statue of the saint in hopes of a cure.

HAEMORRHOIDAL DEFINITION

Haemorrhoids (in Greek *haema* means blood and *rhoos* means flow) are used not so much for the 'normal' vascular anal cushions which have been described as part of the normal continence mechanism in anal closure, but which are reserved for the abnormal dilatation of the haemorrhoidal plexus protruding into the anal canal lumen and reaching beyond the height of the normal anal columns of Morgagni. The English term 'pile' most likely comes from *Pila* (Latin) meaning a ball to describe the palpable external component. Morgagni attributed their presence to increased pressure due to the human upright posture that gets increased in those having constipation and during pregnancy, resulting in vascular pelvic congestion with defecation and causing prolapse, localised trauma, and bleeding. In this sense, haemorrhoids should be considered as non-normal components of human anatomy.

By this definition, there are three valid states of haemorrhoids whereby they are part of the normal vascular cushions, part of the protruding dilated haemorrhoidal plexus, or a definitive disease/disorder. The position of typical haemorrhoids, classically in the 3, 7, and 11 o'clock positions as examined in the lithotomy position, was initially described by Sir Ernest Miles as part of the division of the right main branch of the superior rectal artery into anterior and posterior branches and the left undivided branch of the left superior rectal artery. Others described haemorrhoids in a different manner away from English tradition, where Cruvelhier compared their structure to erectile or cavernous tissue and Virchow regarded them as similar to cavernous haemangiomata demonstrating arteriovenous communications consistent with other erectile soft tissues and explaining the bright red blood lost clinically.

Despite its frequent occurrence, the aetiology of the haemorrhoidal disease remains controversial. Some correlative pathogenic factors have been proposed including constipation, advancing age, socioeconomic status, pregnancy, occupation, physical activity, and obesity. The multiplicity of potential aetiologic factors, however, suggests that no single theory adequately explains the pathogenesis of this common disorder.

Some important contributing factors include:

- **Diet:** Rich, low-residue diets often necessitate prolonged straining of the abdominal and pelvic musculature. It has been suggested that a typical Western diet that is rich in processed food and lacking in fibre directly contributes to haemorrhoids. In this respect, haemorrhoids are rare in less-developed African countries where the diet is rich in roughage and fibre. As the population in these countries changes their diet to include more processed foods, the incidence of haemorrhoids has been shown to increase. Spicy, colon-irritating foodstuffs can also lead to exacerbation of haemorrhoidal disease with correlations with excessive consumption of alcohol or caffeine where an excess of lactic acid in the stool or excessive use of dairy products, like yoghurt, can cause irritation and where reducing such consumption can bring relief.
- **Straining bowel movements due to constipation or hard stools:** One theory proposes that it is the pushing force of stool, especially a hard stool, that when passes through the anal canal, drags the haemorrhoidal cushions downward. Another factor suggests that with age or an aggravating condition, the supporting tissues anchoring the haemorrhoidal region to the underlying muscle of the anal canal deteriorate.
- **Diarrhoea:** The most frequent occurrence of diarrhoeal disorders in patients with the haemorrhoidal disease when compared with the total population suggests that these disorders may be related to or share a common set of aetiologic risk factors. The mechanism by

which diarrhoea leads to haemorrhoidal disease, however, remains unclear. It is hypothesised that loose or frequent stools may result in prolonged contraction of the anal sphincter to maintain continence of faeces.

- **Lifestyle:** The lifestyle modifications, which include excessive time spent on the toilet, poor toileting habits like reading while in the toilet or multiple cleaning attempts or rushing to complete a bowel movement may be contributory. The Western style toilet is another association for haemorrhoids as it encourages excessive straining. Hurrying can also lead to excessive straining and increase pressure on the rectal veins. Regular tobacco use and smoking negatively affect the digestive system and are thought to exacerbate haemorrhoidal symptoms. Equally, insufficient sleep is also associated with excessive straining.

- **Severe coughing:** A chronic cough from asthma, smoking, or any chronic lung disease is associated with an increased risk for haemorrhoids.

- **Pregnancy and childbirth:** It is very well known that during pregnancy and the puerperium, certain anatomical, hormonal, and physiological changes take place in the pelvis where changes in the levels of oestrogens, progesterone, gonadotropins, corticosteroids, thyroid function, and proteins may be associated. Pregnancy and vaginal delivery predispose women to develop haemorrhoids related to these hormonal changes and due to increased intra-abdominal pressure, it has been estimated that between 25% and 35% of pregnant women are affected by this condition. The anorectal vascular dilatation and enlargement along with the laxity of the peri-anorectal structures as well as the increased intrapelvic pressure during labour are also important secondary factors in the causation of haemorrhoids before and during childbirth with these effects being most important during the final trimester. Here, precipitating factors will include an irregular diet, lack of exercise, pushing of the bowel to the periphery by the enlarged uterus, and release of the hormone 'Relaxin'; all these contribute to constipation and straining during or after pregnancy. Third-trimester symptomatology is commonest when venous engorgement is greatest in the pelvis and when dehydration may lead to relative constipation with most symptoms alleviating after delivery. Acute thrombotic events requiring a localised (limited) incision or excision can be safely performed during pregnancy when indicated.

- **Heredity:** It is also possible to inherit a tendency to develop haemorrhoids with many cases of haemorrhoids running in families. There is little objective data where genetic predisposition may be associated with weak rectal vein walls and valves, which contribute to haemorrhoidal development at an earlier age.

- **Colonic malignancy:** The association between anorectal malignancy and haemorrhoidal disease is well described where there have been significant associations observed among primary anorectal cancer, cancer in situ, benign neoplasms of the anus and anal canal, and anal neoplasms of uncertain behaviour.

- **Toileting habits:** The style of the modern toilet lamentably encourages straining with some commercial toilet elevation devices designed to provide perineal support and reputed to treat patients with evacuatory difficulty, chronic anal fissure, and haemorrhoids. Many people admit to reading while sitting on the toilet, adding undue pressure to the anal veins. It is also suggested that cigarette smoking during bowel movements may worsen haemorrhoids and lead to episodes of bleeding.
- **Hepatic disease:** Portal hypertension also represents a potential well-recognised risk factor although there is no real epidemiological difference in the rate of haemorrhoidal disease in cirrhotics with portal hypertension and age-matched normal.
- **Obesity:** As obesity increases rectal vein pressure, it has been associated with haemorrhoids where poor muscle tone or poor posture can exacerbate pressure on the rectal veins. Although faecal seepage is more prevalent in morbid obesity, there is limited data concerning the effects of morbid obesity, and there is no apparent association between haemorrhoidal prolapse and a grossly overweight status.
- **Elevated resting anal pressure:** More recent studies show that patients with haemorrhoids tend to have a higher resting anal canal tone than age-matched normal suggesting that the sphincter muscle of the anal canal becomes tighter than average even when one is not straining.
- **Loss of rectal muscle tone:** Haemorrhoids are more likely with increasing age as the anchoring tissues of the haemorrhoidal cushions weaken and stretch with ageing. Faulty bowel functions due to overuse of suppositories, laxatives, or enemas results in increased straining during bowel movements.
- **Occupation:** People who exert themselves strenuously at work or stand or sit in fixed positions for extended periods of time are most often afflicted. Horseback riding, drivers, and pilots are more likely to suffer from the haemorrhoidal disease.
- **Posture:** One cause of haemorrhoids could simply be the erect position the humans attain, wherein all the blood cephalad to the rectum puts pressure on the rectal and anal areas.
- **Medications or substances 'causing' haemorrhoids:** Few drugs, medications, substances, or toxins have been found to be associated with haemorrhoids, although the list of such presumptive medications is long and includes prescription, over-the-counter supplements, herbal, and alternative treatments.
- **Miscellaneous causes:** Nutritional deficiencies, climatic conditions, anxiety/depressive psyche, senility, endocrine influences, cardiac decompensation, spinal cord injury, rectal surgery, anal intercourse, and specific anal infections are just a few other potential causes and associations that have been mentioned in the pathogenesis of haemorrhoids.

THE VASCULAR ANATOMY OF THE ANAL CANAL

The arteries of the rectum and anal canal include the superior, middle, and inferior haemorrhoidal arteries and at times a branch from the middle sacral and vesicle arteries. These form the internal and external haemorrhoidal plexus formed by the three main arterial vessels. The internal haemorrhoidal plexus is located above the dentate line, and the external haemorrhoidal plexus is located peripherally at the anal verge. The superior haemorrhoidal arteries originate from the inferior mesenteric artery and are the terminal branches of the superior rectal artery. Additional blood supply is received from the middle haemorrhoidal artery, arising from the internal iliac artery and the inferior haemorrhoidal artery originating from the internal pudendal artery. There are several variations in the contribution of blood supply to the haemorrhoidal plexus.

The superior haemorrhoidal veins come up in the plexus of veins in the submucosal tissue of the anal canal and the lower rectum. This plexus is in free communication with the circular veins around the anal orifice. Through this communication, the portal and systemic venous circulations are connected; a fact that explains the frequency of combined external and internal haemorrhoids. This communication between the internal and external venous plexus makes it unlikely that portal vein obstruction leads to haemorrhoidal disease. This plexus of veins ends in the superior haemorrhoidal veins that run up under the mucous membrane along with the corresponding arteries and which perforate the muscular coat of the rectum a few inches above the anus. Congestion of the plexus and varicosity can occur following a muscular compression of these veins by prolonged straining during defecation. Like other veins of the portal system, these veins are also devoid of valves, resulting in congestion and dilatation. The external haemorrhoidal plexus consist of small subcutaneous veins, which drain the margin of the anus. They are situated in the immediate proximity of the subcutaneous band of the external anal sphincter. An arteriovenous plexus is created between the terminal branches of the superior rectal artery and the superior, middle, and inferior rectal veins.

THE NATURE OF HAEMORRHOIDS
AND THEIR PATHOPHYSIOLOGY

The pathogenesis of haemorrhoids and their separation from the normal vascular anatomy remain controversial topics.

Internal haemorrhoids, which to a varying extent are varicosities of the superior haemorrhoidal plexus of veins, can be divided into two main types—vascular and mucosal. Vascular piles occur most commonly in young people, especially men where the bulk of the 'pile' is seen as a dark-blue dilated venules, which can be seen clearly through the thin mucous membrane. Mucosal piles, often seen associated with pregnancy and in older people, appear to consist mainly of thickened mucous membrane only. These two types of haemorrhoids have a different aetiology. Vascular piles develop in the presence of a normal anal sphincter and are caused by straining during defecation. These piles involve the superior haemorrhoidal plexus, which are situated at the opening of a muscular funnel-like structure formed by the pelvic diaphragm and the anal sphincter. Straining during defecation raises the intra-abdominal pressure and at the same time, the anal sphincter relaxes, resulting in a pressure gradient.

Somewhat surprisingly, the exact pathophysiology of the haemorrhoidal disease is still poorly understood. As haemorrhoids and anorectal varices are separate entities, the older concept that haemorrhoids were simply varicose veins of the anal canal has been discarded. The accepted theory currently is that of the sliding anal canal lining proposing disintegration or a deterioration of the supportive anal cushion network so that haemorrhoids are in effect a pathological state of abnormal downward displacement of the anal cushions resulting in venous engorgement. These are anatomically related to the standard haemorrhoidal locale (with minor intervening cushions) with associated pathological changes which include abnormal venous dilatation, vascular thrombosis, fibroelastic and collagen degeneration, and frank rupture of the subepithelial muscular support structure (the so-called mucosal suspensory or Treitz's 'ligament').

More recently, a series of immunohistochemical and molecular biological changes has been demonstrated in haemorrhoidal tissues assessing morphological specialised soft-tissue degradation.

In haemorrhoidal disease, the anal cushions show significant structural impairment, retrograde changes of the cavernous vessels, and hypertrophy, as well as distortion, rupture, and looseness of Treitz's muscle along with injury of the mucous membranes.

These findings are accompanied by microstructural vascular changes with thickening of the tunica media of smooth muscle cells located in the subepithelial space and dilated thin-walled submucosal arteriovenous plexus which may lead to a smooth muscle 'sphincter-like mechanism' in the arteriovenous plexus. This is typically designed to reduce arterial inflow and facilitate normal venous drainage from the region.

Whereas many physicians and almost every layperson consider haemorrhoids to be a pathologic condition, the presence of haemorrhoidal tissue is 'physiological' and represents a part of the anal continence mechanism. The haemorrhoidal tissue is described as a vascular cushion embedded in a rich and complex stroma of connective tissue and smooth muscle fibres situated within the anal canal. This complex fulfils several specific functions. The three cushions in the anal canal provide maintenance of anal continence, (in part) contributing 15–20% of the resting anal pressure and protecting the sphincter mechanism during evacuation forming a compressible lining and facilitating closure of the anal canal. The smooth muscle acts as a supportive structure, forming a fibro-elastic network within the plexi. The vascular structure in these cushions (called the corpus cavernosum recti or the plexus haemorrhoidal) is nourished by a complex structure of blood vessels. According to these concepts, almost everyone would develop haemorrhoids as they grow older where they are considered normal parts of human anatomy and should be regarded as pathologic only if they become symptomatic or grow enormous.

The important parts of haemorrhoids include the lining, the blood vessels surrounded by a connective tissue stroma, and the anchoring system so that they are covered by mucosa (internal haemorrhoids) or by anoderm (external haemorrhoids). While in this view haemorrhoids are considered as a normal physiological structure, the question is raised as to why they become sufficiently 'diseased' to cause symptoms. Several mechanisms have been suggested to explain the onset of haemorrhoidal disease.

The Mechanical 'Sliding and Lining' Theory

Treitz was the first to describe the anchoring connective tissue and smooth muscle deriving partly from the longitudinal conjoined muscle and partly from the internal sphincter spreading into the submucosa of the anal canal. These descriptions originally outlined how the meshwork layers acted as a supporting scaffold for the haemorrhoidal venous plexus supplementing the mucosa itself and preventing it from prolapsing into the anal canal during defecation. Treitz described the thickening of the anal submucosa as 'cushions' with a constant tri-radiate configuration without any specific correlation to the arterial anatomy. This theory corresponds to our clinical experience where 'haemorrhoids' are considered a muco-anal prolapse rather than a primary vascular pathology. It is notable that the prolapse may involve only a single cushion, or it may be circumferential.

The laxity of the anchoring system of the haemorrhoidal cushion results in greater mobility of the haemorrhoids, which can then move downwards during situations where the intrarectal pressure is raised. At the maximal point, the suspensory ligament and the anchoring tissues are ruptured, and the internal haemorrhoids are permanently prolapsed at the anal verge. Laxity of support tissue also enables distension of the vascular component with a resultant increase in the size of the haemorrhoids. This mobilisation and distension results in fragmentation of the mucosa covering internal haemorrhoids and leads to bleeding that does not come from the vascular structures of the haemorrhoidal cushion but rather from the vessels of the mucosa. This evidence would suggest that haemorrhoidal disease is merely the outward manifestation of their downward displacement (Figure 6.1).

The Haemodynamic Theory

Thomson illustrated that the presumed enlargement of the haemorrhoidal veins was normal. He emphasised that the haemorrhoidal venous plexus is present from birth and can be found in every adult as a normal part of the human anatomy. Where it was thought that elevation of the venous pressure results in the development of haemorrhoids and where internal haemorrhoids may be caused due to the backflow of venous blood, it was postulated that this backflow could be the result of increased intra-abdominal pressure. The distension of haemorrhoids could be enhanced by vascular stasis secondary to impaired venous return either by mechanical obstruction due to defecation difficulty or because of stagnation of faeces in the rectal ampulla. The venous drainage may also be impaired due to the failure of the internal anal sphincter to relax during defecation. In this regard, few sphincteric abnormalities have been shown on conventional anorectal manometry in patients with symptomatic haemorrhoids with the commonest being resting sphincter hypertonia.

If haemorrhoids are indeed manifestations of localised vascular disturbance, few of the alterations seen in these lesions are processes

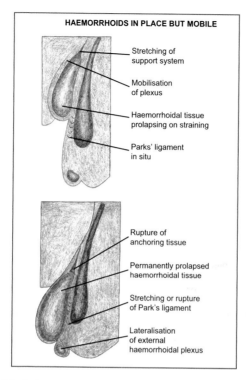

Figure 6.1 Pathophysiology of haemorrhoidal disease.
Illustration: James Oinam.

that are found to be influenced by mast cells in other pathological sites. Enzymes, consisting mainly of tryptases and chymases, can also promote vascular breakdown or vessel wall weakness, leading to tortuosity and revascularisation. Platelet-derived activating factor enhances thrombocyte aggregation and local vasodilatation.

CLINICAL PRESENTATION OF HAEMORRHOIDAL DISEASE AND HAEMORRHOIDAL COMPLICATIONS

Patients suffering from any symptoms related to the anus frequently, often incorrectly, assume that their symptoms are due to haemorrhoids. It is a well-quoted saying amongst physicians that 'nearly every lesion around the anus is liable to be called "piles" by the patient and not infrequently by the referring doctor also'; a practice, which still prevails. It is essential to define specifically the presenting symptoms of the patient to detect any possible abnormalities which are not related to haemorrhoids.

The exact incidence of haemorrhoids the world over is unknown as estimates vary with an overall underestimation. In the United States, around 1.6 million prescriptions for anorectal preparations are written annually where the cost of treating benign anal diseases exceeds $2 billion per year. The German National Insurance Fund spends €38 million yearly for ointments and suppositories whose use is not supported by any scientific data.

The five cardinal symptoms of haemorrhoids are:

- **Bleeding:** It is the most common symptom of haemorrhoids described in the literature besides prolapse. In those who elect for surgery, there is only a weak correlation between the severity of symptoms and the objective grade of prolapse. The symptoms in each patient can vary over time especially concerning the intensity of bleeding. Bleeding occurs specifically in connection with defecation and is painless. The blood is never incorporated in the stool but is seen as stains on the stool or the toilet paper and occasionally colouring the toilet seat with frank spurting often being reported by the patient. A prolapse of the cushions will give an impaired venous return and venous stasis if not reduced. This can cause inflammation of the cushions with the erosion of the epithelium also resulting in bleeding. Rarely, the blood may stagnate in the rectum with the presence of clots and dark red blood in the stools. In a study assessing the role of flexible sigmoidoscopy as part of a single setting in patients who present with typical bleeding (bright red, post-defecatory, painless, and without an associated family history of colorectal polyps or carcinoma), it has been suggested that although some cases may include proctosigmoiditis as an undiagnosed condition that these patients should not be spared full colonoscopic examination despite the classic 'benign' nature of the bleeding. Of course, bleeding from haemorrhoids may cause anaemia with its attendant symptoms.
- **Anal pain:** In general, although the populace believes that haemorrhoids are naturally painful, it is mostly a complication (usually thrombosis) that results in pain in complicated haemorrhoidal disease. Having said this, however, pain is present as a symptom in almost half of the patients. Pain in haemorrhoids has a distinct character. It is related to the prolapse and relieved when the prolapse is digitally reduced. Acutely thrombosed and prolapsed haemorrhoids are associated with rather severe pain where thrombosis of external haemorrhoid (a painful perianal haematoma) acts as a 'five-day wonder' where immediate release under local anaesthesia provides immediate relief and where symptoms gradually abate over five days. The thrombosed internal haemorrhoid provides a hard aspect which extends internally into the anal canal and which is often associated with a degree of gangrenous change (Figure 6.2).
- **Soiling:** Mucoanal prolapse disrupts the closing mechanism of the anal canal. There is a difference between faecal soiling due to anal incontinence from weak sphincters and the mucous soiling due to the mucosal prolapse. The mucous discharge (soiling) may occur during daily activity and in between defecations. It may be responsible merely for a feeling of dampness at the anal verge, or a discharge staining clothing and an irritating, burning perianal sensation.

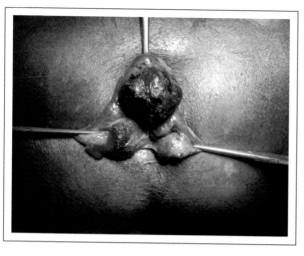

Figure 6.2:   Acutely thrombosed internal haemorrhoid.
Courtesy: Pravin Jaiprakash Gupta.

- **Pruritus:** Anal pruritus is related to irritation of the perianal skin. Without a functional cushion valve sealing the anal canal, chronic exposure to moisture from the mucous discharge will cause anal irritation. This mucous with microscopic stool contents can be a cause of a localised dermatitis resulting in pruritus ani, which becomes a vicious cycle associated with scratching that is worse at night. Skin tags can cause a moist environment in their folds also contributing to the irritation. Pruritus may also develop because of contact dermatitis secondary to the application of haemorrhoid ointments that contain local anaesthetics and topical steroids.
- **Prolapse:** The fragmentation of the connective tissue that supports the anal cushions results in descensus. A single cushion can prolapse, or there may be a total circumferential prolapse. The prolapse may be minor with spontaneous reduction or manifest, requiring digital replacement. Prolapse may occur after prolonged standing, sneezing, coughing, and walking or even on passing flatus. Prolapse may be associated with a feeling of discomfort, described as a desire to defecate, a sense of fullness in the perineum or anus or perineal heaviness. A few patients express a feeling of swelling or heaviness during rectal emptying, although it may be difficult to attribute this symptom to haemorrhoids if it is not possible to reproduce the prolapse at the time of examination.
- **Anal incontinence:** Symptoms of incontinence are potentially more frequent in patients with haemorrhoidal prolapse because the prolapsed cushions typically contribute to the mechanism of anal closure. There are reports describing the presence of impaired continence before the surgical treatment of haemorrhoids usually in those with circumferential prolapse.

EXTERNAL HAEMORRHOIDS

External haemorrhoids may cause symptoms in two main ways. First, acute thrombosis of the underlying external haemorrhoidal vein may occur presenting with specific symptoms. Acute thrombosis is related to a particular event such as straining with constipation, a bout of diarrhoea, physical exertion, or a change in the diet (Figure 6.3). These are acute, painful events where pain results from rapid distension of innervated skin by the clot and the response to surrounding oedema. The pain lasts 5–14 days and resolves with a resolution of the thrombosis. With this resolution, the stretched anoderm persists as excess skin or as a troublesome skin tag in some cases. External haemorrhoids can also cause hygiene difficulty where excess skin folds and tags can mechanically interfere with cleansing and ablution. This can particularly occur in the postpartum period.

Haemorrhoids might present with a range of complications that may be either acute or chronic. At times, some of these complications can be life threatening. Although these states are discussed above, they are also mentioned in this section on complications.

Common complications of haemorrhoidal disease include:

- Haemorrhage leading to anaemia
- Squamous metaplasia
- Strangulation
- Thrombosis
- Suppuration

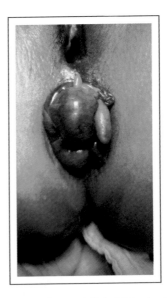

Figure 6.3   The thrombosed external pile (painful perianal haematoma).
Courtesy: Pravin Jaiprakash Gupta.

- Fibrosis
- Gangrene
- Ulceration
- Portal pyaemia
- Haematomas

Haemorrhage

Haemorrhoidal bleeding (haematochezia) may occur as drip or as a jet with or without clots occasionally independently of defecation. Chronic blood loss leads to anaemia with chronic bleeding over an extended period. As a rule, the process is so insidious that patients are not aware of symptoms and often tend to omit significant symptoms unless specifically interrogated.

Squamous Metaplasia and Other Mucosal Changes

These may develop over the haemorrhoidal mucosa due to repeated trauma with prolapse. Damage to the surface could lead to ulceration, inflammation, bleeding, infection, stromal hyperplasia, and ultimately, squamous metaplasia.

Strangulation

Following the prolapse, internal haemorrhoids are gripped by the external sphincter. The impeded venous return leads to congestion, which is associated with considerable pain and distress. Usually, this episode occurs after straining at stool where the haemorrhoids become entrapped due to increased internal sphincter tone, resulting in oedema, thrombosis, and ultimately necrosis. These haemorrhoids may need immediate reduction as progressive venous engorgement and incarceration of the acutely inflamed haemorrhoid leads to thrombosis and infarction.

Thrombosis

Acute thrombosis is usually associated with symptoms of swelling with a lump and severe, persistent pain. The haemorrhoids become dark purple or black in colour and feel solid to the touch. They are associated with oedema of the anal margin that apparently extend into the anal canal with persistent tenderness and often, mild systemic symptoms.

Gangrene

Gangrene of haemorrhoids occurs when the strangulation is sufficiently tight to constrict the arterial supply. The resulting sloughing is often superficial and localised. Occasionally, haemorrhoid sloughs off, leaving an ulcer, which heals gradually. Massive gangrene may rarely lead to portal pyaemia.

Superficial Ulceration

This may follow strangulation with thrombosis in patients with tight sphincters. Should the congestion and oedema be sufficient to compromise the blood flow to the superficial areas of the mucous membrane and skin, ulceration will ensue. Left unattended, the natural course of events is one of slow resolution over a period of weeks.

Suppuration

Though fortunately uncommon, it results from infection within a thrombosed haemorrhoid. Throbbing pain is followed by perianal swelling, and a perianal or submucous abscess may occur. The suppurative process can also be a result of injection sclerotherapy, cryodestruction, electrosurgical ablation, or banding of the haemorrhoids.

Fibrosis

Following thrombosis, internal haemorrhoids may be converted into a fibrous tissue. The fibrous tissue is initially sessile, but often becomes pedunculated and constitutes a fibrous (or fibroepithelial) anal polyp, which is white in colour. The appearances macroscopically and microscopically resemble the fibrous anal polyp noted when an anal papilla hypertrophies in association with a chronic anal fissure. Fibrosis in external haemorrhoid may also be associated with prolapse of an associated internal haemorrhoid.

External Haemorrhoidal Thrombosis

External haemorrhoids present caudal to the dentate line that develops because of distension and distortion of the external haemorrhoidal venous system.

Leukoplakic Changes

Repeated trauma, prolapse, and manual reduction may induce leukoplakic changes in the haemorrhoidal skin.

Portal Pyaemia

Extensive gangrene may lead to portal pyaemia (pylephlebitis) and even a liver abscess, which are fortunately rare events. It may also occur following emergent haemorrhoidectomy or following rubber band ligation and injection sclerotherapy.

APPROACH TO HAEMORRHOIDS

A meticulous examination of the anorectum is often inadequately performed in clinical practice. Careful inspection and experienced diagnostic examination skills complement a detailed history. The history as it pertains to haemorrhoids should ascertain whether the patient has felt and reduced any protrusions, whether symptoms occur during or after defecation or at night, features of incontinence or faecal seepage, bleeding frequency and volume, if mucous is expressed with stools or between bowel movements, and whether anal or pelvic pain is associated with the passage of stool.

Classification of Haemorrhoids

A classification, gradation, or degree of haemorrhoidal disease is of interest as it directs treatment. It is also important to ascertain grade-specific treatment modalities to compare more scientifically

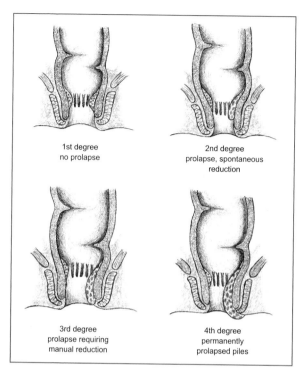

1st degree
no prolapse

2nd degree
prolapse, spontaneous
reduction

3rd degree
prolapse requiring
manual reduction

4th degree
permanently
prolapsed piles

Figure 6.4 Stages or grades of haemorrhoids.
Illustration: James Oinam.

outcomes and recurrence rates. There are several classification systems for haemorrhoids although data concerning the correlation between the symptoms of haemorrhoids and their grade of the disease has been relatively poorly documented (Figure 6.4). The commonest used classification was that described by John Goligher, who graded haemorrhoids from Grade 1 to Grade 4 although this system fails to factor in the severity of symptoms. Haemorrhoids emanating from the dentate line are internal with those below designated as external, thus leaving a mixed category. They may exist at the classic locales as primary left lateral, right posterior, and right anterior, or between these areas as secondary or circumferential variants.

Grade 1

- **Morphology:** Small haemorrhoids
- **Symptoms:** Intermittent bleeding, no prolapse
- **Additional features:** None, except some pain
- **Visual appearance:** Minor, but definite increase in the size of the cushions as observed by proctoscopy
- **Typical age group (years):** 20–45

Grade 2

- **Morphology:** Intermediate haemorrhoids
- **Symptoms:** Prolapse during straining but spontaneously returns; frequent bleeding, sometimes profuse
- **Additional features:** Anal itching (pruritus ani) and occasional skin tags
- **Visual appearance:** Moderate increase of individual masses that prolapse during straining
- **Typical age group (years):** >30

Grade 3

- **Morphology:** Large haemorrhoids
- **Symptoms:** Prolapse that needs manual aid to be returned into the anal canal bleeds frequently and often profusely
- **Additional features:** Anal itching (pruritus ani), discomfort, and skin tags
- **Visual appearance:** Major increase in the size of the cushions and prolapse
- **Typical age group (years):** >40

Grade 4

- **Morphology:** Enormous haemorrhoids
- **Symptoms:** Permanent prolapse, profuse bleeding, bloodstains on the underwear even without a bowel movement
- **Additional features:** Severe pain, anal itching, severe discomfort, soiling, and skin tags
- **Visual appearance:** An extreme increase in size, visible skin tags, and secondary haemorrhoids may develop between the classical sites
- **Typical age group (years):** >50

The classification system used today could be improved by including the external components as a separate entity. It is simple and precise to use classification of anodermal, haemorrhoidal, and mucosal prolapse as an alternative, which could be valuable in several ways. Mucosal prolapse is evident in patients who digitally reduce the prolapse and is easily diagnosed by directly asking the patient about this requirement. Anodermal prolapse is visible as anal tags and polyps on surgical inspection so that treatment aims to remove both of these features with a before-and-after record of this accomplishment. There is currently no specific quality of life data about haemorrhoidal management that would guide surgeons as to the success of the treatment modalities (conservative and operative) in the alleviation of specific symptoms.

Although the term haemorrhoidal disease has been in use for a few years, it clearly establishes that, for a long time, the word 'haemorrhoid' was, in essence, a misnomer used to describe a series of anorectal symptoms and signs that often have nothing to do with the original meaning of the term. The classical physical findings were bleeding, thrombosis of the internal haemorrhoidal plexus, prolapse of the anal cushions, or a combination of these so that some researchers proposed classifying haemorrhoidal disease as bleeding, prolapsing, thrombotic and mixed, thus aiming at a more rational symptom-based treatment rather than an established grade or appearance of the anus. Of course, the haemorrhoidal disease must be differentiated from rectal mucosal prolapse, complete rectal prolapse, a pedunculated rectal polyp, anal cancer and other anal neoplasms, a fibrous anal polyp, a perianal abscess, condyloma accuminata, perianal Crohn's disease, proctitis, pruritus ani, anorectal varices, and a rectal cavernous hemangioma.

THE MANAGEMENT OF HAEMORRHOIDS

The range of reported conservative treatments for haemorrhoidal disease is legion, where treatment varies from dietary and lifestyle modification right through to radical surgery dependent upon the degree and severity of symptoms. As it is suggested that the shearing action of hard stool during straining may damage the anal cushions and lead to symptomatic haemorrhoids, there is extensive literature assessing the introduction of fibre where its use has shown that persistent symptoms are reduced by about 50% overall in treated cases, although there is no evidence that fibre reduces the symptoms from prolapse, pain, or itching. Patients may expect, in simple, non-complicated cases, some form of response after a six-week period of fibre use so that these treatments (whether used naturally incorporating psyllium seeds or ispaghula husk or if used as synthetic fibre supplements) are integral to combined strategies of management.

These are usually complemented by lifestyle changes with an increase in oral fluid intake, a reduction in the consumption of dietary fats, regular exercise, improvements in anal hygiene, and an abstinence of excessive straining or reading on the toilet as well as the avoidance of medications which induce constipation or diarrhoea. It is accepted that diet has a pivotal role in causing and preventing anorectal diseases. However, fruits and vegetables are an essential part of our dietary intake; thus, their role as a fibre for the prevention of colorectal diseases remains controversial.

There are other particular advantages of fibre intake for haemorrhoidal patients, including improvement in coronary heart disease, cerebrovascular disease, hypertension, diabetes, hypercholesterolaemia, and obesity with gastrointestinal benefit in reflux, peptic ulceration, and diverticulosis are believed to aggravate symptoms of anal disorders. Capsicum is also known to be harmful where there is some experimental data to show that red chilli powder in human volunteers causes a considerable increase in the DNA content of gastric aspirate and suggests exfoliation of the surface epithelial cells, although the exact mechanism by which chillies influence colonic and rectal physiology is not well documented. Capsaicin, a pungent principle of hot red pepper, can excite and later dysfunction a subset of primary afferent neurones producing rectal hyperalgesia in patients with irritable bowel syndrome and result in accelerated gut transit while increasing the frequency of stool.

An important component of a safe and efficient therapy for haemorrhoids that are often ignored is the use of plant and nutritional therapies. Several botanical extracts like *Aesculus hippocastanum*, *Ruscus aculeatus*, *Centella asiatica*, *Hamamelis virginiana*, and bioflavonoids have been shown to improve capillary flow, microcirculation, and vascular tone as well as strengthen the perivascular connective tissue.

Also, the low compliance or complications associated with treatments including hydrotherapy, mechanical compression therapy, and diet and lifestyle changes facilitate oral dietary supplementation of this type an attractive alternative. An extensive literature has accrued using a series of phlebotonic (venotonic) oral agents, which were first described for use in patients with varicose veins and chronic venous insufficiency with oedema. These increase venous capacity, decrease capillary permeability, and facilitate lymphatic drainage with associated anti-inflammatory properties.

The use of oral flavonoids as a part of haemorrhoidal management, in particular, is prominent in Europe and Asia usually using a micronised purified flavonoid fraction (MPFF–Dalton). This is available in doses comprising 90% diosmin with 10% hesperidin. They have also been shown to have vasculoprotective effects and are antagonists to proinflammatory mediators. They also act as antagonists of the biochemical mediators of acute inflammation. Of this group of agents, daflon is typically used with a loading dose of three 500 mg tablets twice daily for the first four days and then two tablets twice daily for the following three days, with an objective assessment of the clinical severity of proctorrhagia, anal discomfort, pain, and anal discharge and with particular benefit in pregnant women who present with symptomatic haemorrhoids.

Another venotonic agent, calcium dobesilate that is used in diabetic retinopathy, impairs platelet aggregation and improves blood viscosity where its use in combination with a fibre supplement results in substantial reduction in bleeding from acutely symptomatic oedematous haemorrhoids. Another agent, which has been used in haemorrhoids, is diosmin, which is a potent inhibitor of prostaglandin and thromboxane synthesis, inhibiting leukocyte activation, migration, and adhesion and improving venous tone, increasing lymphatic drainage, and protecting the capillary bed microcirculation.

Diosmin produces a noticeable decrease in plasma levels of endothelial adhesion molecules to reduce neutrophil activation and provides protection against microcirculatory damage. The annual herb, *Euphorbia prostrata*, has flavonoids, phenolic acid, and tannins as its principal agents where preclinical studies with its dried extract have suggested an anti-haemorrhoidal activity. The oligomeric proanthocyanidins found in grape seed extract alleviate and prevent haemorrhoidal symptoms by inhibiting the collagenase enzyme that can damage the blood vessels of the walls of the anal canal in haemorrhoids.

Ointments, Creams, and Suppositories

A range of ointments and creams are available that contain local anaesthetics, mild astringents, or steroids. These agents may be used to provide short-term relief from anal discomfort, but they lack evidence to support their regular use. They hardly have any effect on the underlying pathological changes in the haemorrhoidal cushions. A continuous application can cause eczema and sensitisation of the anoderm; rectal absorption can lead to systemic side effects.

The role of the topical haemorrhoid preparations is to provide temporary relief from haemorrhoidal discomfort and prevent further irritation. It should also provide shrinkage of the swollen haemorrhoidal tissue and prompt soothing relief from painful burning, itching, and discomfort.

Ointments containing belladonna to alleviate sphincter spasm and silver nitrate to promote healing, opiates, xylocaine, amethocaine, and cinchocaine to relieve pain have all been in use. These compositions can be introduced either with the finger or via a short rectal bogie to ensure widespread application over the affected part of the anus. Recent reports of the topical application of Solcoderm, ketanserin gel, a mixture of 5% prilocaine and 5% lidocaine, or a combination of policresulen and cinchocaine have shown excellent symptomatic relief in anal pain.

Other topical agents used include sucralfate, metronidazole, and topical glyceryl trinitrate 0.2% in those patients with haemorrhoids and sphincter hypertonia. Others have suggested benefit in these latter patients for pain management with L-arginine and 0.25% oxethacaine chlorhydrate in post-surgical cases. Topical nifedipine or 1% isosorbide dinitrate has also been recommended for the conservative treatment of thrombosed external haemorrhoids. The commonly available PREPARATION H® has been designed to induce vasoconstriction within haemorrhoid (Pfizer, USA) and contains 0.25% phenylephrine, petrolatum, light mineral oil, and shark liver oil.

The phenylephrine has preferential vasoconstrictive effects on the arterial side of haemorrhoid and differs from the other agents that may be considered protectants. These agents may be supplemented naturally where a mixture of honey, olive oil, and beeswax has been found to be clinically useful in the treatment of some patients with haemorrhoids reducing bleeding and relieving itching without any real risk of side effects. The author, however, rarely recommends topical medications in the form of suppositories, creams, enemas, or foams for the treatment of haemorrhoids with most patients volunteering that they are ineffective by the time they are referred.

For the treatment of acutely inflamed piles, a conservative approach may include bed rest in a Trendelenburg's position, administration of a liquid diet, stool softeners, antibiotics, and anti-inflammatory drugs along with warm Sitz baths and the local application of glycerine and magnesium sulphate paste. In this respect, local anodermal cooling treatment (the Anuice device) has also been advised for symptomatic cases. The anodermal blood flow, which is exposed to cooling, of healthy subjects is regulated not only by nervous mechanisms but also by humoral mechanisms. Based on the Lewis reaction (cold vasodilatation), it is suggested that the short-time cooling of the anoderm can be used as a conservative therapy for symptomatic haemorrhoids. The device available is a plastic cylinder 6 cm in length and 15 mm in diameter, with a broader base, which contains a mixture of glycols as a gel and which can be frozen for 4 hours in the freezer of a home refrigerator. The introduction of this device into the rectum lowers the temperature of the surrounding tissues while it thaws, usually within 5–10 minutes. The device is inserted twice daily and expelled after 3–5 minutes.

Outpatient (Office) Haemorrhoidal Management

A majority of patients with symptomatic haemorrhoids can be successfully treated by minor procedures and can avoid the need for extensive surgical interventions. Treatment is often aimed at relieving symptoms rather than improving the appearance of the anal canal so that the management is for symptomatic disease and based upon the designated grade. Patients with haemorrhoids can be distinguished into two groups: (1) young people, usually men, whose chief symptom is bleeding and anal discomfort, and (2) older patients or women, in whom prolapse is the principal complaint. It has been suggested of late that a procedure aiming at relieving anal spasm is most logical for patients with anal pain and bleeding while fixation of the mucosa is most appropriate for patients with prolapsing piles.

Interventional outpatient procedures are performed in the office to treat Grade 1 haemorrhoids unresponsive to conservative methods discussed earlier and for second- and third-degree haemorrhoids. Treatment is directed at the base or pedicle of haemorrhoid, which lies above the dentate line. If performed correctly, these procedures are almost painless. Various office procedures like injection sclerotherapy, ablation using various forms of heat, rubber band ligation (RBL), and haemorrhoidal artery ligation are aimed at restoration of the prolapsed or congested haemorrhoids back into the anal canal by submucosal fibrosis and fixation. The consensus on proposing appropriate treatment options relies on the following issues:

- The aim of treatment should be the induction of fibrosis to replace the haemorrhoidal cushions back to their normal position.
- Internal haemorrhoids are treated with office procedures.
- Haemorrhoids need not be dealt with unless they produce symptoms.
- Only those advanced grades of haemorrhoids in which there has been an extensive fragmentation of the supportive connective tissue need be treated surgically.
- Treatment should be modified depending on the stage of the haemorrhoids.

Injection Sclerotherapy

The extension of the use of sclerotherapy designed to induce local vascular thrombosis to haemorrhoidal treatment resulted from the utilisation of a range of sclerosants for varicose veins in other locales. The twentieth century saw a revival of different medicaments including carbolic acid, perchlorate of mercury, sodium carbonate, and salicylates as well as quinine and urea, polidocanol, ethanol, n-dodecane, hypertonic saline, fibrin foam, biotrol, epinephrine, tetracycline, ethoxysclerol, and sotradecol foam and finally with the development in the 1940s of sodium tetradecyl sulphate. In China, there has been an established trend to use a longer lasting inflammatory agent aluminium potassium sulphate and tannic acid (ALTA), which has also been advocated for larger degree haemorrhoids using a four-step injection technique.

The treatment of internal bleeding haemorrhoids by the submucosal injection of 5% phenol in almond (or cottonseed/arachis) oil was introduced by Morley in the United Kingdom in 1928. There is a debate about the volume of sclerosant to be used although all agree that two or three sites may be injected at a single proctological sitting. The method is highly technique-dependent where too superficial injection may result in a white mucosa and ultimate mucosal necrosis, and too deep infiltration may lead to delayed deep-seated perirectal sepsis. The traditional view is that if the injection is submucosally placed correctly, the mucosa overlying haemorrhoid will 'balloon forward' into the mouth of the proctoscope and small vessels coursing over haemorrhoid will become more prominent and visible in what is referred to as the mucosal 'striate' (Figure 6.5). The sign shows the technique of injection.

There have been considerable complications reported with this technique; particularly, if repeated, which may include pain (if the injection site is too low or too deep), excessive bleeding (usually in vascular haemorrhoids in patients on anticoagulant therapy), and the development of submucosal or more extensive perianal sepsis. Mucosal ulceration may ensue in some cases with delayed haemorrhage or sepsis. In some cases, injection of the anterior haemorrhoidal complex has been associated with prostatitis and even haematuria and haematospermia or rectovaginal/rectourethral fistula.

Antibiotic prophylaxis is advised before sclerotherapy in patients with valvular heart disease or in those who are immunocompromised. Rarely, life-threatening complications have occurred including chemical hepatitis and hepatic abscess (due to systemic absorption of phenol), as well as rectal necrosis, rectal perforation, necrotising retro peritonitis and necrotising perineal sepsis.

Rubber Band Ligation (RBL)

The technique of band ligation for haemorrhoidal treatment was first described by Barron in 1963. The technique has been well described with application of the rubber (elastic or latex) bands above the dentate line after grasping the haemorrhoid and then firing the band. Because of the requirement of someone to hold the proctoscope for two-handed banding, a suction band ligator was developed for single-handed use. Many commercial devices with screw release mechanisms are now available for such single-handed purpose. The band serves two purposes—it reduces the excessive bulk of the disrupted anal cushions and encourages adhesion of haemorrhoid distal

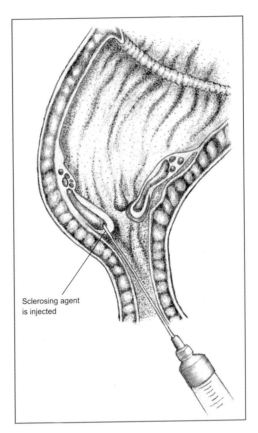

Sclerosing agent
is injected

Figure 6.5   The technique of injection sclerotherapy.
Illustration: James Oinam.

to the band to the underlying internal sphincter through an inflammatory reaction. Figure 6.6 shows the technique of RBL.

The original paper recommended that only one haemorrhoid
should be treated at a time with three weekly intervals between
bands. Assessment of this technique showed that the standard piles
could be safely banded in a single sitting without undue pain. This is,
however, controversial, with relatively insufficient data where some
have found that pain is more severe as is a recurrent disease when
multiple sites are banded at a single sitting.

The addition of local anaesthesia with bands does not appear to
influence the incidence of significant reported pain where the disposition of the band clearly above the dentate line to incorporate
haemorrhoid that could be surrounded by the band is critical for
a response. Patients should be warned that the band may fall off,

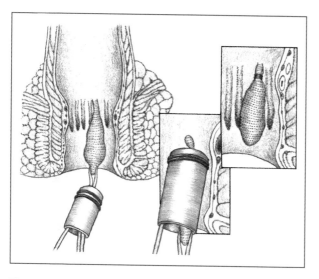

Figure 6.6 The technique of rubber band ligation.
Illustration: James Oinam.

and they may visualise it in the toilet bowl if it is too superficially placed, or that they can get delayed haemorrhage. It is contraindicated for use in anticoagulated cases, and although rare, serious complications including perirectal sepsis, urinary difficulty, and even liver abscess have been reported. It will appear that patients taking clopidogrel are at substantial bleeding risk if RBL is performed during therapy. RBL remains the commonest office ambulatory haemorrhoidal treatment currently available. Although patients should expect recurrence over time, RBL may be effectively repeated on Grade 1/2 haemorrhoids with an expectation of surgery in only 10% of treated patients overall.

Facts about Rubber Banding of Haemorrhoids

- Before applying the band, the operator should carefully assess by judging through the proctoscope as to which part of the pile to grasp for optimum effect. Selection of the correct site enables the maximum amount of disrupted tissue to be banded without encroaching upon the sensitive anoderm.
- A second 'polypoid' area of haemorrhoid can be raised from the same pile if it is too bulky for one application, or the originally banded part can be further augmented by pulling the first one back into the banding device and incorporating a further 'polyp' of tissue beyond it, like two beads on a string.
- High banding to reduce the chance of pain is not required, as no extra discomfort from bands placed on the actual prolapsing mucosa has been noticed.

- Banding should be avoided within three weeks of a patient's trip abroad.
- Most patients are in moderate discomfort afterwards. However, local anaesthetic injection or scissor division of the band may relieve excessive pain from an inadvertently low band. Although specialised hook devices for band division are available, they are difficult to apply directly to patients with pain and the author has not required their use in over 30 years of clinical proctology. Excessive pain is due to inappropriately low placement of a band.
- Four quadrant local anaesthetic infiltrations in the submucosa at the upper part of the anal canal result in complete relaxation and maximal mucosal redundancy of the anal canal. It provides an excellent exposure enabling an accurate and multiple applications of rubber bands.
- If the application of the first band causes discomfort then repeated sessions of single banding are advised.
- Constipation can be a likely factor to complicate the outcome of RBL. It is better not to attempt to have a bowel movement for the next 24 hours after band ligation and patients are advised against immediate straining at stool.
- No rectal medication such as enemas, suppositories, or creams should be used immediately after the procedure.

Complications of Rubber Band Ligation

As many as one-quarter of patients undergoing the procedure are unable to carry out their normal activities on the day of the procedure, and a significant proportion has fainting spells. The complications, especially pain, occur even if it is ensured that the bands have been applied at the appropriate site. Minor complications include haemorrhoidal thrombosis, band displacement, band-related abscess, mild bleeding, and mucosal ulceration. Major complications include urinary retention, delayed massive rectal bleeding, pelvic sepsis, and perianal abscess.

Overall, severe complications are uncommon with one study showing that 2% had minor pain, 1% band slippage, and <1% urinary retention. Patients should be warned that pain might start several hours after the procedure but that it is usually controllable with simple analgesics. It may last up to 48 hours in some cases. Minor post-procedural bleeding is common and may occur late up to 5–10 days after the RBL as the mucosa sloughs. However, the technique may be safely performed in HIV-positive patients.

Heat and Cold Therapy

The application of heat (as well as cold) has been well described for the treatment of haemorrhoids. The popular form of this type of treatment is infrared photocoagulation (IRC) using a specialised applicator where mechanical pressure and radiation energy are applied simultaneously to ablate the blood supply to the haemor-rhoidal mass.

This method was first described by Neiger in 1977 and updated in 1989. Infrared radiation (light transformed into heat) causes protein coagulation and evaporation of intracellular water over an area of approximately 3 mm and to a depth of 3 mm, which is immediately visible as a white spot at the point of application with the formation of a coagulative eschcar. Over the course of the next one to four weeks, a small ulcer will develop, which heals by cicatrisation, reducing the blood flow to haemorrhoid followed by a tethering of the mucosa to the underlying tissues. The apparatus (Redfield Corporation, NJ, USA) produces infrared radiation from a 14 V Wolfram-halogen projector bulb surrounded by a gold-plated reflector and focused by a photoconductor. The tip of the instrument is protected by a polymer-coated cap designed to prevent adherence to the underlying tissues. The power supply unit has a built-in timing device that allows variation in the duration of radiation so that a one-second pulse is used for treatment. The infrared probe is applied to the base of haemorrhoid at the site normally used for injection sclerotherapy with at least three points of spot welding being produced at the pedicle of each haemorrhoid. The probe is angled through 90° in a clockwise direction for subsequent application where up to six points may be coagulated per haemorrhoid along the base and somewhat depending on its size. The device is shown in Figure 6.7.

Endoscopic IRC is a modified form of infrared radiation generated by a control box and applied with a flexible, fibre optic light guide

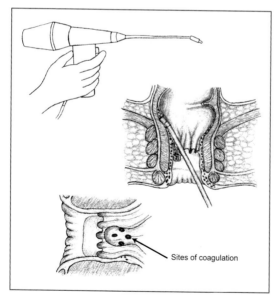

Sites of coagulation

Figure 6.7 The infrared photocoagulation procedure.
Illustration: James Oinam.

(Precision Endoscopic Infrared Coagulator™); this technique may provide better visibility and simultaneous endoscopic treatment of haemorrhoids during colonoscopy. It has overall been suggested that IRC, when compared with injection sclerotherapy, may be more efficient at increasing the proportion of symptom-free patients early who present with non-prolapsing haemorrhoids, although there is variability in the reported haemorrhoidal degree. This effect disappears at one and up to four years of follow-up. It is unknown whether IRC increases the proportion of those patients where they would rate themselves as improved and so this evidence is of low quality overall. Further outpatient treatment is required significantly more often following photocoagulation although with relatively few patients coming to haemorrhoidectomy over one year of follow-up.

There are several recommended technical aspects of the IRC technique.

- It is quicker and easy to use by a single operator. The method is technically straightforward, convenient, and can be applied in both in- and outpatient clinics.
- The equipment is portable, handy, and long lasting, thus need little care and maintenance.
- The anatomical results suggest that the progression of haemorrhoids is not arrested. Thus, late recurrences are common and require repeated treatment sessions. However, even when repeated several times, it does not cause significant difficulty in its application and may achieve clinical success.
- RBL is more painful when compared with IRC, but their short-term clinical results are similar. Infrared photocoagulation gives its best results in early grades of haemorrhoids (Grades 1 and 2) only.
- Too high or too low application will be ineffective or painful.
- Five days of treatment combining flavonoids and photocoagulation has been found to be significantly effective in controlling bleeding in patients with Grades 1 and 2 internal haemorrhoids in comparison to each treatment used individually.
- Complications reported with the use of photocoagulation include post-treatment bleeding, which is rarely severe. Patients on antiplatelet agents should be advised to discontinue therapy for seven days before treatment. Pain may be produced if photocoagulation is performed close to the dentate line. Rarely, the wound at the application site may become infected.

There are some other reported techniques, which require further trailing against standard therapies. These include laser surgery, bipolar haemorrhoidal diathermy, radiofrequency ablation, and haemorrhoidal atomisation. Of the lasers, the neodymium-doped yttrium aluminium garnet (Nd:YAG), the CO_2, and the diode lasers have been used to coagulate first-degree and second-degree haemorrhoids using a flat contact probe. The laser probe is applied around haemorrhoid in a rosette fashion similar to that used for infrared coagulation. The power used is between 5 and 10 W for 2–3 seconds using a coaxial water flow. The Nd:YAG laser is prohibitively expensive and overly powerful, sometimes destroying muscle tissue without any benefit substantiated by controlled clinical trials. A range of lasers has been used for haemorrhoid treatment although this type of therapy has largely come and gone.

Direct current electrotherapy (or haemorrhoidolysis) uses a direct current technique, which has been popularised by gastroenterologists and was transferred to haemorrhoid management in the 1980s. In this technique, direct current therapy (Ultroid Technologies, Florida) is applied with a hand-held probe. It has been claimed that all degrees of haemorrhoids are amenable to this therapy. A grounding plate is placed on the patient's thigh, and direct current is applied through a probe placed via a proctoscope with the probe held in place for 10 minutes. The probe is initially placed on the mucosa over the haemorrhoid base, and the current is increased to 2 mA slowly to the maximum tolerable level where it is gently pushed through the mucosa into the haemorrhoidal tissue.

The current is then increased to 10–16 mA on average. Given the time involved in treatment, it is seldom possible to treat more than one haemorrhoid at each outpatient visit. At subsequent visits, the remaining haemorrhoids are similarly treated and if necessary, any pile that has not resolved after one treatment is re-treated. A randomised and crossover trial of direct current electrotherapy found no difference between medical therapy and the use of this modality in the alleviation of symptoms or the need for surgery.

Griffith et al. from Nottingham, England described a bipolar probe called the Bicap® (Santa Barbara, CA) to treat Grade 1 and Grade 2 haemorrhoids. The basis of using bipolar coagulation is to induce tissue destruction, ulceration, and ultimately fibrosis by local application of heat. Bipolar diathermy is applied via a proctoscope using a hand-held probe controlled by a foot switch. The probe is placed directly on to haemorrhoid above the dentate line where tissue coagulation occurs almost immediately when the probe is activated.

All visible haemorrhoidal tissue is treated at each session, but care is taken to avoid circumferential injury. Bipolar diathermy has the advantage of multiple applications to the same site as it produces little further penetration of the tissues due to changes in the electrical properties of the resultant eschar. Bipolar diathermy produces smoke during haemorrhoid treatment, which may obscure the operator's view.

Radiofrequency ablation (RFA) is a comparatively new but expensive approach where a ball electrode is connected to an RFA generator for direct contact vaporisation. The radiofrequency generating unit utilises a disposable probe on which an electrical current is flowing between two flat electrodes (positive and negative) which are aligned at the tip. Activating the unit for 2 seconds in three or four areas of the same haemorrhoid complex efficiently coagulates the vessels. In the radiofrequency ablation and coagulation technique, a ball electrode is used to coagulate the whole pile mass by gently rotating the electrode over the haemorrhoid. The power of the radiosurgical unit is adjusted to produce shrinkage and a gradual change of the haemorrhoid until it takes on a dusky white colour (so-called blanching), which indicates satisfactory coagulation necrosis.

Radiowaves use much lower temperatures than classic diathermy with less collateral thermal damage, resulting in less postoperative pain as well as providing an almost bloodless operating field with a shortened coagulating time. The aims are similar to other contact therapies for the creation of a reduction of the vascular surface area of haemorrhoid and secondary haemorrhoidal fixation. It has had some reported complications including acute urinary retention, thrombosis, and perirectal infection. Although painless as a therapy, there does appear to be a high incidence of recurrent bleeding reported. It has been suggested that RFA may reduce the hospital stay in those with larger (third-degree) haemorrhoids so treated with reduced reported pain when this treatment is opted for in selected cases.

Haemorrhoidal atomisation uses an innovative waveform of electrical current where a specifically designed electrical probe slices out or vaporises one or more cell layers of the applied tissue, reducing the haemorrhoids to minute particles of fine mist or spray that are immediately vacuumed away. The haemorrhoids are essentially disintegrated into an aerosol of carbon and water molecules. Results are similar to those reported with laser removal of the haemorrhoids but with a less bleeding with the atomiser. The cost of the atomiser is much less. The procedure can be used for haemorrhoids of Grades 1, 2, and 3 without the need for the hospital stay and comparative published data is awaited. Presently, this treatment is offered exclusively in Arizona, USA.

A final area of conservative treatment used for haemorrhoids, which were popular, but which fell away because of poor healing and excessive menorrhoea, was Cryotherapy. Cryosurgery, which was originally described by Lewis in 1969, induces cellular destruction by the rapid freezing followed by rapid thawing of the haemorrhoidal tissue. Liquid nitrous oxide and carbon dioxide are used to produce freezing where liquid nitrogen circulates through a system of tubes cooling the tip of the cryoprobe to freezing temperature. For internal haemorrhoids, freezing is performed for 1–3 minutes, while for external haemorrhoids freezing is for 2–4 minutes.

Following the freezing, the haemorrhoids swell and become red and start melting and discharging, which at the beginning is serosanguinous and becomes purulent later. The discharge lasts for about two weeks to decrease gradually after that. Although a popular method 20 years ago, cryosurgery has fallen out of favour because of the pain as the cryoball approaches the mucocutaneous junction. Comparative studies have shown that cryosurgery can be more painful than other medical surgeries. Furthermore, the open wound can occasionally become infected. Also, for as much as a couple of weeks after surgery, patients can have an abnormal rectal discharge with a relatively foul odour, which may require the use of absorbent pads. The overall incidence of residual haemorrhoids with this technique is high, ranging between 25% and 50% of all of them.

Newer and Innovative Treatment Options for Haemorrhoids

HET™ bipolar ablation: HET™ bipolar system is a new tissue ligation device for the treatment of symptomatic Grades 1 or 2 internal haemorrhoids. It is a modified anoscope with built-in tissue ligating bipolar forceps, a light source, and tissue temperature monitoring mechanism. The haemorrhoid pedicle is clamped with incorporated tissue forceps and ablated with bipolar energy to obscure haemorrhoidal vasculature.

The HemorPex procedure: The HemorPex System is a single-use device, which is based on the principle of dematerialising haemorrhoidopexy. This technique can be performed without anaesthesia or with local anaesthesia, and allows the patient to return immediately to his activities. The procedure is indicated for prolapsing types of haemorrhoids, especially second and third degree. The device is made of two parts. One is a fixed part, which remains in contact with the anoderm and the sensitive mucosa of the anal canal, and the second is a rotating operative part, which includes the window through which the suture stitches are made on haemorrhoid.

Doppler-guided haemorrhoidal laser procedure (HeLP™): The HeLP™ procedure utilises lasers and doppler assistance for completing the process. First, a proctoscope is passed into the anal canal, to which is attached a disposable doppler probe. It identifies the branches of the superior haemorrhoidal arteries above the dentate line. Then, focalised laser energy is applied using the fibre hand piece to each one of the submucosal branches of the haemorrhoidal artery to lead to photocoagulation.

THE SURGERY OF HAEMORRHOIDS

Elective surgery is advised for symptomatic third-degree haemorrhoids not responding to banding or for fourth-degree haemorrhoids as well as for cases of patient preference and where other anorectal procedures may be performed *en passant*. By a rough estimate, one can say that about 10% of patients suffering from haemorrhoidal disease will require some or other form of surgical intervention.

Much of the historical information available on haemorrhoid surgery is anecdotal in nature. Haemorrhoidal ligation and excision (akin to the Milligan-Morgan haemorrhoidectomy) are attributed to Hippocrates where in his *Corpus* he discusses needle transfixion and ligation with a prescription for the prevention of anal stenosis in always recommending leaving some haemorrhoidal tissue behind. Celsus (25 BC–AD 14) also described the ligation-excision procedure and its complications, as did Galen, who reported on the surgical management of gangrenous cases. The base of any surgical procedure for the haemorrhoids encompasses elimination of the prolapsing vascular cushions alone or in combination with a relocation of the squamous epithelium. It is as good as reconstructing the anal canal in an attempt to reduce blood flow with the excision of prolapsing tissue.

In the United Kingdom, the Milligan-Morgan procedure is still considered the gold standard of haemorrhoid surgery and regarded by far the most acceptable open procedure for advanced grades of symptomatic haemorrhoids. Unlike some of the more minimalist procedures developed to reduce peri- and post-operative pain, the advantage of the formal excisional open technique is the ability to expose the internal anal sphincter and divide formally the adhesions between this sphincter and the anal cushion complex which are always present, even in children.

The inherent disadvantage of the technique was the tendency to be disrupted unless the V cut on the skin was very small (or in some cases like the smaller anterior haemorrhoid, there was no skin cut at all), that the defect in the skin left after excision was often larger than one had planned. It was deemed essential that due care was taken to leave intact at least 8–10 mm of anal mucosa and the skin between the classical haemorrhoidal wounds as skin bridges for epithelialisation and in the prevention of a cutaneous anal stenosis. Moreover, this still represents the main key to success in performing a Milligan-Morgan style haemorrhoidectomy.

There are few long-term follow-up studies after Milligan-Morgan haemorrhoidectomy where an older report by Seleznieff and colleagues from Marseille showed a 2.9% incidence of clinical stenosis on a retrospective assessment of patients at 15 years. Anal stenosis is even more likely to occur if the haemorrhoidectomy were performed as an emergency for strangulation (although one performs an isolated excision of involved haemorrhoid here rather than a formal haemorrhoidectomy).

In the Ferguson approach described in 1952, the haemorrhoid is elevated so that the involved anoderm and skin are excised, the pedicle ligated, and the skin is closed with a running absorbable suture. The same procedure is performed in the Milligan-Morgan technique; however, the difference is that the skin is left open to granulate. Although excisional haemorrhoidectomy is the most efficient treatment for haemorrhoids with a low (but definitive) rate of recurrence when compared with other modalities, debate in the literature has focused on variations in technique, examining the use of scissors or diathermy and the utilisation of vascular sealant devices such as the LigaSure™ or the harmonic scalpel as well as decisions regarding anaesthetic supplementation (pudendal nerve blockade) or whether day-case haemorrhoidectomy could be safely conducted.

Today, many surgeons excise the pedicles using monopolar diathermy, reducing bleeding where traction of the skin tag and pedicle permits dissection in a plane that preserves the subdermal fascia continuous with the fascia covering the internal anal sphincter. One of the major drawbacks, which have driven out the new haemorrhoidal surgery, is a post-operative pain after the Milligan-Morgan and Ferguson approach with the new techniques designed to reduce immediate and delayed post-operative pain along with hospital stay, resulting in a more rapid return to work.

LigaSure™ Haemorrhoidectomy

The recent Cochrane analysis by Nienhuijs and de Hingh in 2009 asserted an advantage for LigaSure™ over other techniques because of reduced immediate post-operative pain without an increase in adverse operative side effects on the function where they postulated that minimal thermal injury could be achieved using a bipolar electrothermal sealing device. In contrast to diathermy or electrocautery, this device uses a very high-frequency current providing haemostasis by denaturating collagen and elastin in the vessel wall and adjoining connective tissue, with no evidence of thermal damage (Figure 6.8).

Recent advances in instrumental technology and the use of various energy sources have provided new alternatives for the technical aspects of excisional haemorrhoidectomy. These include the bipolar scissors (dissecting scissors that incorporate a bipolar cautery device), radiofrequency, and ultrasonic waves. The use of an ultrasonic device (Harmonic scalpel) has also been compared in one study to LigaSure™ where the harmonic scalpel (UltraCision, Ethicon Endo-Surgery, Inc., Cincinnati, OH) was associated with more immediate post-operative pain and a longer operative time for the achievement of haemostasis.

The harmonic scalpel vibrates at 55,500 Hz per second, with the blade travelling 50–100 microns per stroke cutting by two mechanisms. At the first instance, ultra-speed vibrations disrupt hydrogen bonds within the protein structure and form a coagulum that seals blood vessels up to 5 mm in diameter. As against the electrosurgery, there is minimal tissue desiccation, char formation, and the zone of thermal injury. A second cutting mechanism is that of cavitational fragmentation in which low-density tissue is broken, leading to separation of anatomic tissue planes. Another effect is brought about by vaporising fluids through cavitational bubbles that are produced at a low (37°C) temperature, minimising thermal injury and associated energy transfer. Moreover, because the instrument operates

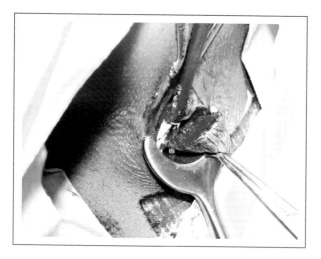

Figure 6.8 The technique of LigaSure™ haemorrhoidectomy.
Courtesy: Pravin Jaiprakash Gupta.

at temperatures less than 100°C, it is associated with less undesirable tissue trauma. The use of harmonic scalpel inflicts minimal lateral thermal injury, and this is believed to be the reason for diminished post-operative discomfort.

Haemorrhoidectomy has also been performed with a laser as the excisional device. The energy of the Nd:YAG laser can penetrate water and be absorbed by the tissue, inducing a thermal effect, which damages tissue and results in photocoagulation. The initial enthusiasm for this approach has been tempered by the cost component of the device where there is no available evidence supporting it as a technique with reduced pain, bleeding, or operative time and the procedure is not currently employed in most proctology units.

The Milligan-Morgan procedure has been well described and standardised where the trainee surgeon can find an adequate discussion of the technique in most operative surgery texts. Briefly, the external haemorrhoid is grasped with an artery forceps clamp and then the internal haemorrhoid is clamped with a second forceps. Lateral traction away from the anus causes the anal mucosa to be visible up to the mark of the dentate line to facilitate the placement of the second clamp. Each haemorrhoid is exposed in this manner so that a tri-radiate appearance is created holding the clamps at each point with a towel grasp. By drawing the clamp outward in the anal canal by the pressure of an index finger, a V-like cut is made in the skin of the anus, ending approximately at the dentate line. The mucosa and submucosa containing the haemorrhoidal tissue are dissected, leaving the internal sphincter (which is deliberately sought and separated) untouched. The haemorrhoidal plexus, which now swings free on its pedicle, is then transfixed tightly above the proximal clamp and is resected.

The suture is left long for assessment at the end of the procedure and to determine the adequacy of the transfixion. Bleeding at the apex of a vascular pedicle can be controlled by a running suture. Care is taken to leave intact at least 8–10 mm of anal mucosa and the skin between the wound of the haemorrhoidal cushions for purposes of regeneration and sensorial continence. Finally, any redundant skin is trimmed, and the wounds external to the anal canal are left open. Insertion of an Eisenhammer speculum assesses the individual pedicles for haemostasis and the wounds at the anal verge, which can be a source of significant post-operative bleeding.

Although both methods (open and closed) are successful forms of treatment, in theory, wound closure should offer quicker healing, but this has not been shown continually in comparative studies; particularly, if there is a post-operative complication. In this respect, wound dehiscence after excision of three piles will prolong healing after closed surgery. It would appear that closed haemorrhoidectomy also offers no advantage regarding post-operative pain, but when performed carefully it may lead to less pruritus and discharge in the post-operative period during the initial stages of healing. In the past, other methods were used *en passant* with haemorrhoidectomies (however performed), such as preliminary anal dilatation and combined lateral internal anal sphincterotomy; however, these have been abandoned because of reported increases in the risk of incontinence and soiling.

Other types of haemorrhoidectomy are now briefly considered as the colorectal surgeon may encounter patients who have undergone these procedures.

Submucosal haemorrhoidectomy (Parks' procedure): This procedure (formerly called a submucous haemorrhoidectomy) was developed in the 1950s by Parks, who published details and results of the technique in 1959 where his concept was to reduce post-operative pain as well as diminish post-operative anal stenosis. For this procedure, scissors are used to excise a small diamond of anal epithelium around a haemostat grasping haemorrhoid.

The incision is carried on cranially for 2.5 cm, forming two mucosal flaps on either side, which are each clasped with further haemostats and submucosal dissection is commenced to detach the haemorrhoidal plexus from the underlying internal anal sphincter muscle and overlying mucosa. This dissection is continued into the rectum, where the resulting broad base of tissue is suture-ligated and divided. The mucosal flaps are then allowed to fall back into position. The same procedure is carried out on the other haemorrhoids. The submucosal aspect of the procedure is bloodier and more time consuming than a standard Milligan-Morgan haemorrhoidectomy. Parks in his original description expressed concern that the mucosal flaps may be associated with more recurrence although he stated that he had not seen this in over 300 cases performed. Review of this technical paper does not, however, reveal any specific patient data.

The Whitehead haemorrhoidectomy: Since its first description in 1882, the Whitehead haemorrhoidectomy has earned a maligned repute as a radical procedure for circumferential prolapsed haemorrhoids. This process ensures excision of entire haemorrhoid bearing area of the anal canal as a tubular segment, where the entire edge of rectal mucosa is then sutured circumferentially to the skin of the anal canal. This technique has been useful in bleeding haemorrhoids or circumferential prolapse and gangrenous or strangulated haemorrhoids; however, the approach has been criticised because it is time-consuming and causes considerable blood loss, disturbed continence, and most importantly an ectropion of the rectal mucosa and stricture formation that leads to troublesome mucosal leakage and discharge. This operation has been abandoned and now stapled haemorrhoidectomy or haemorrhoidopexy are the preferred options for circumferential haemorrhoids. Although the colorectal surgeon will still see this complication (usually as mucosal ectropion) either completely or in part (*forme fruste*) which may require secondary reconstruction and more recent modifications, such as a circular incision, an anodermal flap graft, or a sliding skin flap graft have been developed to reduce the risk of complications associated with the primary Whitehead method. Nonetheless, the results largely remain unsatisfactory.

It is probably artificial to discriminate between circumferential haemorrhoidal prolapse and rectal mucosal prolapse, and both (although there may be differing anorectal physiology) can be treated similarly. Several procedures have been used as local plications for circumferential haemorrhoids, which in today's day and age might be more readily treated by stapled haemorrhoidopexy.

One of these is the Gant-Miwa procedure; it's traditionally combined with a Thiersch procedure for the perineal treatment of troublesome mucosal, rectal prolapse, which could, in theory, be used for the treatment of circumferentially prolapsed haemorrhoids. The procedure is not performed in the West being developed in the 1960s in Japan. Plication in a quadrant fashion of prolapsing haemorrhoidal tissue has been in practice for a long time and is tailored to the patients' haemorrhoids where Farag described his 'pile suture' in the 1970s using three interrupted sutures to obliterate the haemorrhoidal mass. The results of this rather conservative approach to mucosal prolapse seem justified. This sort of reefing of the mucosa may also be performed as a purse string type suture as advocated by Shafik and also may be carried out by initial vertical mucosal cautery followed by a reefing of the muscularis as a cauterisation-plication procedure similar to an internal Delorme's operation for rectal prolapse. This latter technique has been described by Olfat El-Sibai, but in the author's opinion it does not offer any specific advantage over a conventional Delorme's mucosectomy, which can also be used for circumferential haemorrhoidal prolapse.

Doppler-guided haemorrhoid artery ligation (DGHAL): This technique, also known as transanal haemorrhoidal dematerialisation, provides selective ligation of the arteries supplying the haemorrhoids after ultrasound identification. The procedure can be performed on ambulatory patients under local anaesthesia using a specialised anoscope incorporating a doppler's head. The superior haemorrhoidal arteries are identified under the guidance of the arterial doppler sound and then ligated or reefed through a window located just above the doppler's head. Although rapid (taking about 30 minutes) with minimal pain, it is associated with a moderately high recurrence rate necessitating combination with haemorrhoidal mucopexy designed to control prolapse. For this purpose, a running suture beginning at the apex of the haemorrhoidal pedicle continues down to the dentate line and is then tied back to the apex to lift the haemorrhoidal tissue back into anatomic position. The technique remains somewhat controversial. First, anatomically, as Felix Aigner and colleagues from Austria, who have conducted several studies on the anatomic variations of the haemorrhoidal arteries, show that the arteries supplying the haemorrhoidal cushions are at a more distal level than located by the doppler so that they cannot adequately be ligated during the process with the arterial ligator.

This has been echoed by other studies. In one study, the macroscopic arterial branching patterns were examined in human pelvis impregnated in epoxy resin showing additional branches of the superior rectal artery which were coursing in the outer layers of the rectal wall and entered into the rectum just above the levator ani to supply the corpus cavernosum recti. The constant submucosal arterial course as postulated originally by Sir Ernest Miles is relatively rarely observed with a significant variation in the entry points of the distal muscular branches. The implication of this work was that the DGHAL technique might miss feeding vessels and be relatively ineffective in the longer term. In an anatomic work done by Avital and colleagues from Israel, in 135 patients 6–8 terminal branches were located with three-quarters of the cases being located at all the odd-numbered clock positions around the anus. It has been suggested by a group from Singapore that an extra aberrant fourth superior rectal arterial branch is detected in the left anterior 1 o'clock position requiring ligation.

Second, the haemorrhoid artery ligator device has a wide diameter, which is thought to have a dilating effect when inserted, which might reduce the resting pressure and improve the venous outflow of the haemorrhoidal cushions. Further anatomic studies has shown that haemorrhoids are arteriovenous cushions whereby ligating the main vessels, the smaller haemorrhoidal vessels will then hypertrophy over time. These anatomical studies also show that during the process of ligation, not all of the arteries are found and ligated raising concerns about the procedural efficacy in the absence of a coincident mucopexy.

In a recent study from the Cleveland Clinic in Ohio, Ursula Szmulowicz assessing the outcome of four different surgeons treating 96 patients and followed for 15 months on average where a mucopexy was also performed in 87 of the cases, had a residual haemorrhoid rate of 20% with 13.5% requiring further haemorrhoid treatment. The majority of the recurrent/residual disease occurred within the early learning curve of the surgeons.

Stapled haemorrhoidopexy: In 1998, Antonio Longo first presented this 'procedure for prolapsing haemorrhoids' (PPHs), also known as the stapled haemorrhoidopexy, as a new treatment. Since then it has dominated European and world proctology as a significant surgical treatment for Grades 3 and 4 haemorrhoids with particular modification of the technique towards selective resection in China. Despite concerns regarding very specific procedural-related morbidity, it has been shown to be a cost-effective treatment with a decrease in operating room time and hospital stay, which provides an incremental social cost benefit. It is performed using a transanal stapler which has since been considerably modified to reduce the prolapse by the excision of a circumferential ring of insensitive mucosa 2–3 cm above the dentate line resulting also in a secondary benefit through a shortening or hitching of the prolapsed mucosa as well as providing an arterial interruption in a manner similar to DGHAL (Figure 6.9). The aim of its introduction was to simplify haemorrhoidectomy when indicated and reduce pain. The further argument is that the normal haemorrhoidal tissue returned to its usual place may assist in post-haemorrhoidectomy anal closure and support continence.

The indication for the PPH technique would be equivalent to other forms of surgery; however, the author feels that this procedure is not suitable for Grade 4 prolapse.

The general feeling is that in Grade 4 prolapsing cases with a significant external component where a manual style haemorrhoidectomy is most suitable and has the greatest chance of a lower recurrence rate when compared with a combined stapled plus skin

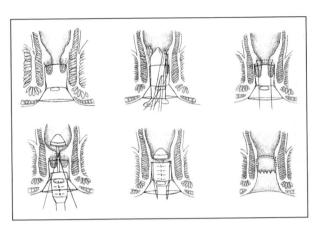

Figure 6.9 The stapled haemorrhoidopexy procedure.
Illustration: James Oinam.

tag excision technique. It is, however, accepted that the enthusiasm of the proctologist will govern the use of these devices as does the long-term recurrence rate and the complication rate. On the one side are great enthusiasts who are guided by international guidelines and can quote their conversion rates and complications while on the other hand, are those who have expressed concerns concerning worrisome and even serious life-threatening complications. Another view is that there is a place for stapled haemorrhoidopexy, but not in the majority of patients, and it should be used for Grade 3 haemorrhoidal prolapse that is either circumferential or where there are secondary Grade 3 components without any associated external element. These types of patients are relatively uncommon.

There have been more than 25 randomised controlled trials comparing stapled haemorrhoidopexy with conventional haemorrhoidectomy although most have been of small sample size. Early, small randomised trials compared stapled haemorrhoidopexy with traditional excisional surgery showing the former to be less painful with quicker recovery. These reports also suggested a better patient acceptance and a higher rate of day-case procedures with the stapled PPH technique. The control of haemorrhoidal symptoms was equivalent between techniques. As stated, much of the completed randomised trials are too small to make definitive conclusions without achievable long-term functional outcome after stapled haemorrhoidopexy. Also, there have been reports of serious complications such as severe pelvic sepsis, rectal obstruction, rectal perforation, and staple line dehiscence following the new technique along with a serious post-defecation proctalgia syndrome in some cases which some have referred to as the post-PPH syndrome.

An extension on a 2006 Cochrane review performed by Lumb et al. in 2010 analysed comparisons between the PPH and the excisional techniques assessing 22 studies with follow-up periods ranging from

6 to 56 months. The combined data showed less ongoing symptoms after PPH, although bleeding was more common as were prolapse symptoms, pruritus, post-operative soiling, faecal urgency, and persistent skin tags. Pain in most studies was considerably less, as was anal stenosis with post-PPH cases more likely to have recurrent haemorrhoids during follow-up and a higher haemorrhoidal reoperation rate.

In an analysis of 29 randomised controlled trials, Laughlan et al. recently showed a higher rate of recurrent prolapse after PPH haemorrhoidectomy when compared with both the Ferguson and the Milligan-Morgan techniques, with less perioperative bleeding but more long-term recurrent bleeding although long-term data are lacking. This finding, in general, would represent the worldwide view that stapled techniques are easier and quicker with less post-operative pain but in some non-randomised series subject to systematic analysis and meta-analysis reported that the incidence of recurrent prolapse and bleeding requiring secondary treatment and surgery is moderately high.

Summary of these meta-analyses and systematic reviews shows several key points:

- Stapled haemorrhoidopexy is clearly superior in the area of immediate perioperative pain although there is considerable heterogeneity in the studies.
- PPH is associated with a higher but not statistically significant reoperative rate for haemorrhoidal problems in the stapled group.
- The stapled group had significantly fewer cases of anal stenosis requiring treatment in the meta-analysis.
- PPH has a higher incidence of temporary and persistent faecal leakage after the procedure.
- There appears to be no difference in standard post-operative complications (for example, post-operative haemorrhage, urinary retention).
- There are no deleterious effects of PPH on anorectal manometry.
- Residual skin tags are more frequent following PPH.

Despite these interpretative difficulties, most studies suggest that recurrent disease requiring intervention is more prevalent in those stapled cases followed over time when compared with more traditional excisional techniques. The data currently, however, does not support the use of a PPH in a day-case setting although many units practice DC PPH operations.

Cost analysis shows that additional stapler costs are offset by savings in operating time and hospital stay and less post-operative wound care. Clearly, costs are not going to prohibit the stapler use. It is equally accepted that the rate of re-intervention will reflect the number of Grade 4 cases initially admitted in each study even when these may be considered relative contraindications to stapled procedures.

The decision currently to perform a stapled haemorrhoidopexy will be based on the patient preferences (providing full informed consent of the complications of the procedure), an analysis of potential post-operative pain benefits (particularly where haemorrhoids are circumferential), situations where there is not a major external component that disturbs the patient and their anal hygiene, the estimated likelihood of recurrence re-intervention over time and on the surgical preference and training.

The right data about this procedure (and its variants) will simply not be known until large adequately powered randomised controlled trial data are available. Despite the inherent biases in the available data, patients must be informed of the current information concerning long-term recurrence with these stapled technologies.

Moreover, we still do not know enough hard data concerning how recurrences and other complications after stapled haemorrhoidopexy should be treated, whether the stapled procedure can be safely repeated, or what other available treatment modalities are required.

POST-OPERATIVE COMPLICATIONS IN HAEMORRHOID SURGERY

Despite the variety of haemorrhoidectomy techniques, most complications encountered post-operatively are similar. These include post-operative pain, bleeding, continence disturbance, sepsis, and anal narrowing (stenosis), although there is a novel range of new disorders specific to stapled haemorrhoidopexy that should form part of the informed consent along with very specific complaints following particular types of haemorrhoidectomy such as the Whitehead procedure. Most of these complications are inherently preventable by specific attention to a technique employed for the individual procedure performed.

Pain

The pain associated with haemorrhoidectomy often is a source of anxiety both for the patient and the surgeon as both would anxiously await the first in-hospital bowel action as this issue governs the length of hospital stay. A perfect agent that alleviates pain after haemorrhoidectomy but is limited and its side effects remain to be identified. Post-operative pain after haemorrhoidectomy has three likely primary components:

- Discomfort from the surgical incision in the uniquely sensitive anoderm and perianal skin
- The reflex spasm of the involuntary anal sphincter
- Incarceration of smooth muscle fibres and mucosa in the transfixed vascular pedicle and epithelial denudation of the anal canal.

Other less prominent causes include bacterial fibrinolysis and defecation stress.

As has been discussed above, the use of high current diathermy or another alternate source of energy to excise the haemorrhoidal tissue reduces early post-operative pain. These devices probably cause some thermal injury to the nerve endings adjacent to the wound to induce analgesia. Use of these techniques also helps in achieving good haemostasis and clarity of the operating field, minimising injury to the internal sphincter. Good haemostasis and the avoidance of an intra-anal pack or pedicle fixation sutures will also reduce post-operative discomfort.

The phenomenon of comparatively late (or persistent) pain, however, is more mysterious in some cases and where in particular, it may form part of what some have referred to as a post-PPH syndrome. After conventional haemorrhoidectomy, late onset pain is experienced during the first few weeks after surgery and is most excruciating in the post-defecation period where a spasm of the internal sphincter seems to play an important role. Reduction of the anal pressure is necessary to lessen the spasm of the internal sphincter and interrupt a vicious pain-spasm circle. Methods to reduce the sphincter spasm by disruption of the internal sphincter fibres, or a gentle anal stretch, or a formal lateral internal sphincterotomy have mixed effects in the literature and are avoided because of concerns regarding long-term continence although they may be used in a small minority of patients with post-haemorrhoidectomy fissure with success.

Other approaches to reducing the anal sphincter pressure include the caudal injection of bupivacaine into the epidural space, the use of trimebutine as well as topical EMLA cream (lidocaine 2.5% and prilocaine 2.5%), topical metronidazole, and topical sucralfate. Specifically, as mentioned, botulinum toxin injection into the internal anal sphincter after haemorrhoidectomy has been reported to be effective in reducing maximum resting pressure, the overall time of healing and post-operative pain both at rest and during defecation. Further, the use of *Plantago ovata* after open haemorrhoidectomy has been found to reduce pain, tenesmus, and post-operative hospital stay. Analgesia has also been produced by bilateral pudendal nerve block using a nerve-stimulator. Analysis of the large list of pharmacological and surgical manipulative techniques shows that it is clear that the quest to relieve post-haemorrhoidectomy pain will likely continue.

Chronic pain has been a particular worrisome feature after PPH stapled haemorrhoidopexy, and it should be an important part of the informed consent if this procedure is contemplated. There is some evidence in patients with obstructed defecation who are about to undergo the STARR (Stapled TransAnal Rectal Resection) procedure that up to half the patients will decline the procedure if they are informed that chronic pain may ensue in some cases.

Severe chronic proctalgia after PPH is rarely reported but in our colorectal referral practice, this presentation is not rare. The incidence of chronic pain has a range of 1.6–31% in the studies that report this complication with pain being described as post-defecatory or associated somewhat separately with urgency. The aetiology of this pain is debatable where it has been suggested that it is related to striated muscle incorporation in the doughnut although it may be present without muscle incorporation. Chronic pain has also been attributed to persistent haemorrhoidal disease; sphincter spasm, rectal contraction, or high anal resting pressures, as well as suture/staple line dehiscence, a post-operative anal fissure, anorectal sepsis, or retained staples. In the latter circumstance, the novel procedure called 'agraffectomy' (from the French agrapphes 'staples') which requires the manual refashioning of the anastomosis and the excision of the staple line, has been advocated although a more conservative approach using transanal electrostimulation or transanal injections of steroids and local anaesthetic may also be attempted, though without improvement in a significant number of cases.

Fissures are fortunately uncommon after all forms of haemorrhoidectomy and take place in about 2% resulting from the trauma of a forceful insertion of the stapler into a spastic anal canal in teenage boys. There is no significant difference between PPH and conventional excisional haemorrhoidectomy in the incidence of a post-operative anal fissure in the latest reviews.

Bleeding

Post-haemorrhoidectomy secondary haemorrhage is rare but widely recognised post-operative complication of all forms of haemorrhoidectomy. It may occur several days after an operation in 0.6–5.4% of cases. Left undetected or not promptly treated, it may be life threatening because of cardiovascular decompensation with circulatory collapse. The cause of this haemorrhage is unclear in some cases although like all haemorrhage it is divisible into reactionary and secondary. Clearly, a failure to provide adequate haemostasis at the time of surgery is associated with a risk; particularly, if adrenaline is used locally for reactionary haemorrhage. Among the several factors that appear to play a role in this complication are an infection, faulty surgical procedure, trauma, and defecation with excessive straining as well as recent anti-platelet therapy where it has been suggested that male patients are more likely than female patients to develop post-haemorrhoidectomy secondary haemorrhage.

Both of these main types of haemorrhage are different in clinical presentation and management. Goligher attributed delayed or secondary haemorrhage specifically to sepsis, believing that the haemorrhoidal pedicle might become infected with subsequent softening and erosion of the arterial wall. He described delayed haemorrhage as internal or concealed and caused by a disruption of a clot in the vessel, which was neither secured or, more commonly, by a slough of tissue exposing a large vessel.

It is also believed that mass ligation of the pedicle with the inclusion of large amounts of tissue may create a greater risk of sloughing with subsequent bleeding that is an argument for diathermy haemorrhoidal excision. In this type of haemorrhage, patients should be instructed to report to the emergency department if they notice a trickle of dark and fresh blood from the anus or passage of large amounts of clotted blood. At the emergency room, after initial resuscitation, the bleeding should be confirmed by a rectal examination. An accurate history of the timing and the amount of the episodic bleeding should be recorded. The amount of bleeding is estimated by asking the patient or measured at the emergency room if the bleeding is persistent.

When the diagnosis of secondary haemorrhage is confirmed, and intravenous fluid resuscitation is administered, sedatives are given to relieve pain and anxiety. Blood transfusion depends on upon the amount of bleeding and the haematocrit. The treatment of post-haemorrhoidectomy secondary haemorrhage is controversial. One-half of these cases will have ceased bleeding spontaneously without any treatment other than bed rest. Given this fact, once the vital signs of the patient are stable, they should be taken to the operation room for examination under anaesthesia. The blood and clots inside the rectum should be urgently evacuated; else most patients will feel the urgency, continue to defecate blood intermittently, and complain of persistent haemorrhage from the anus. The usual treatment of those patients taken to the operating room is simple diathermy, the application of topical thrombostatic agents and antibiotics. The base of a bleeding pedicle may be sutured.

This type of bleeding is separated from that of reactionary haemorrhage, which can be massive. In the latter patients, there are two primary sites of bleeding. One is a small usually arterial bleeder from the skin of the anal verge. The other is a bleed from a major pedicle. Extensive literature has been described concerning packing of the rectum in these patients. It is the author's view that as the rectum is a distensible organ that tamponade cannot be satisfactorily achieved by packing and that all of these patients should be taken back to the operating room with full resuscitation. Although a range of packing agents have been described including those containing adrenaline combined with ice-cold water, a 23 G Foley balloon catheter suspended over the bed rail with tamponade using a leveraged glove half filled with water, an anal plug, or topical Gelfoam®.

It is anticipated that up to 15% of these patients may experience further intermittent bleeding and septic complications after their emergent treatment. Overall, rectal bleeding after PPH required readmission within two weeks in 5.6% of over 3,000 cases reported from Singapore. Bleeding after PPH may occur immediately or after about 10 days. Some specialised cases result in a rectal wall haematoma, which can be progressive and require a formal rectotomy and drainage. Bleeding with PPH is more likely to occur for fourth-degree haemorrhoids, anorectal varices or for thrombosed haemorrhoids where bleeding is the principal cause after a PPH for reoperation. Like manual haemorrhoidectomy, prevention is better than cure where attention to operative detail assists in avoiding post-operative bleeding. The surgeon should avoid manual overstretching of the staple line, use a PPH-03 or a TST stapler (as these use smaller staples that are more haemostatic), tighten the gun sufficiently as per any endoanal staple gun, and can use a perioperative endoanal sponge. Evidence would suggest that the risk of bleeding after a PPH procedure decreases with operative experience.

Urinary Retention

Urinary retention is a common post-operative complication after haemorrhoidectomy that increases hospital stay. Patients over 50 years of age have a significantly higher incidence of hesitancy in micturition than younger patients, with men twice as likely as women to have urinary retention following anorectal surgery. This effect of male gender can be explained by the anatomic differences in the urethra and the presence of pre-existing benign prostatic hyperplasia. Urinary complications after haemorrhoidectomy result from nervous reflexes originating from the anus and determined by the operative trauma and rectal discrimination. Adrenergic stimulation that causes reflex inhibition of the detrusor muscle and bladder outlet contraction secondary to anal distension and pain may play a role. Several strategies have been advocated for the prevention of post-operative urinary retention. Patients should be asked to void immediately before surgery. The use of parasympathomimetics and alpha-adrenergic blockers, the restriction of perioperative fluid intake, pain control, Sitz baths, and the use of local anaesthesia have all been advocated. Recently, outpatient haemorrhoid surgery, which reportedly decreases patient anxiety, has been found to reduce urinary retention. It is recognised that psychological factors come into play in some cases where a scientific study assessing spontaneous micturition and which assessed urethral sphincter electromyography, showed that the mere manoeuvre of sitting in a warm bath aided micturition and initiated a reflex urethral sphincter relaxation in the post-haemorrhoidectomy setting.

Data from Zaheer et al., reporting a 34% incidence after haemorrhoidectomy of urinary difficulty, confirmed that age and male gender were the principal risk factors and that prior urinary obstructive symptoms were not an independent risk factor. Others have suggested that diabetes mellitus, the need for post-operative narcotic analgesia, and more than three haemorrhoid masses are independent risk factors for post-operative urinary hesitancy. The risk is not increased with epidural anaesthesia if there is a judicious fluid restriction.

Incontinence and Urgency

The rate of tenesmus or urgency after PPH is probably under-reported although it is likely to diminish with the use of the wider stapler as those result in less early anastomotic oedema and stenosis. This should decrease the reported early but resolvable evacuatory difficulty combined with urgency, which correlates with initial anastomotic compliance. In one study by Ortiz and colleagues, tenesmus affected half of the patients who underwent PPH for fourth-degree haemorrhoids one year after surgery. This rate fell to 25% after six months of follow-up in another study and was not a feature of Milligan-Morgan haemorrhoidectomy.

Manometric studies after PPH have shown minimal changes in fundamental parameters, although in hypertonic resting cases, stapled haemorrhoidopexy reverts resting sphincter pressures to normal. There may be pre-existing factors that are exacerbated by haemorrhoidectomy and that are associated with post-operative incontinence. These can include cases with Grade 4 prolapse. The use of endoanal retraction and the possibility of occult sphincter defects may be contributing factors. A low-placed staple line may lead to faecal soiling after PPH or fragmentation of the internal sphincter in multiparous females after the forceful introduction of the device. It may be that some patients unsuited to a PPH because of a risk

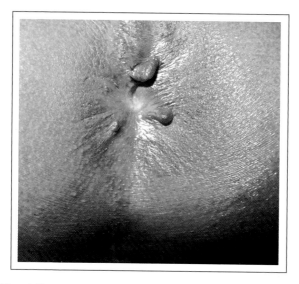

Figure 6.10: Anal stricture following haemorrhoid surgery.
Courtesy: Pravin Jaiprakash Gupta.

of post-operative soiling are somewhat predictable by demonstration of pre-operative rectal hypersensitivity. It is also important not to forget that some cases of soiling may be due to post-operative faecal impaction.

Anal Stenosis

Anal stenosis is an uncommon but disabling condition, which is preventable in both manual and stapled haemorrhoidectomy. Anal stenosis usually results from haemorrhoidectomy carried out over-zealously without the required technical knowledge (Figure 6.10). When there are multiple haemorrhoids, the loss arising from such operative procedures leaves only minimal portions of intact elastic anal tissues. With progressive healing, fibrous scar tissue proliferates and contracts the anorectal outlet, and when healing is complete, a narrow, foreshortened, inelastic stenotic orifice is left which can be exacerbated by secondary infection, ischaemia, and foreign body reaction. Anal stenosis leads to increasing constipation, a reduction of stool volume and shape, abdominal cramps, and rectal bleeding. Anal examination under general anaesthesia is recommended to evaluate the stricture and choose the appropriate surgical reconstructive technique.

Residual Skin Tags

Careless grooming of redundant skin after completion of a manual haemorrhoidectomy can result in oedematous perianal skin tags that persist after complete epithelisation of the wound. When they are excessive, cleansing of the perianal region after defecation can be difficult and troublesome where soiling and pruritus can result requiring a secondary aesthetic anal procedure. As expected, skin tags requiring definitive treatment are more frequent following a stapled procedure.

The Whitehead Deformity

This is largely preventable by avoidance of drawing the mucosa towards the anal verge, but although the Whitehead operation has largely disappeared, it may also result from a zealous mucosal advancement anoplasty. The clinical result is a mucosal ectropion with persistent mucous discharge that is extremely troublesome to the patient. The treatment is akin to that of an anal stenosis with the advancement of skin towards the anal canal after separation from the sphincter apparatus. An alternative procedure described by Rand to provide skin coverage to the anal canal after haemorrhoidal mucosectomy has not been adopted.

Specific Complications Attributable to Stapled Surgery

The introduction of stapled haemorrhoidopexy introduced some neo-syndromes, some of which were severe and even life threatening. Some of these were particularly peculiar to the technique of stapled haemorrhoidopexy and are now preventable such as rectovaginal fistula, the rectal pocket syndrome, and complete rectal obliteration. The rectal pocket develops from a partial slippage of the purse string resulting in a diseased pouch in the lower rectum, resembling a diverticulum that accumulates faecal material and which can mimic a perianal abscess. The condition is treated by opening the pouch for internal drainage. Total rectal obliteration is, fortunately, rare and is due to an erroneous placement of the purse string suture and firing outside of the purse string to create a blind pocket, which requires complete refashioning of the anastomosis and even a colostomy. A mixture of severe septic complications has been reported which are all, fortunately, rare including inadvertent rectal perforation, severe pelvic sepsis, progressive rectal haematoma with rectal obstruction, and complete anastomotic dehiscence. Overall, as the indications for PPH and TST haemorrhoidectomy have become more crystallised with the added knowledge of higher recurrence rates with stapled technology when compared with manual haemorrhoidectomy, there has been a decrease in the use of PPH amongst the members of the Italian Colorectal Clubs (the SICCR), from 26% to 20% of haemorrhoidal surgeries in the consecutive years.

Specific Management of External Haemorrhoidal Disease

External haemorrhoids have already been discussed briefly. External haemorrhoids grow from the ectoderm and are placed distal to the dentate line. These haemorrhoids are sensitive to pain, touch, temperature, and pressure as they are enveloped by stratified squamous epithelium and have somatic sensory innervations from the inferior rectal nerve. They may be painful, and are often accompanied by pruritus ani or itching, swelling, and burning. They occur more commonly in young and middle-aged adults than in older adults and typically occur in association with internal haemorrhoids.

Thrombosed external haemorrhoids are one of the most frequent anorectal emergencies. They are associated with swelling and intense pain and accompanied by internal sphincter hypertonicity. External haemorrhoids may suddenly become thrombosed in an otherwise healthy adult. When there is engorgement of distended haemorrhoidal vessels and acute swelling of these vessels, blood pools in the perianal space with clot formation. Persons with external haemorrhoidal thrombosis present with pain on standing, sitting, or defecation. The body may slowly absorb the thrombosis during several weeks. During resolution, the thrombosis may erode through the skin and produce bleeding or drainage. The tissues may be further traumatised by hard bowel movements and by increased pressure from straining. The pain and swelling may be intense and even incapacitating for the first several days. Symptoms may last for up to four weeks, but usually resolve within a week. The pressure in the pelvic floor from diarrhoea, constipation, straining during defecation, pregnancy, delivery, lifting heavy objects, and the like are the common etiologic factors. A significant number of patients complain of frequent straining at defecation, and almost one-fifth of them may have a previous 'external haemorrhoid' in their history.

Although it has been suggested that there is no apparent association with pregnancy, Abramovitz et al. reported that thrombosed external haemorrhoids were observed in 8% of women during pregnancy and in 20% of women during the postpartum period. The left lateral and dorsal quadrants of the anal verge are the most common sites for the occurrence of this disease. As part of the differential diagnosis, sudden onset of anal pain without the presence of thrombosed haemorrhoid should suggest investigation for an alternate cause, such as an inter-sphincteric abscess or anal fissure where as many as 20% of patients with haemorrhoids will have concomitant anal fissures. Large external haemorrhoid-like lesions may, in fact, be granulomatous inflammatory masses of undiagnosed Crohn's disease. Currently, accepted treatment alternatives consist of conservative and surgical approaches. Conservative therapy includes a combination of anal hygiene, tub baths, dietary changes, and stool softeners to encourage soft stools along with oral and topical analgesics. A recently published trial comparing topical therapy with lidocaine alone to lidocaine plus nifedipine ointment 0.3% for the treatment of acutely thrombosed external haemorrhoids found that the addition of nifedipine was more efficient. Equally, a small series has extolled the virtues of immediate botulinum toxin use.

The operative indications are severe pain, necrosis, or perforation of the overlying skin, and persistent bleeding after perforation of the overlying skin. An anatomically based method involves a circumferential incision over the thrombosed haemorrhoidal sinus with the removal of the thrombi from the involved veins. The procedure can be smoothly performed under local anaesthesia, and only few will need general anaesthesia. The thrombosed external haemorrhoid is excised, starting perianally and dissecting into the anal canal continuing to the dentate line. Complete excision avoids the potential development of a hypertrophied anal papilla with impaired wound healing. The wound is left open for healing by secondary intention, and the specimen is submitted for histopathology. Patients are advised to take Sitz baths and change the wound dressings accordingly. Post-operative analgesia is attained with oral non-steroidal anti-inflammatory agents. The dictum that surgery is always the answer has been recently questioned by a German group that employed an entirely conservative policy of simple dry cleaning and analgesics, suggesting that on prospective assessment of 72 cases, two-thirds were asymptomatic on follow-up.

External haemorrhoids are not composed of single veins but rather of a venous plexus so that when there is a thrombosis, there are multiple clots. A single radial incision may open only one or two veins and leave several thrombi in place so that the patient continues to have symptoms. The thrombosis may involve a significant portion of the circumference of the anus, and total excision may result in a large wound that heals slowly. The proposed circumferential incision opens across the plexus and removes the clots from all the veins without leaving a large wound. While the majority of patients who are treated conservatively will experience resolution of symptoms over a period, it will nevertheless be prudent to go ahead with excision of external haemorrhoidal thrombosis that results in more rapid symptom resolution, a lower incidence of recurrence, and longer remission intervals in comparative studies.

An anal skin tag is a fold of skin arising from the anal verge that is the requiem or result of thrombosis of external haemorrhoid. The frequency increases in women especially at the beginning of the second decade and in men particularly in the fourth decade of life where 80% of all women and 60% of all men have skin tags. The size of the skin tag increases as the person becomes older with women having bigger skin tags on average than men. The commonest location of the skin tags is in the region of the 12 and the 6 o'clock positions in lithotomy. The treatment of external skin tags is rarely surgical.

CHALLENGES WITH HAEMORRHOIDS IN SPECIAL SITUATIONS

Haemorrhoids in the Ante- and Postpartum Period

Pregnancy and the puerperium predispose to symptomatic haemorrhoids, being the most common anorectal disease at these times. Symptoms are usually mild and transient and include intermittent bleeding from the anus along with pain. Hormonal variations during pregnancy result in an increase in the elasticity of the perianal, anorectal, and recto pelvic structures with relative sphincter and pelvic muscle hypertrophy and pelvic vessel dilatation, congestion, and hypertrophy that result in a pelvic blood volume increase of up to 25% above average. This effect is maintained until childbirth and rapidly decreases to near normal towards the tenth day after labour. In the absence of these physiological changes, the anorectal tissues would be significantly damaged during normal childbirth. The anorectal vascular dilatation, enlargement, and the laxity of the peri-anorectal structures, as well as the increased intra-pelvic pressure during labour, are important secondary factors in the causation of various anal lesions before and during childbirth.

Most haemorrhoidal disease in pregnancy is underestimated by obstetricians, often precluding patient access to possible medical and surgical or rehabilitative treatments designed to correct eventual dysfunction related to the delivery. In this regard, it has been estimated that between 25% and 35% of pregnant women are affected by haemorrhoids with symptoms presenting most commonly in the second and third trimesters. The worst symptoms are usually reserved for the third trimester at the time of greatest pelvic pressure with associated periods of constipation and dehydration. Acute haemorrhoidal crisis can also occur with irreducible prolapse, thrombosis, and protracted pain along with external haemorrhoidal thrombosis.

Treatment during pregnancy is mainly directed at the relief of symptoms, especially pain control. Laxative treatment for patients with dyschezia during childbirth and the postpartum period significantly decreases the occurrence of anal lesions in the postpartum period. The conservative management includes stimulants or depressants of the bowel transit, dietary modifications, local treatment, and phlebotonics, which are discussed earlier in this chapter. For many women, symptoms will resolve spontaneously soon after birth and so any corrective treatment is usually deferred although Khubchandani has reported successful haemorrhoidectomy during pregnancy. Most forms of the condition can be successfully treated by increasing the fibre content in the diet, administering stool softeners, increasing liquid intake, anti-haemorrhoidal medications, analgesics, and training in toilet habits. The best treatment is cold bathing of the anal region with cotton-wool pledges and replacement of the haemorrhoids should they prolapse. Some women prefer natural and herbal approaches where relief may be obtained with oral rutosides, *Centella asiatica*, hidrosmine, disodium flavodate, grape seed extract, or French maritime pine bark extract, each of which can decrease capillary fragility and improve the microcirculation in venous insufficiency disorders.

More aggressive therapies used in other haemorrhoidal disease are reserved for patients who have persistent symptoms after one month of conservative therapy either during pregnancy or in the postpartum period although the latter should be delayed for at least three months, if possible. Once the true haemorrhoidal disease develops, correction should be performed before a subsequent pregnancy. The acute haemorrhoidal crisis should have a short period of conservatism in pregnancy but be followed because of septic risk with surgery directed at removing only the symptomatic, complicated, or gangrenous area. One should note that haemorrhoids are not the only cause of rectal bleeding in pregnancy and that the physician should properly confirm the diagnosis and exclude other colonic causes where appropriate before initiating any treatment. Equally, thrombosed external haemorrhoids during pregnancy should be treated as per the non-pregnant population. Risk factors appear to include traumatic and late delivery, as well as the delivery of a large baby and a prolonged first stage of labour.

Haemorrhoids in Children

Haemorrhoids in children are uncommon. There is almost no evidence of the presence of haemorrhoids in children who were examined for sexual abuse or in the perianal findings at postmortem. The most common cause of haemorrhoids in young children is portal hypertension with a higher incidence of both haemorrhoids and rectal varices with extrahepatic disease. The occurrence and severity of haemorrhoids are related to the number of previous oesophageal sclerotherapy sessions. A strong family history of such illness and a history of constipation may be contributing factors to initiate this rarity. In children, the differential diagnosis includes rectal prolapse or prolapse of a rectal polyp. These lesions may not be visible when the child is anaesthetised because of lack of straining. A 20 F Foley catheter with a 30 mL balloon can be inserted into the rectum with gentle traction to demonstrate haemorrhoids at an examination under anaesthetic (EUA). Therapy consists of correction of constipation and, where appropriate, treatment as per adults with sclerotherapy, photocoagulation, or banding.

Haemorrhoids in the Elderly

While haemorrhoidal disease is seen quite frequently in the middle-aged patients, its frequency goes on decreasing after 65 years of age. The diagnosis of symptomatic haemorrhoids may pose a problem in elderly patients as may their treatment if there are coincident medications such as anticoagulants. Surgery in this group may reveal problems of anal closure and affect continence and independence. Anecdotally, pain appears less in the elderly after banding where there is less sphincter hypertonia. Haemorrhoidectomy is not contraindicated with the proviso that all haemorrhoidal tissue is sent for pathology.

Haemorrhoids in Association with Ulcerative Colitis

Haemorrhoids can be associated with ulcerative colitis and appear to be one of the complications of diarrhoea caused by the disease. The patient may complain of passing bright blood on defecation and erroneously may be treated as a case of haemorrhoids by injection or even may undergo a haemorrhoidectomy. The symptoms would persist, and it is not uncommon to find that the patient has a distal form of ulcerative colitis, which manifests as bleeding without diarrhoea. When severely prolapsed haemorrhoids occur during an actual attack of ulcerative colitis, the chances of complications are high. It would be wise to manage them conservatively until the ulcerative colitis is quiescent and then to carry out haemorrhoidectomy along the usual guidelines. Both surgical and conservative treatment of haemorrhoids in patients with ulcerative colitis appears to have a low complication rate.

Haemorrhoids and Crohn's Disease

Perianal Crohn's disease is covered elsewhere in this book. Specifically, haemorrhoids in Crohn's disease have been traditionally contrasted with haemorrhoids presenting with ulcerative proctosig-moiditis. It has always been suggested that haemorrhoidectomy in Crohn's disease is often complicated and may result in proctectomy or diversion. Further, the treatments available for active Crohn's proctitis were limited. It is the author's experience that haemorrhoidectomy if indicated in patients with quiescent Crohn's disease or active perianal disease is quite safe. This view has been supported by Wolkomir and Luchtefeld, who concurred that the different surgeries and treatments were safe if the Crohn's disease elsewhere was inactive.

Haemorrhoids in HIV-positive Patients

A series of anorectal disorders are now widely recognised as one of the most common complications occurring in HIV-positive patients. There seems to be a common belief that anorectal surgery in an HIV-positive patient is an invitation to disaster. Early reports describing outcomes of HIV-positive patients undergoing anorectal procedures have published quite a serious problem in wound healing and excessive perioperative morbidity. Few other reports, however, have demonstrated that a prudently selected management will result in high rates of symptomatic relief. One can expect satisfactory wound healing after haemorrhoid surgery without excessive morbidity and mortality particularly if the CD4+ counts are within the normal range.

The burden of haemorrhoidal disease to the health service is enormous. It would appear that the most durable and acceptable results of conservative treatments are achieved currently with RBL. If patients come to surgery, traditional haemorrhoidectomy is favoured as either an open or a closed technique with some advantage for diathermy and the LigaSure™ device with a reduction in stapled haemorrhoidopexy because of delayed recurrence, particularly where the original haemorrhoids were large. The place of DGHAL combining a mucopexy even for larger haemorrhoids requires more research to define better its actual place. Despite the universal nature of haemorrhoids, there is little comparative operative data with established treatment options and accepted outcomes. It is hoped that these newer, better-designed trials will provide high-quality data that could direct therapy by disease presentation and severity.

CLINICAL PEARLS

- Haemorrhoids are the most common cause of anorectal bleeding, but can also present as pruritus or a mass on examination. Internal haemorrhoids occur above the dentate line, and external haemorrhoids occur below the dentate line. Internal haemorrhoids are classified as Grades 1–4 based on the degree of prolapse.

(Cont'd)

- Only a third of patients with symptomatic haemorrhoids seek medical help.
- Current guidelines recommend a minimum of anoscopy and flexible sigmoidoscopy for bright red rectal bleeding.
- There is still no consensus on optimal treatment. Improvements in our understanding of the anatomy of haemorrhoids have prompted the development of new and innovative methods of treatment.
- The most appropriate treatment is tailored to the individual patient.
- A classification orientated therapeutical regime offers high healing rates with a low rate of complications and recurrences.
- Conservative treatment consists of dietary and lifestyle modifications and medications like flavonoids and calcium dobesilate.
- Standard interventional procedures in outpatient treatment are injection sclerotherapy, rubber band ligation, and infrared coagulation.
- Among the surgical options for prolapsed haemorrhoids, formal haemorrhoidectomy using newer devices like radiofrequency and ultrasonic waves now compete with stapled haemorrhoidopexy, which is less painful and allows shorter convalescence but may have a higher recurrence rate and needs further long-term evaluation. Other popular methods include the doppler-guided haemorrhoidal artery ligation and LigaSure™.

SUGGESTED READINGS

Abramowitz L, Batallan A. Epidemiology of anal lesions (fissure and thrombosed external hemorrhoid) during pregnancy and post-partum. *Gynecol Obstet Fertil*. 2003 Jun;31(6):546–9.

Aigner F, Bodner G, Conrad F, Mbaka G, Kreczy A, Fritsch H. The superior rectal artery and its branching pattern with regard to its clinical influence on ligation techniques for internal hemorrhoids. *Am J Surg*. 2004; 187:102–8.

Aigner F, Bodner G, Gruber H, et al. The vascular nature of hemorrhoids. *J Gastrointest Surg* 2006; 10:1044–50.

Ambrose NS, Morris D, Alexander-Williams J, Keighley MR. A randomized trial of photocoagulation or injection sclerotherapy for the treatment of first- and second-degree hemorrhoids. *Dis Colon Rectum*. 1985; 28:238–40.

Avital S, Itah H, Skornick Y, Greenberg R. Outcome of stapled hemorrhoidopery versus doppler-guided hemorrhoidal artery ligation for grade III hemorrhoids. *Tech Coloproctol*. 2011;15:267–71.

Awojobi OA. Modified pile suture in the outpatient treatment of hemorrhoids: a preliminary report. *Dis Colon Rectum*. 1983;26:95–7.

Chew SS, Marshall L, Kalish L, et al. Short-term and long-term results of combined sclerotherapy and rubber band ligation of haemorrhoids and mucosal prolapse. *Dis Colon Rectum*. 2003;46:1232–7.

Chung YC, Hon YC, Pan AC. Endoglin (CD105) expression in the development of haemorrhoids. *Eur J Clin Invest*. 2004;34:107–12.

Diurni M, Di Giuseppe M. Hemorrhoidectomy in day surgery. *Int J Surg*. 2008; 6(Suppl 1):S53–5.

Farag AE. Pile suture: a new technique for the treatment of haemorrhoids. *Br J Surg*. 1978;65:293–5.

Faucheron JL, Gangner Y. Doppler-guided hemorrhoid artery ligation for the treatment of symptomatic hemorrhoids: early and three-year follow-up results in 100 consecutive patients. *Dis Colon Rectum*. 2008; 51:945–9.

Giordano P, Nastro P, Davies A, Gralante G. Prospective evaluation of stapled haemorrhoidopexy versus transanal haemorrhoidal dearterialisation for stage II and III haemorrhoids: three-year outcomes. *Tech Coloproctol*. 2011;15:67–73.

Griffith CD, Morris DL, Ellis I, et al. Outpatient treatment of haemorrhoids with bipolar diathermy coagulation. *Br J Surg*. 1987;74:827.

Gupta PJ. Radiofrequency coagulation versus rubber band ligation in early hemorrhoids: pain versus gain. *Medicina*. 2004; 40:232–7.

Han W, Wang ZJ, Zhao B, et al. Pathologic change of elastic fibers with difference of microvessel density and expression of angiogenesis-related proteins in internal hemorrhoid tissues. *Zhonghua Weichang Waike Zazhi*. 2005; 8:56–9.

Kairaluoma M, Nuorva K, Kellokumpu I. Day-case stapled (circular) vs. diathermy hemorrhoidectomy: a randomized, controlled trial evaluating surgical and functional outcome. *Dis Colon Rectum*. 2003; 46:93–9.

Laughlan K, Jayne DG, Jackson D, et al. Stapled haemorrhoidopexy compared to Milligan-Morgan and Ferguson haemorrhoidectomy: a systematic review. *Int J Colorectal Dis*. 2009;24:335–44.

Lumb KJ, Colquhoun PH, Malthaner R, et al. Stapled versus conventional surgery for hemorrhoids. *Cochrane Database Syst Rev*. 2006;(4):CD005393.

MacRae HM, McLeod RS. Comparison of hemorrhoidal treatments: a meta-analysis. *Can J Surg*. 1997;40:14–7.

McLemore EC, Rai R, Siddiqui J, Basu PP, Tabbaa M, Epstein MS. Novel endoscopic delivery modality of infrared coagulation therapy for internal hemorrhoids. *Surg Enodsc*. 2012;26:3082–7.

Milito G, Caddedu F, Muzi MG, Nigro C, Farinom AM. Haemorrhoidectomy with LigaSure™ vs. conventional excisional techniques: meta-analysis of randomized controlled trials. *Colorectal Dis*. 2010;12:85–93.

Neiger A. Infrared-photo-coagulation for hemorrhoids treatment. *Int Surg*. 1989;74:142–3.

Nienhuijs S, de Hingh I. Conventional versus LigaSure™ hemorrhoidectomy for patients with symptomatic Hemorrhoids. *Cochrane Database Syst Rev*. 2009;1:CD006761.

Reese GE, von Roon AC, Tekkis PP. Clinical evidence: haemorrhoids. *Dig Syst Disorders*. 2009;01:415.

Ross NP, Hildebrand DR, Tiernan JP, Brown SR, Watson AJM. Haemorrhoids: 21st-century management. *Colorectal Dis*. 2012: 14:917–9.

Shafik A. A new concept of the anatomy of the anal sphincter mechanism and the physiology of defecation. IV. Anatomy of the perianal spaces. *Invest Urol*. 1976;13:424–8.

Tan EK, Cornish J, Darzi AW, Papagrigoriadis S, Tekkis PP. Meta-analysis of short-term outcomes of randomized controlled trials of LigaSure™ vs. conventional haemorrhoidectomy. *Arch Surg*. 2007;142:1209–18.

Zaheer S, Reilly WT, Pemberton JH, et al. Urinary retention after operations for benign anorectal diseases. *Dis Colon Rectum*. 1998;41:696–704.

Zbar AP, Guo M, Pescatori M. Anorectal morphology and function: analysis of the Shafik legacy. *Tech Coloproctol*. 2008;12:191–200.

Chapter 7

Anal infections

Anorectal abscess and fistula are common pathologic findings, which have been described from the beginning of medical history. About 6–10 anal gland orifices reside along the dentate line. These glands extend through the submucosa, pierce the underlying muscularis, and often track to the inter-sphincteric groove. Faecal bacteria are exposed to these glands, and an acute perirectal abscess develops when the orifice is occluded. A fistula-in-ano represents the chronic version of this infection. Pain in the perianal region, fever, and difficulty to void constitute the classic triad of perineal sepsis. Its most common reason is advanced cryptoglandular infection resulting in a necrotising perineal infection. An anorectal abscess is the acute inflammatory process that often is the initial manifestation of an underlying anorectal fistula. Anal gland infection or cryptitis can lead to abscesses that are perianal, ischiorectal, inter-sphincteric, and supra levator.

AETIOLOGIC CONSIDERATIONS

The known fact underlying all anal infections is the invasion of anal ducts and glands and regional tissues by pathogenic bacteria.

Anal crypts are tiny grooves intervening the anal papillae at the proximal end of the anal canal, that is, the mucocutaneous junction. The crypts are small mucous glands that function to lubricate, and they are arranged in a circle near the upper end of the anal canal. They look like pockets in a coat devoid of flaps or covers. The orifice or mouths of these pockets project upwards on to the rectum, and they are within the grasp of the sphincter muscles. Before the bowel movement, the sphincter muscles contract and squeeze out a little drop of lubricating mucous from each of these crypts.

Cryptitis occurs when these crypts become inflamed, and the mucosal lining of their roofs becomes denuded. Possible causes of cryptitis can be one of the following:

- Frequent watery stools may cause trauma or deposits in the crypts
- Direct trauma from large hard stools
- Inflammation from adjacent structures
- External sources of infection, such as parasites or foreign bodies

Because of their delicate nature and position in the anal canal with the openings upwards, the crypts are easily injured (usually by hard particles in the stool). It turns out to be one of the most common sources of infection in the anal canal and rectum. In one such case, they stood in columns and appeared erythematous and oedematous on proctoscopic examination. In many instances, both crypts and papillae are present. Irregular bowel movements, laxative abuse, spicy foods, and other types of mucosal irritation are few other causative factors. A possible sequel is that as one of the papilla becomes inflamed and swollen, it attracts faecal matter to accumulate in the crypts where they can trigger widespread inflammation. These are most commonly found in the area of the posterior commissure of the anal canal. Either faecal matter or other infectious material gathers in the crypt to begin the formation of an abscess.

The discomfort of cryptitis is usually of the sharp burning variety. The sphincters may go in a state of spasm causing further pain. At other times, the symptoms of cryptitis may be milder in the form of a feeling of heaviness, uneasiness after the bowel movement, a dull rectal ache, or aching in the hips and legs. Cryptitis at times can become quite painful, and yet it may go undiagnosed. It is usually labelled as a case of proctalgia of unknown origin.

Anal papillae, which are also called as papillitis hypertrophicans, anal fibroma, or 'cat tooth' are the fine points of projections at the mucocutaneous junction of the extreme upper end of anal canal skin (Figure 7.1). Small papillae usually remain asymptomatic. A hypertrophied anal papilla may be associated with pain and, at times, bleeding at defecation may be encountered in infancy. Bleeding into a hypertrophied anal papilla can cause sudden rectal pain. At times, the papilla may be trapped by contraction of the sphincter mechanism after defecation. Histologically, the papillae are made up of an oedematous, loosened up, fibrotic connective tissue in parts, with raised capillary contents. Occasionally, acanthosis and broadened disk epithelium may be visible, but they never proceed to malignant degeneration. At times, a swollen red papilla is encountered with dull pain and a purulent discharge from the associated crypt. This condition is termed as 'papillitis' associated with 'cryptitis'. The hypertrophy of the existing anal papillae is a result of a chronic inflammatory process

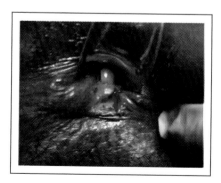

Figure 7.1   Hypertrophied anal papilla.
Courtesy: Pravin Jaiprakash Gupta.

associated with fibrotic proliferation within the limits of the linea
dentata, the distal rectal mucosa, and the anorectal zone.

THE ANAL GLANDS

The anal glands are located at the bottom of the anal crypts and situated at the level of the dentate line. Usually, there are about 6–8
such glands, which extend down into the internal sphincter and up to
and including the inter-sphincteric groove. Blockage of these glands
causes stasis with bacterial overgrowth, and results in the formation of abscesses, which are located in the inter-sphincteric groove.
These abscesses have different ways of emergence, the most common being a caudal extension to the anoderm (perianal abscess) or
through the external sphincter into the ischiorectal fossa (ischiorectal
abscess). Occasionally, the spread can mount up superiorly the inter-
sphincteric groove and then to the supra levator zone or in the submucosal plane. When the abscess is evacuated either by surgery or
of its own, the persistence of the septic foci and epithelisation of the
draining tract may occur and lead to a fistula-in-ano.

The role of the anal crypt, duct, and gland system in the
pathogenesis of the anorectal disease is rigorously investigated,
and it is established that the crypt orifices serve as 'funnels' along
which infection is led into anal ducts and glands (Figure 7.2). It is a
well-known fact that these glands play a crucial and important part
in the origin of infectious anorectal lesions, although all the possible
intermediary processes are not entirely known.

The transmission of an infection through the system of anal glands
is seen by various microscopic changes, which ultimately leads to its
clinical manifestations. Microscopic findings illustrate that localised
cellulitis-involving duct and gland structures constitute an early stage
in the process. Initially, a single gland gets involved in the suppurative
process, then the adjoining tissues and other glands. The severity of

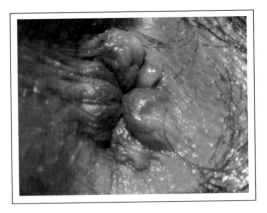

Figure 7.2   Anal inflammation.
Courtesy: Pravin Jaiprakash Gupta.

infection depends not only on the number of glands present, but also on the place and the depth of penetration. It is likely that the spread of infection to these tissues is metastatic in nature, where the infection is carried indirectly by way of lymphatic channels and blood vessels.

In clinical practice, anorectal inflammatory disease by the complexity of aetiologic patterns cannot be considered a single disease. Furthermore, it may manifest in more than one form in the same patient (Figure 7.3). For convenience, an anorectal infectious disease can be grouped into two types—direct and indirect; the classification depends on upon the avenue of infection, that is, the direct diseases like suppuration, abscess, and fistulous disease. Indirect disease includes hypertrophy of anal papillae and contracture or stenosis of the anus.

Haemorrhoids, which are comprised of arteriovenous structures and supportive tissues, are in close relationship with the anal ducts and glands, and like other tissues, they too are vulnerable to infection through their supporting tissues. Inflammation of these vascular cushions produces sudden swelling followed by congestion, and occasionally rupture, resulting in haemorrhoidal thrombosis—also known as a thrombotic pile. A self-limited manifestation of this process is the single or multiple external thrombotic haemorrhoids.

Even though a patient may have symptoms indicating anal pathology, complete history must be taken and thorough physical examination must be performed. The cardinal symptoms of anorectal infection are an alteration in bowel habits, pain, bleeding, swelling, purulent discharge, and loss of weight.

Pain due to anorectal inflammation is usually localised and usually a dull aching or throbbing. Acute anorectal pain, which causes a patient to consult promptly a physician, suggests ulceration, infection, or thrombosis of the regional vessels.

Acute progressive swelling with pain, malaise, fever, and leucocytosis indicates abscess formation. On the other hand, a sudden

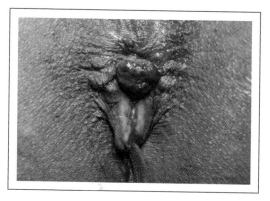

Figure 7.3 Infected granuloma.
Courtesy: Pravin Jaiprakash Gupta.

appearance of a localised swelling with pricking sensation and pain near the anal margin indicates haemorrhoidal thrombosis, which may be associated with regional infection.

Anoscopic examination under direct or indirect lighting is best accomplished by using an open-end anoscope with a removable obturator. The presence of hypertrophied anal papillae, which may assume a polypoid appearance, can be noted. One can also observe anal gland infection by squeezing purulent exudates from the mouth of the crypt with the margin of the scope. The internal opening of a fistula also may be detected, and on a few occasions, this impression may be confirmed by gentle probing.

Differential Diagnosis

Even with the most meticulous office examination, it is impossible to estimate the magnitude of all the infective processes involving the anorectal canal. The final analysis in every extremely painful condition is to examine under regional anaesthesia in the operating theatre where surgical treatment can be carried out if required.

Infectious pyodermia or hidradenitis suppurativa involving the perianal cutaneous surfaces is characterised by sinus formation with the joining of superficial abscesses involving integumental areas where the apocrine sweat glands predominate. This process, however, does not affect the gland duct system (Figure 7.4).

Pilonidal cyst and sinuses, considered as a differential diagnostic problem, must be viewed with their possible association with abscess and fistula formation involving the posterior part of the anal margin. A direct continuity may exist between these two lesions in one person.

Haemorrhoidal varicosities associated with oedema and swelling accompanying variable degrees of acute thrombosis may be difficult clinically to be differentiated from acute inflammatory disease with abscess formation. It is important that an exact diagnosis is established, may be under regional anaesthesia if necessary, to avoid an extension of the infection.

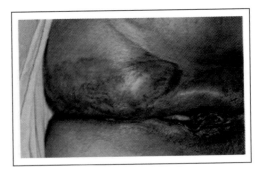

Figure 7.4 Perianal suppurations.

Courtesy: Pravin Jaiprakash Gupta.

Treatment

Sub-mucous anal canal abscesses are preferably opened with a cautery, with bevelling of edges, excision of secondary fistulous processes, and dependent drainage to the anal verge. Using rubber drains and avoidance of gauze packing minimise pain and are adequate if surgical drainage has been completed. If one is sure that this abscess is an acute manifestation of a fistula, no sooner the infection has been checked by incision and drainage, the patient should undergo a planned fistulectomy at the earliest.

HUMAN PAPILLOMA VIRUS INFECTION

Anogenital papillomavirus infection is the most common sexually transmitted disease (STD) and is increasing in incidence. In many of the gastrointestinal disorders, HPV infection can undergo a progressive transformation of normal cells to dysplasia and ultimately to invasive anal malignancy.

This susceptibility is even more prominent in men who are homosexual or in immunocompromised patients. The duration of HPV infections in the majority of healthy individuals is short lived. Most infections clear in a very short time and may go unnoticed.

Other risk factors recognised to increase the incidence of HPV include immunosuppression, women with a history of cervical disease or neoplasia, organ transplant patients, patients with a history of anogenital warts, men and women having more than ten female sex partners, human immunodeficiency virus (HIV) infection, cigarette smoking, previous exposure to STDs, and radiation therapy.

PATHOPHYSIOLOGY OF THE HUMAN PAPILLOMAVIRUS VIRUS

The HPV virus has a great affinity for the transitional zones of the tissues like the cervix and the pectinate line of the rectum around the squamous-columnar junction (SCJ) epithelium. The HPV virus hits the basal membrane stem cells. It is at this place where virus replication occurs.

Clinical Presentation and Examination

The standardised anatomic description is critical to communicate the findings adequately on physical examination. The following four distinct regions have been proposed for description:

- Skin: It is 5 cm away from the anal opening with local examination.
- Perianal (anal margin): It is within 5 cm of the anal opening (Figure 7.5).
- Anal canal (intra-anal): Not visible; needs anoscopy to be examined.
- Transformation zone: Above the dentate line/squamous columnar junction.

Symptoms

In the beginning, patients may report a wide range of symptoms that could be vague, moderate, or severe. Symptoms may include

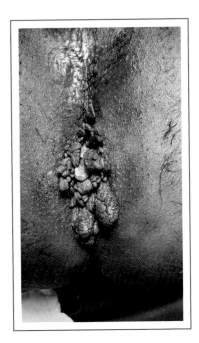

Figure 7.5   Ano-perianal warts.
Courtesy: Pravin Jaiprakash Gupta.

pruritus, anal discharge, tenesmus, changes in bowel habits, discomfort, fissures, lumps, or fistulas.

Condyloma acuminata (meaning knuckle or knobs and pointed or tapered) can be easily identified.

The clinical appearance can be apparent and more evident with swelling, irregular scaling, white or pigmented plaques, flaking or oozing in the anal area.

Anogenital warts can be described in these three ways:

- Classical: Look like cauliflower, acuminata-like knuckles or horny with pointy edges
- Smooth: Exophytic, papulous appearance with hill-like, raised edges
- Flat: Non-exophytic, plaques that may require high-resolution anoscopy for identification

Evaluation of patients should comprise a full proctological examination that consists of inspection, palpation, anoscopy, and sigmoidoscopy. Some clinician may augment their examination with anal cytology or high-definition anoscopy using acetic acid or lugol's solution. One can add HPV-deoxyribonucleic acid (DNA) testing and endorectal ultrasound before biopsy in patients with lesions suspicious for invasion.

Differential Diagnosis

It is presumed that perianal Bowen's disease and high-grade AIN 3 have a common aetiology of types 16 and 18 HPV. Many other perianal pathologies might have a skin appearances that can look alike and should be ruled out include herpes, Paget's disease, secondary syphilis, condyloma lata (flat skin lesions), reactive atypia in squamous metaplasia, squamous hyperplasia, molluscum contagiosum (condyloma subcutaneum), haemophilus ducreyi, and chanchroids. A correct diagnosis should be substantiated by a biopsy.

Treatment

The treatment of HPV depends on several factors. These include the extent and location of disease, atypia, and patient-related factors. Possibly, the easiest way of breaking this down is by dividing the patients into two groups. One group comprises those patients who are at low risk of developing anal cancer. These patients have normal immune systems and do not show dysplasia on biopsy of their anal lesions. Patients in the other group are those who are more vulnerable to develop anal malignancy, comprising patients with dysplasia on biopsy and/or a compromised immune system. If the approach is considered in these terms, the risks, advantages, treatment options, and follow-up workup of the patients become easier to consider.

It is rare to find a benign disease progressing to dysplasia if the patient is immunocompetent. For such patients, the most important feature of their ailment is its extent. For patients having a limited disease, local excision that fulfils a pathologic evaluation and removal of the lesion in total is what is needed. The choices for therapy are extensive. Treatment is multimodal, which includes excision, destruction with cryotherapy, trichloroacetic acid (TCA), electrocautery, CO_2 laser, or infrared coagulation. In minor recurrences, topical application of podophyllotoxin or imiquimod has been shown to be effective as well.

Local excision and destruction using electrocautery have been shown to be safe without significant risk of anal stenosis. The advantage of this approach is that it allows one to evaluate the anal canal under anaesthesia and potentially complete therapy in one sitting. Gynaecologists have employed laser treatment with excellent results as well. Others have utilised infrared coagulation to attain success. For smaller lesions, treatment in the office with TCA or cryotherapy has the advantage of being quick, easy to conduct, and inexpensive.

About topical home therapy, the choicest options are imiquimod and podophyllotoxin. These applications have the advantage of avoidance of surgical procedures and, in turn, surgical complications. In addition, these topical agents have the ability to treat large areas without any significant collateral damage. For reasons unknown, women have been found to respond better to immunotherapy with topical imiquimod than men. While comparing imiquimod and podophyllotoxin, it is found that cure rates are almost equal, but the side effects were more severe with the latter. Topical therapy could be more appropriate for patients with extensive disease as excision or

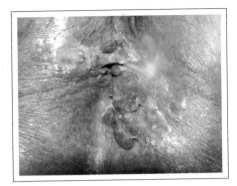

Figure 7.6 Dysplasia with malignant transformation.
Courtesy: Pravin Jaiprakash Gupta.

destruction of such lesions could be quite morbid or may require a staged procedure.

One must understand that a significant percentage of patients may be non-responders to imiquimod or podophyllotoxin.

Treatment options for patients with dysplasia on biopsy and those with immune system compromise are not very different from those with more benign disease except for the addition of high-resolution anoscopy. In the absence of a high-resolution anoscopy, patients having a large circumferential lesions may be subjected to frequent random circumferential biopsies and exhaustive non-targeted destructive therapies (Figure 7.6).

It is produdent to wear condoms and avoid sharing sexual or genital objects. Smoking should be given up if one is infected; it will have an advantage while dealing with an HPV infection.

ANORECTAL INFLAMMATORY DISEASE

Inflammation of the mucosal aspect of the rectum is termed as proctitis while anusitis means inflammation of the anal canal. Affections in these areas can cause varied symptoms including itching, burning, pelvic pressure, rectal bleeding, or foul-smelling discharge. The difference between proctitis and anusitis is not quite apparent, as the aetiology and the management of anusitis and proctitis are similar.

The variable aetiologies include infectious organisms (for example, gonorrhoea, salmonella, and shigella), inflammatory bowel disease, non-infectious causes like radiation, ischaemic, diversion, and idiopathic causes. Proctitis can occur in both the acute and chronic settings and cause significant anorectal complaints.

It can also develop from Crohn's disease or ulcerative colitis. It can be initiated by a STD (such as syphilis, Chlamydia trachomatis infection, gonorrhoea and cytomegalovirus infection), or herpes simplex virus infection, especially among homosexual men. Viral infections like the Herpes simplex virus or Cytomegalovirus can also lead to proctitis.

Patients with ulcerative colitis may initially present with proctitis. Also, patients treated with radiation therapy have a chance of developing chronic radiation proctitis. This percentage is related to the dose of radiation received. Infectious causes come from Clostridium and Salmonella species. Other unusual causes of proctitis include diversion, ischaemia, and radiation.

The patient may present with rectal bleeding, which is bright red in colour and is persistent, but rarely severe. The bleeding may persist for several weeks or longer. Changes in bowel habits may occur, like a decrease in volume with increase in mucoid contents. Patients complain of mild diarrhoea along with a lot of mucous. The mild diarrhoea is the most common complaint. Patients may report tenesmus or faecal urgency. While severe diarrhoea is uncommon, constipation may occur if there is an acute inflammation. Patients may also be having abdominal cramps that are caused by the inflammation within the pelvis.

While taking the patient's history, pertinent questions should include a personal history of inflammatory bowel disease, travel history, profession, sexual history (including questions regarding anal intercourse), and pelvic radiation. It is important to note the patient's HIV status as well. Obtaining a list of medications consumed (for example, non-steroidal anti-inflammatory drugs [NSAIDs], antibiotics) is also important. A family history of inflammatory bowel disease (IBD) or other gastrointestinal diseases is crucial.

A physical examination may be unremarkable. Abdominal tenderness may be felt in IBD, infectious colitides, and ischaemic proctitis. A digital rectal examination is painful due to tenderness. In such situations, an evaluation under anaesthesia is required.

The indications for therapy vary according to the aetiology of the proctitis. The first-line therapy in such patients is medical treatment. Surgical intervention is needed if the medical therapy does not work or any dysplasia is seen on biopsy specimens, and in case of cancer. Selective antibiotics are the best treatment for proctitis caused by a specific bacterial infection. When proctitis is caused by the use of an antibiotic that destroys healthy intestinal bacteria, one may prescribe metronidazole. When the cause is radiation therapy or idiopathic, anti-inflammatory drugs such as hydrocortisone or mesalamine may provide relief. Various formulations like an enema or a suppository are available. Some corticosteroids are available in a foam preparation that can be inserted with a cartridge and plunger. In the case of poor response, other anti-inflammatory drugs such as sulfasalazine may be taken orally and per rectally. If these treatment modalities do not reduce the inflammation, formalin may be applied directly to the lesion or oral corticosteroids may be used. Surgery has no role in proctitis secondary to an infectious aetiology. The goal of therapy is to remove the infection that is causing the inflammation. On occasions, profound sepsis may require a surgical resection as a life-saving manoeuvre. Few reports have achieved a good result with a laser or argon plasma coagulation.

CLINICAL PEARLS

- Infection in and around the anus is a common proctological disorder, often responding to conservative approaches but may require surgical treatment. The pathogens responsible for such infections are mixed aerobic and anaerobic organisms.
- Now a cryptoglandular theory causing suppuration and abscess formation is widely accepted. A majority of the perianal abscesses are the result of an infection originating in the anal crypts and extend into the anal glands in the intersphincteric plane. It may track downwards further to form a perianal abscess.
- No specific indication is laid down regarding culture of the as antibiotics are infrequently used. Few studies, however, have concluded that the likelihood of a fistula increases manifold if gut-derived organisms like *Escherichia coli* and *Bacteroides fragilis* are seen in the pus.
- Perianal abscess is not rare in a child and is found exclusively in boys and systemic signs of sepsis are surprisingly absent. Suppuration is common in adults. Antibiotics are not needed for the operation, unless marked cellulitis, immunosuppression, valvular heart disease, signs of systemic infection, or diabetes exist.

SUGGESTED READINGS

Buchan R, Grace RH. Anorectal suppuration: the results of treatment and the factors influencing the recurrence rate. *Br J Surg*. 1973;60:537–40.

Charles J, Miller G, Fahridin S. Perianal problems. *Aust Fam Physician*. 2010;39:365.

Daling JR, Sherman KJ, Hislop TG, et al. Cigarette smoking and the risk of anogenital cancer. *Am J Epidemiol*. 1992;135:180–9.

Daling JR, Weiss NS, Hislop TG, et al. Sexual practices, sexually transmitted diseases, and the incidence of anal cancer. *N Engl J Med*. 1987;317:973–7.

Meislin HW, Lerner SA, Graves MH, et al. Cutaneous abscesses. Anaerobic and aerobic bacteriology and outpatient management. *Ann Intern Med*. 1977;87:145–9.

Nicholls RJ, Dozois RR (eds). *Surgery of the Colon and the Rectum*. New York: Churchill Livingstone;1997.

Parks AG. Pathogenesis and treatment of fistula-in-ano. *Br Med J*. 1961;1:463–9.

Pfenninger JL, Zainea GG. Common anorectal conditions: Part I. Symptoms and complaints. *Am Fam Physician*. 2001;63:2391–8.

Vernon SD, Holmes KK, Reeves WC. Human papillomavirus infection and associated disease in persons infected with human immunodeficiency virus. *Clin Infect Dis*. 1995;21(1):S121–4.

Whitehead SM, Leach RD, Eykyn SJ, Phillips I. The aetiology of perirectal sepsis. *Br J Surg*. 1982;69:166–8.

Chapter 8

Anorectal abscess and fistula

Suppuration in and around the anus and anal fistulas are the disease processes that have their basis of understanding and treatment firmly rooted in the anatomic design of the anal canal. They, at a time, are fraught with potential for disastrous complications. One needs a careful, cautious, and meticulous care for the diagnosis and treatment of the fistulous abscesses to result in favourable outcomes in most cases.

Perirectal and perianal abscess are the commonly encountered problems in surgical practice. Timely and appropriate treatment is needed to prevent severe morbidity and mortality. Recognition of the complex perirectal abscess from the perianal abscess is necessary to avoid long-term complications.

PATHOPHYSIOLOGY

Anal abscess develops from infection of the mucous-secreting anal glands, which opens into the anal crypts. Obstruction of the duct is believed to be the initiating cause of infection. The suppuration can then extend to involve the perianal spaces that are filled with fatty areolar tissue, and offer little resistance to infection. These areas include the perianal, ischiorectal, inter-sphincteric and deep postanal space, which connects the ischiorectal space on each side posteriorly. Occasionally, the supra levator spaces are also involved. The infection may be limited to one space or in combination with one another.

The pathogenesis of anal fistula and abscess is believed to be derived from infection within one of the anal crypt glands located at the level of the dentate line. Recent anatomical dissection has provided a new glandular classification system revealing that the largest number of fistulae lie in the right lower quadrant in association with the largest recognisable fraction of anal glands, although prior theories that all inter-sphincteric fistulae develop as a result of inter-sphincteric sepsis have been challenged by dissections of acute cases that showed an inter-sphincteric connection or locale in only 25% of acutely infected cases. Despite this view, the cryptoglandular theory as advanced independently by Parks and Eisenhammer is still widely accepted. Eisenhammer postulated that an intramuscular gland became infected which was then unable to drain spontaneously into the anal canal. This was supported by Parks, who found cystic dilatation of the anal glands in 8/30 consecutive fistulae dissected, suggestive of a primary inter-sphincteric site of sepsis.

Perirectal abscess is a mix of aerobic and anaerobic polymicrobial infection. Bacteroides fragilis is the predominant anaerobe. Various common bacteria include the E. coli and those of the genera

Proteus, Bacteroides, and Streptococcus. These organisms are derived from the skin, bowel, and, rarely, the vagina.

A variety of disease states is associated with the development of an abscess; these include trauma, Crohn's disease, carcinoma, radiation fibrosis, Hodgkin's disease, and immunocompromised states. Infectious organism includes Gonococcus, Chlamydia, Actinomyces, Streptococcus, Bacteroides, and Proteus species; E. coli, Staphylococcus aureus, Herpes, Lymphogranuloma venereum, and Mycobacterium tuberculosis.

While it is hard to locate the extent of a perirectal abscess, a perianal abscess is easily palpable (Figure 8.1) and not accompanied by fever, leukocytosis, and sepsis in the immunocompetent patient.

Perirectal abscess is fraught with the formation of fistula in almost 25–50% of cases. It can further be complicated with bacteraemia and sepsis, especially in immunocompromised patients. Fournier's gangrene has occasionally been reported.

Anatomy

The two major muscular groups found in the anorectum include the inner muscle group, which is circular smooth muscle, and becomes hypertrophied distally to develop into the internal sphincter muscle. This cone-shaped structure is enveloped by a second set of muscles called the external sphincter muscles. It starts distally and advances into the anal canal, and is composed of the subcutaneous, superficial, and deep sections, followed by the puborectalis.

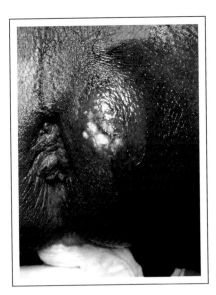

Figure 8.1 Perianal abscess.
Courtesy: Pravin Jaiprakash Gupta.

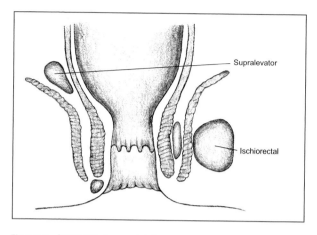

Figure 8.2   Locations of anorectal abscess.
Illustration: James Oinam.

The puborectalis is also the level of what is anatomically described as the anorectal ring. This anatomic and somatic muscle is important; it has been described as the 'core to continence'. Division of the ano-rectal ring and the puborectalis will lead to anal incontinence. Above the puborectalis lies, the levator muscles, that is, the iliococcygeus and pubococcygeus.

The anatomical space between the external and the internal anal sphincter is called the inter-sphincteric space. This area contains few anal glands and obstruction of the glands with an accumulation of faecal and foreign debris is blamed for initiating stasis, bacterial accumulation, and chronicity for the development of an anorectal abscess. The anatomical spaces that can spread the abscess include the inter-sphincteric, ischiorectal, and the pararectal space above the levators (Figure 8.2).

Differential Diagnosis

The different types of perianal abscesses are Bartholin's gland cyst, sebaceous cyst, hidradenitis supprativa, tuberculosis, and inflamma-tory bowel disease.

INCIDENCE

No racial predilection has been found. Males are more frequently affected than the women are with a male-to-female predominance of 2:1 to 3:1. A perianal abscess can affect any age groups, from infants to elderly persons. The peak incidence is in the third and fourth decades of life.

History

The history is critical in leading the physician to consider the diagnosis. Dull aching or throbbing pain in the perirectal or perianal area is present in 99% of patients. The pain is most severe while sitting and just before defecation when the rectum is full; the pain decreases after defecation but persists between bowel movements. In the advanced situation, the patient is not able to sleep. Perianal abscess presents with more localised pain. The pain often worsens as the abscess increases in size. Coughing, sneezing, and straining aggravate the pain. Rectal or perirectal drainage of pus, fever and chills, dysuria, constipation, and anorexia may follow.

Physical Examination

One can palpate a tender, fluctuant mass at the anal verge (perianal abscess) or on rectal examination (perirectal abscess). A perirectal abscess can be extensive and can spread to an area distant from the anal verge (Figure 8.3), yet only a diffuse, tender mass may be palpable through either the rectal wall or the overlying skin. The overlying skin may look normal or inflamed depending upon the depth of the suppurative focus. The patient is febrile, localise erythema may be noted. Purulent discharge per anus may be seen or found during digital rectal examination or anoscopy. Signs of sepsis may be viewed in the form of toxaemia. In a neglected case, septicaemia may ensue.

Causes

Reasons of a perirectal abscess are believed to be a blockage of the perianal gland duct with resultant infection, rupture, and abscess

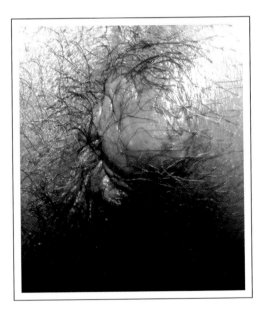

Figure 8.3 Ischiorectal abscess.

Courtesy: Pravin Jaiprakash Gupta.

formation. Risk factors include immunosuppression, diabetes, Crohn's disease, ulcerative colitis, pregnancy, tuberculosis, and foreign body.

Other causes include cancer, actinomycosis, lymphogranuloma venereum, radiation, and leukaemia-lymphoma. Traumatic causes of fistulous abscesses include implement, enemas, prostatic surgery, episiotomy, and haemorrhoidectomy.

Investigations

Routine laboratory studies cannot be used to exclude the diagnosis of perirectal abscess. One should always keep the possibility in mind, and reliance on historical and physical findings is imperative. Complete blood counts may show leukocytosis. However, this study may produce normal results, and leukocytosis is not diagnostic.

Imaging Studies

- Plain radiographs are rarely helpful. A chest radiograph yields the most benefit; especially, if free air is seen under the diaphragm, or if chest pathology mimicking abdominal pathology is found.
- CT may be used to determine the existence and anatomy of a perirectal abscess and should unresolve recrudescent liberally. Whereas, ultrasonography may be useful in the diagnosis of submucosal and inter-sphincteric abscesses, CT can detect a deeper abscess and is, therefore, more useful.
- Endoanorectal, transperineal, and transvaginal ultrasonography may be used to determine the existence, extent, and location of an abscess. Ultrasonography is an accurate, painless, and cost-effective method for documenting perirectal and perianal fluid collections, fistulas, or sinus tracts, and it can be performed at the bedside.
- MRI is useful in identifying deep abscesses and helpful in detecting granulation tissue, which may be useful in detecting fistulae.

Confirmation of Diagnosis

If the diagnosis of a perianal or perirectal abscess is in doubt, aspiration with an 18-gauge needle may be performed. Aspiration of pus confirms the diagnosis.

Adequate analgesia before aspiration is mandatory. However, ultrasonography, computerised tomography (CT) scan, and MRI are more comfortable methods of confirming or excluding the diagnosis and should be used if available.

Treatment

All abscesses must be drained. There is no conservative treatment for anorectal abscess unless a gross contraindication. A small, superficial perianal abscess can be drained in the office. Adequate analgesia should be obtained. Conscious sedation may be considered for controlling pain and making the procedure as humane as possible. The patient may be discharged home after appropriate wound care with instructions for Sitz baths and routine follow-up care.

Conscious sedation should only be used if the physician is trained and when the isolated perianal abscess is not associated with deeper, perirectal abscesses.

Perirectal abscess must be treated in the operating room so that the most suitable anaesthesia can be given, and the abscess, any fistula, or other complication may be dealt with definitively. The site of a deep-seated abscess must not be mistaken for a superficial perianal abscess. Inadequate debridement of a perirectal abscess may result in increased morbidity and even mortality. Debridement of perirectal abscesses should not be performed.

Drainage of Abscess in the Operation Room

The optimal treatment of ischiorectal abscesses is incision and drainage often followed by fistulotomy under general anaesthesia in the operating theatre.

The performance of an extensive and complete surgical procedure by a consultant with accurate anatomical knowledge of the region is imperative to avoid serious complications. Such a treatment results in a lower recurrence rate. Intravenous antibiotics may be used as preventive or therapeutic measures in patients who are immunocompromised, in those who appear septic, or in those who have heart valve abnormalities or prostheses.

The goal in treating any abscess is to make an incision to surgically release the pus and remove any dead tissue and then to keep the surgical incision open by the use of a drain. In the case of a perianal abscess, the procedure involves sterile preparation, adequate analgesia, incision, and drainage often facilitated by irrigation of the abscess cavity, an abrupt disruption of any loculations, debridement of any accessible necrotic tissue, and placement of a drain.

The abscess cavity should not be packed wherever possible. The rationale behind this is to leave the surgical incision open so that pus and other material can drain. If a pack is used, using a limited amount of gauze is important, that is, just enough to keep the wound open. Packing the wound with tape gauze will harm than any good. In fact, it may worsen the prognosis by creating a large foreign body that may become a nidus of infection. This nidus could perpetuate the infection and cause the abscess to enlarge, spread to other areas, erode into vessels or the peritoneal cavity, and, occasionally, it could cause sepsis and death.

Expecting Best Outcome

When the diagnosis of the perirectal abscess is made or is being entertained, a timely consultation with a surgeon is utmost necessary. Timely and appropriate surgical intervention will avoid more serious complications such as an extension of the abscess or serious systemic infection. The proper surgical treatment of perirectal abscess is complex and painful and, therefore, should not be undertaken in the outpatient department. The choice is between general or spinal anaesthesia whichever is appropriate for the patient.

A newer technique includes endoscopic ultrasonographic-guided drainage of deep pelvic abscesses with stent placement for drainage of pus.

Medication

Antibiotics are unnecessary in otherwise healthy individuals. The practitioner should provide appropriate empiric intravenous antibiotic coverage for patients who are elderly or immunosuppressed, patients who have co-morbidities, patients with a heart valve abnormality or prosthetic valve likely to benefit from antibiotic prophylaxis or those in whom infection has become systemic. Predisposing or co-morbid factors may guide empiric antibiotic selection.

Round the clock analgesia is necessary for pain control and may be given orally or via intravenously, in conjunction with anaesthetics if needle aspiration or incision and drainage (I&D) of an abscess is performed.

Anti-anxiety medication may be needed in individual patients who are apprehensive about needle aspiration, imaging studies, or surgery.

Post-operative Management

The patients should report immediately for any unusual symptoms, including persistent pain or fever. After inpatient surgical treatment, a surgeon should carefully monitor patients because of the frequent occurrence of fistula or recurrence of the abscess. Provide adequate outpatient analgesias such as codeine with acetaminophen or an oxycodone-containing compound. Outpatient antibiotics may be indicated and are best chosen according to the culture and sensitivity of pathogens derived from the abscess.

Complications

These include fistula formation, bacteraemia, and sepsis, including seeding of the infection to other areas by haematogenous spread. Fournier's gangrene (Figure 8.4), epidural abscess, and death have been reported. However, with adequate treatment, the prognosis is excellent.

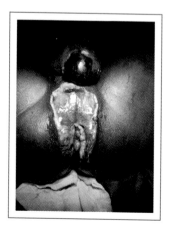

Figure 8.4 Pararectal abscess with Fournier's gangrene.
Courtesy: Pravin Jaiprakash Gupta.

Iatrogenic Problem

Certain problematic area surrounds the treatment of anorectal abscess. These include delayed diagnosis, misdiagnosis, or failure to diagnose, resulting in a complication or death. Inadequate treatment or failure to refer for adequate surgical debridement may result in a complication or death. Aspiration, hypoxic injury, or death could result because of inadequate airway management with the use of conscious sedation and overzealous packing of a perirectal abscess cavity-causing inadequate drainage, extension of suppurative process or recurrence.

FISTULA-IN-ANO

A fistula-in-ano is a hollow tube-like structure with granulation tissue inside and connecting a primary opening within the anal canal to a secondary or external opening in the perianal skin. While secondary openings may be multiple but they will always be from the same primary opening.

Frequency

The male-to-female ratio is 2:1, and the mean age of patients is 38.3 years.

Aetiology

Fistula-in-ano is mostly caused by a previous anorectal abscess. Anal canal glands that are situated at the dentate line provide the path for infecting organisms to reach the intramuscular spaces.

Fistulas can also develop following trauma, radiation therapy, actinomycoses, tuberculosis, Crohn's disease, anal fissures, carcinoma, and chlamydial infections.

Pathophysiology

Following surgical or spontaneous drainage of these abscesses in the perianal skin, at times, a granulation tissue-lined tract is left behind, which causes recurrent symptoms. Multiple series have shown that the formation of a fistula tract following anorectal abscess occurs in almost 40% of cases. Recent anatomical dissection has provided a new glandular classification system revealing that the largest number of fistulae lie in the right lower quadrant in association with the largest recognisable fraction of anal glands, although prior theories that all inter-sphincteric fistulae develop as a result of inter-sphincteric sepsis have been challenged by dissections of acute cases that showed an inter-sphincteric connection or locale in only 25% of acutely infected cases. Despite this view, however, the cryptoglandular theory as advanced independently by Parks and Eisenhammer is still widely accepted.

Eisenhammer postulated that an intra-muscular gland became infected which was then unable to drain spontaneously into the anal canal. This was supported by Parks, who found cystic dilatation of the anal glands in 8/30 consecutive fistulae dissected, suggestive of a primary inter-sphincteric site of sepsis.

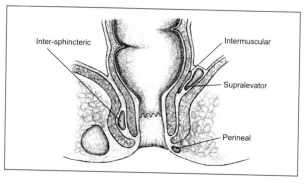

Figure 8.5 Sites of extension of abscess to cause anal fistula.

Illustration: James Oinam.

Anatomy

To clearly understand the classification system for fistulous disease, a thorough understanding of the pelvic floor and sphincter anatomy is always a prerequisite.

The external sphincter complex is a striated muscle and is under the voluntary control by three of its components. They are the sub-mucosal, superficial, and deep muscle. Its deep segment is continuous with the puborectalis muscle and forms the anorectal ring, which can be palpated upon digital examination (Figure 8.5).

The internal sphincter is a smooth muscle, is under involuntary autonomic control, and in continuation of the circular rectal muscles.

In straightforward cases, the Goodsall's rule can help to anticipate the anatomy of fistula-in-ano. The law states that fistulae having an external opening anterior to a line that passes horizontally through the centre of the anal opening will follow a straight course to the dentate line. However, fistulae with their openings posterior to this line will follow a curved path to the posterior midline. Nonetheless, there are exceptions to this rule like an external opening that is more than 3 cm from the anal verge. It usually originates as a primary or secondary tract from the posterior midline, consistent with a previous horseshoe abscess.

PRESENTATION

History

Patients will give a reliable history of past pain, swelling, and spontaneous or planned surgical drainage of an anorectal abscess.

Signs and Symptoms

Anal and perianal discharge, which could be frank pus or just a thin seepage along with pain, swelling, and a single or multiple external openings (Figure 8.6) are the commonest features. Few exceptional cases may present with symptoms of diarrhoea, bleeding, and skin excoriation due to purulent and irritant discharge may be noticed.

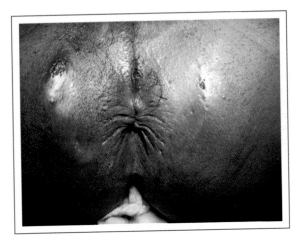

Figure 8.6 A horseshoe fistula with multiple openings.

Courtesy: Pravin Jaiprakash Gupta.

Clinical observation of the perineum and perianal area plus experienced digital assessment is the cardinal component of decision making in simple and complicated perirectal sepsis and is the hallmark of successful treatment. The impression of high or complex (as well as iatrogenic) fistulae is suggested by aberrant locales that bear no particular recognised anatomic patterns or which lie well lateral to the anal verge. In general, the more laterally disposed of the external opening, the greater likelihood that the fistula will be trans- or extra-sphincteric in type. Although it is not inevitable that a perianal abscess will lead to a fistula (namely, that all abscesses have a fistulous origin or connection), those with significant horseshoe components (usually in the retrorectal space) usually have a central fistula opening at the level of the dentate line.

Few patients with a complex fistula may include diverticulitis, inflammatory bowel disease, tuberculosis, steroid therapy, previous radiation therapy for prostate or rectal cancer, or HIV infection. The patient may complain of abdominal pain, weight loss, or change in the bowel habits in these complexities.

Physical Examination

The diagnosis is based mainly on physical examination findings. One should observe the entire perineum, and search for an external opening that appears as a discharging sinus or elevation with granulation tissue popping out. Upon digital rectal examination, spontaneous discharge via the external opening may be apparent or expressible. A gentle digital examination is essential where an internal opening is very frequently palpable as an indurated area along the dentate line in most cases or occasionally as a tangible 'grain of rice' area of induration internally.

A fibrous tract or cord may be felt beneath the skin or digital rectal examination. It will also help in making out any occult focus of suppuration that is not yet drained. An induration in the lateral or posterior induration suggests a deep postanal or ischiorectal extension.

It is prudent and safer that the examiner must determine the relationship between the anorectal ring and the position of the tract well in advance, that is, before the patient is relaxed by anaesthesia. If available, assessment of the sphincter tone and voluntary squeeze pressures should be done before any surgical intervention to delineate whether the anal manometric evaluation is indicated. Anoscopy is usually required to identify the internal opening.

PARK'S CLASSIFICATION OF ANAL FISTULA

The Park's classification system defines fistula-in-ano into four types resulting from cryptoglandular infections (Figure 8.7).

- **Inter-sphincteric**: Its common course is via internal sphincter to the inter-sphincteric space and then to the perineum. Almost 70% of all anal fistulae are of this category.
- **Trans-sphincteric**: Its common course is low via internal and external sphincters into the ischiorectal fossa and then to the perineum. Twenty-five per cent of all anal fistulae are the trans-sphincteric type.
- **Supra-sphincteric**: Its common course is via inter-sphincteric space superiorly to above puborectalis muscle into ischiorectal fossa and then to the perineum. About 5% fistulae fall in this group.
- **Extra-sphincteric**: Its common course is from perianal skin through levator ani muscles to the rectal wall completely outside sphincter mechanism. Less than 1% of all anal fistulae are from this group.

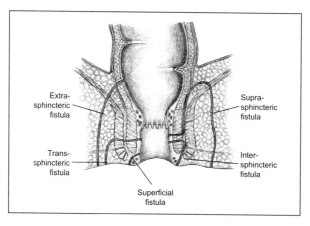

Figure 8.7 Park's classification of anal fistula.
Illustration: James Oinam.

Although widely accepted, Park's classification has its limitations. As the whole emphasis is focused on the inter-sphincteric plane, superficial fistulae are not mentioned which are said to occur in up to 15% of cases. Unlike the current procedural terminology, which is more accurate as far as surgical procedures are concerned, the Park's classification does not mention the subcutaneous fistula. These fistulas are not of cryptoglandular origin but are usually caused by unhealed anal fissures or anorectal procedures, such as haemorrhoidectomy or sphincterotomy.

For low fistulae, the functional significance of whether a fistula is inter-sphincteric or trans-sphincteric is not effectively relevant. Moreover, it is a matter of debate as to what constitutes a high fistula that is treated with excision or incision in individual cases or with formal repair (or other treatments) depending upon the surgical experience. For all intents and purposes, one may regard a fistula as 'high' if it exceeds one-thirds of the coronal length of the anal sphincter although in some multiparous women who may harbour an occult anterior external anal sphincter defect this extent may be excessive and in these cases the surgeon may decide to repair comparatively low fistulae often after initial drainage of coincident abscesses or deployment of a guiding seton. Because of this, the Park's classification, particularly for recurrent fistulae, referred to a tertiary referral centre may not be appropriate.

Current Anal Fistula Terminology

- Subcutaneous
- Submuscular (inter-sphincteric, low trans-sphincteric)
- Complex, recurrent (high trans-sphincteric, supra-sphincteric, and extra-sphincteric, multiple tracts, recurrent) (Figure 8.8)

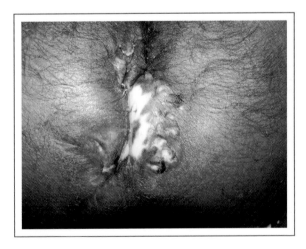

Figure 8.8 A tubercular fistula with multiple openings.
Courtesy: Pravin Jaiprakash Gupta.

Investigation

No specific laboratory studies are required apart from the standard pre-operative investigations that are indicated based on age and co-morbidities. Radiologic studies do not have much to highlight in routine fistula evaluation. They can be helpful when the internal opening is hard to identify or in the case of recurrent or multiple fistulae to search for secondary tracts or missed primary openings. More information can be gathered with a specialised imaging technique called as fistulography. The surgical view regarding the place and type of imaging used in complex fistula-in-ano is somewhat dependent upon individual philosophy as well as upon the availability and expertise of different imaging modalities at one's hospital.

Put simply, the successful operative treatment of fistulae requires the ability to find an internal opening and determine its relationship to the main sphincter complex operatively. While the low types can be readily laid open, the high types require more tailored and specialised treatment. Within successful therapy, it is recognised that the principal determinant of failed fistula surgery is the inability to detect an internal opening. It is acceptable to utilise imaging that has a high sensitivity to assist in the definition of the site of the internal opening and the relationship of any primary or secondary tracts (or collections) to the main sphincter complex and levator floor, although it should be recognised that the exact definition of the subepithelial space (and hence the exact site of the internal opening) is limited in imaging and could only be inferred.

Specific imaging for fistula should be considered when:

- There is unexpected sepsis (particularly when extensive) after conventional drainage,
- Suspicion of an anovaginal or rectovaginal fistula,
- Suspicion of inflammatory bowel disease-related sepsis,
- Sepsis in an immunosuppressed patient cohort (HIV-positivity, post-transplantation, acute leukaemia, selected cases of uncontrolled diabetes mellitus, post-chemotherapy neutropenia or agranulocytosis),
- Suspicion of a malignant fistula,
- Sepsis plus incontinence,
- Sepsis after recent anorectal surgery,
- Suspicion of a high fistula (above one-third of the coronal length of the anal canal),
- Suspicion of supra levator disease or origin, and
- Fournier's gangrene as a presentation of perirectal sepsis.

FISTULOGRAPHY

This is performed by injection of contrast from the external opening or passing a soft catheter up to the internal opening. X-ray images are taken in an anteroposterior, lateral, and oblique view that shows the course of the fistula tract. The accuracy rate varies between 16% and 48%. The procedure is well accepted and requires the ability to visualise the internal opening. Except in the case of recurrent disease, fistulography is no more useful than a careful examination under anaesthesia. This technique should not be used any longer. Although it shows a high accuracy in the detection of an internal opening, the relationship between the fistula and the levator complex cannot be assessed and consequently it does not influence surgical decision-making. One can still see patients presenting to the outpatient clinic with fistulogram that provides no specifically useful information but which have been painful to perform and which risks attendant bacteraemia. This technique has been shown to miss high rectal openings, supralevator, and horseshoe extensions.

Endoanal or Endorectal Ultrasound

This safe and simple procedure helps in the interpretation of the location of the primary internal opening, the anatomy of the primary and secondary tracts and horseshoe formation, and the integrity of the internal and external anal sphincter musculature in simple and complex cryptogenic and Crohn's related anal fistulae. For such studies, a 7- or 10-MHz transducer is passed into anal canal to help define muscular anatomy differentiating inter-sphincteric from trans-sphincteric lesions. A standard water-filled balloon transducer can help evaluate the rectal wall for any supra-sphincteric extension. Few papers show that the addition of hydrogen peroxide through the external opening helps delineate the fistula tract course. This may be useful to help locate missed internal openings. These studies are reported to be 50% better than physical examination alone to help find an internal opening that is hard to localise. Unfortunately, this modality has not been used widely for routine clinical fistula evaluation. Endoanal ultrasound (EAUS) is unable to distinguish recrudescent unresolved sepsis in some cases from perianal scarring. Further, if EAUS is totally relied upon for surgical decision-making, a large associated inter-sphincteric abscess may cause sufficient acoustic shadowing so that an inter-sphincteric fistula will be overcalled as trans-sphincteric, and potentially more sphincter muscle may be divided. Exact resolution with this technique of the internal opening may also be compromised in some cases by air in the rectal ampulla, bubble effects within the anal canal, and variability of transducer strength.

Endoanal sonography has recently been supplemented with improved accuracy utilising three-dimensional software and a post-processing technique called volume rendering mode (VRM) which modifies the opacification, the pixel luminance, and the beam penetration (or thickness of the image) and which filters low-intensity pixels with three-dimensional imagery.

Magnetic Resonance Imaging

Magnetic resonance imaging has shown a high level of accuracy in the definition of both simple and complex sepsis, although it remains limited in its demonstration of the subepithelial disposition of the tract as it leads towards the fistula's internal opening. Its distinct advantage is in the demonstration of a supralevator extension or origin of disease above the pelvic floor as part of its multiplanar capacity, with the use of coronal imaging being of particular value. An additional benefit of MRI is an accurate description of the status of the external anal sphincter and coincident atrophy as a secondary feature of destructive perirectal sepsis. Incorporation of a specified MR classification system for complicated perianal fistulas has shown distinct prognostic value in successful fistula outcome.

It is strongly recommended that given the nature of tertiary referrals that MR imaging should be increasingly used in complicated perirectal sepsis particularly where there is a suspicion of supralevator disease. The earlier use of MR imaging will make a predictive outcome analysis related to surgical success possible.

Computerised Tomography Scan

With the advent of ultrasonography and MRI, the role of CT scan is very limited now. It may be helpful in the diagnosis of perirectal inflammatory disease than looking for fistulae, as it is suitable for delineating fluid pockets that need drainage. A CT scan requires the use of oral and rectal contrast that has their drawbacks. Muscular anatomy is not delineated as well.

Barium enema or small bowel imaging is useful for patients with multiple fistulae or recurrent disease to help rule out inflammatory bowel disease.

Anal Manometry

Sphincter pressure evaluation is helpful in individual patients. If decreased tone is observed with manometry, a surgical division of any portion of the sphincter mechanism should be avoided. Situations like previous fistulotomy, obstetrical trauma, high trans-sphincteric, or supra-sphincteric fistula and very elderly patients may have decreased anal tone.

There are certain situations that demand examination under anaesthesia before subjecting the patient to surgery for an anal fistula; especially, if outpatient evaluation causes discomfort or has not helped delineate the course of the fistulous process. Several recommendations have been described to trace the course of the fistula and, more importantly, identify the internal opening. One can instil hydrogen peroxide, milk, or dilute methylene blue from the external opening to look for the emergence of these liquids from the internal opening. The use of methylene blue is controversial as often obscures the field and makes it difficult to identify the opening. Pull or push on the external opening may also cause a dimpling or protrusion of the involved crypt.

The direction of the tract can be sought by insertion of a blunt-tipped crypt probe via the external opening. If it reaches the dentate line within a few millimetres, one can presume that a direct extension likely exists. Care should be taken not to exert too much force and create false passages.

Anoscopy, Proctosigmoidoscopy, and Colonoscopy

Viewing the anal and rectal canal by one of the scopes may help to detect any associated disease process in the anal canal and rectum. Further colonic evaluation is performed only as indicated.

Differential Diagnoses

These include hidradenitis suppurativa, infected inclusion cysts, pilonidal disease, or bartholin gland abscess in females. None of them, however, communicates with the anal canal.

Treatment

Intervention is indicated in all symptomatic patients. They usually manifest in the form of recurrent episodes of anorectal sepsis. Repeated abscess development is seen as and when the external opening on the perianal skin seals itself.

In an asymptomatic patient, where a fistula is found during a routine examination, no therapy is required.

Medical Therapy

No definitive medical treatment is curative. However, long-term antibiotic prophylaxis and infliximab may play a role in recurrent fistulae in patients with Crohn's disease.

Surgical Therapy

The basis of primary surgery as it applies to fistula-in-ano is the balance between fistula cure at the expense of continence. Although it is accepted that the principal reason for fistula recurrence is the missed internal opening(s) at surgery, it is equally evident that factors that affect continence after such surgery include the surgical technique (fistulotomy vs. fistulectomy), with no clear evidence that manometry is a predictor of continence outcome. Much of the surgical approach towards complex cryptogenic fistula may be translated, defining the extent of disease, usually just draining collections of pus and using the deployment of setons to control recurrent sepsis.

The surgery for cryptogenic fistula-in-ano is represented by a choice of the following:

- Fistulotomy or fistulectomy
- Seton use (cutting/draining/chemical/rerouting)
- Mucosal (endorectal) or cutaneous advancement flaps
- Anoplasty with variations on the management of the internal opening and the use of an internal sphincterotomy
- Fistula ligation (the ligation of inter-sphincteric fistula tract [LIFT] and BioLIFT procedures)
- Fistula ablation: This may be performed blindly or under vision. Here, there is a range of techniques using synthetic glues, anal plugs, the OTSC® fistula Nitinol® clip, the instillation of autologous regenerative adipose cells, the FiLac™ radial emitting laser, and video-assisted anal fistula treatment (VAAFT) procedure.

Fistulotomy or Fistulectomy

These procedures are useful for 85–95% of simple fistulae like the submucosal, inter-sphincteric, and low trans-sphincteric. The prevailing view is that in low fistula-in-ano, fistulotomy (division onto a probe) is more acceptable regarding continence than fistulectomy (fistula excision). Another view is that often in a low fistula, it is desirable to perform a fistulectomy, keeping close to the probe so that there is minimal soft tissue excision, always providing a specimen for histological examination.

It is accepted that data suggest less sphincter damage (based on ultrasonographic measurements of both the internal and external anal sphincter thicknesses) with fistulotomy, however, recent studies comparing a sphincter splitting fistulotomy with a non-sphincter splitting fistulectomy showed no difference in fistula recurrence over the short term but a higher mean resting anal pressure (and continence score) in the group undergoing fistulotomy.

Fistulotomy

After passing a blunt probe into the tract from the external opening and negotiating up to the internal opening, the overlying skin, subcutaneous tissue, and internal sphincter muscle are split opened with a knife or electrocautery to slit open the entire fibrous tract. At superficial levels in the anal canal, the internal sphincter, and subcutaneous external sphincter can easily be divided horizontally to the underlying fibres without affecting continence. However, one has to be cautious if the fistulotomy is performed anteriorly in female patients. If the fistula tract courses deep and high into the sphincter mechanism, it is better to place a seton rather than dividing this sphincter complex. Curettage is performed to remove granulation tissue in the tract base (Figure 8.9).

Supplements to this approach may be made with lay open fistulotomy or core out fistulectomy being supported by definitive repair/sphincter reconstruction, although there are no randomised controlled trials to add the weight of a definite sphincter repair. The further addition one may use with lay open fistulotomy in recurrent cases is formal marsupialisation of the chronic fistula edges. There is some

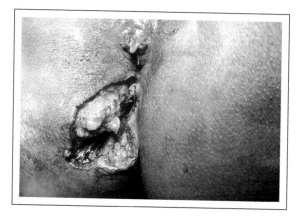

Figure 8.9   Anal fistulotomy wound with a visible tract.
Courtesy: Pravin Jaiprakash Gupta.

data to suggest that healing with marsupialisation is a little faster when compared to the conventional open wound, and the post-operative analgesia requirement appears to be comparatively a little less. Finally, a further supplement of fistulotomy has been the closure of the internal opening with an advancement flap, where most recurrence, if it is to occur, tends to do so within the first year.

It is wise to open the wound out on the perianal skin for a centi-metre or two adjacent beyond the external opening excising the skin that promotes internal healing before external closure. Biopsy from the tract tissue should always be done to rule out any granulomatous lesion as a cause of anal fistulae, such as tuberculosis.

Seton Placement

The actual word 'seton' is derived from the Latin '*seta*' meaning a bristle, where it was initially described by Hippocrates who used stout horsehair wrapped around a lint thread. These setons were advanced alongside directors much as today with the use of what would be equivalent to today's Lockhart-Mummery probes. The use of these setons was as slow cutting devices. The principal use of the seton is to assist in the drainage of pus and debris and reduce the likelihood of further abscess formation. These loose setons are referred to as draining setons. They serve as geographical markers for subsequent definitive treatments including the use of plugs and glues, or in the performance of mucosal advancement anoplasty or LIFT procedures.

The alternative is to slowly tighten the seton in an attempt to cut gradually through the sphincter that becomes traversed like a cheese-wire, stimulating fibrosis as the tightening process occurs but without causing a complete separation of the sphincter musculature so that the tissues are sufficiently held in fibrotic tissue to maintain continence. These latter setons are referred to as cutting setons. The third option is an ancient one where the seton is chemically preserved to ablate the fistula. This caustic chemical seton has historically been given the Indian name of *Ksharasutra* related to a plant derivative. In the Western society, there is little use for chemical setons of these types (the so-called Ayurvedic seton) where a trial of its use by Ho et al. comparing it in low fistulae with simple fistulotomy showed it to be a little more painful with no advantageous effect on wound healing or recurrence.

A variety of different seton materials has been advocated over a prolonged period, with their use dependent upon material availability and surgeon preference. The most commonly used materials are the vascular latex loop, silk, wire, elastic bands, Penrose drains, and nylon or plastic tubing. These approaches have been associated with novel designs for maintaining the seton position and for seton tightening with the most recent being a self-locking cable device. Recently, specialised irrigation devices have been incorporated into the seton tube for use in high complex fistulae with associated abscess cavities, with the irrigation of normal and hypertonic saline as well as with metronidazole gel.

A seton may be tied as an independent device, combined with fistulotomy, or in a staged fashion. This technique is indicated in complex fistulae like high trans-sphincteric, supra-sphincteric, extra sphincteric, or multiple fistulae. In recurrent fistulae after the previous fistulotomy, anterior fistulae in female patients, and compromised sphincter pressures. Patients with Crohn's disease or who are immunosuppressed should also be treated with seton placement.

Setons, apart from giving a visual impression of the amount of sphincter muscle involved, help to drain and promote fibrosis while cutting through the fistula. Setons can be made from large silk suture, silastic vessel markers, or rubber bands (Figure 8.10) that are threaded through the fistula tract.

Setons could be of two types—single-stage seton and two-stage seton. The single-stage seton is passed through the fistula tract around the sphincter complex. It is slowly tightened down and secured with a separate silk tie. Over a period, fibrosis will occur above the seton, as it will cut through the sphincter muscles gradually to exteriorise the tract. The seton is tightened on subsequent visits until it travels the entire tract when it is pulled through. This will take about 6–8 weeks time. A cutting seton can also be inserted through the tract by railroading and without the need for a fistulotomy.

Two-stage seton is called as draining or fibrosing seton. The seton is passed around the same way as the cutting seton; but unlike the cutting seton, this seton is left loose to move freely draining the inter-sphincteric space and promoting fibrosis in the deep sphincter muscle. Once the surrounding wound is healed completely, the seton-bound sphincter complex is divided. The reported eradication of the fistula tract with this technique is about 60–78%.

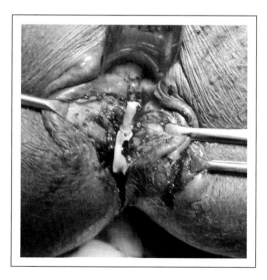

Figure 8.10 Cutting rubber seton in tract.
Courtesy: Pravin Jaiprakash Gupta.

Mucosal Advancement Flap

Mucosal advancement flap is restricted for the use in patients with high chronic fistula though it is suggested for the same disease process as for the use of seton. Advantages include a single-stage procedure with no additional sphincter damage. A disadvantage is a poor success in patients with Crohn's disease or acute infection.

This process involves total fistulectomy, with the removal of the primary and secondary tracts and completes excision of the internal opening. The rectal mucomuscular flap is raised with a wide proximal base (two times the apex width). The muscle defect is approximated with an absorbable suture, and the flap is sewn down over the internal opening without overlapping its suture line on the muscular repair.

Newer Treatment

Recent advances in biomedical and bioengineering have led to the development of many new tissue-adhesive and biomaterials. In few cases, the fistula is closed by the injection of fibrin glue (a solution of the clotting factors fibrinogen and thrombin). This glue acts as a sealant within the fistula, which helps to promote obscuring and healing of the tract.

Due to the least invasive nature, this therapy is associated with decreased post-operative morbidity.

The anal fistula plug has also found a place as a non-invasive technique in few clinical trials. The anal fistula plug is a firm cylindrical structure made of a biomaterial that supports tissue healing. The plug is inserted by drawing it through the fistula tract and suturing it in place. Long-term success rates vary with the methodology but with minimal morbidity can easily be repeated for recurrence. However, the recent report observed that the success rate with this plug is less than 15%.

Ligation of Inter-sphincteric Fistula Tract and BioLIFT™

The introduction of the ligation of inter-sphincteric fistula tract (LIFT) procedure has revolutionised complex and recurrent fistula management even though currently there is no long-term outcome data concerning its success. It takes advantage of ligation of the main tract with curettage, obliteration, and healing of the secondary tracts after disconnection that has previously been noted in the horse-shoe ischiorectal fistula where extensive ischiorectal excisions as a procedure have disappeared in favour of dealing with the principal tract only. The other advantage of this technique is the minimal disruption of normal tissues and sphincter to get to the main tract. The value of this approach will be reliant on the long-term success of the procedure.

The available data concerning LIFT shows that although there appears to be a high initial success, there is a late worrisome recurrence rate that probably is consequent upon the inherent philosophy that does little to the glandular origin of disease and the internal opening. It may well be that a hybrid LIFT with a small mucosal advancement may be more appropriate. A variation on this technique has been proposed in which the LIFT was supplemented with the insertion of a bioprosthetic plug (the so-called BioLIFT procedure). However, at present, the addition of a biosynthetic is not defined, as it requires considerably more dissection than the standard LIFT procedure where sustained healing success over time is critical.

FISTULA ABLATION TECHNIQUES

Some novel fistula ablation techniques have been developed over the recent years designed to eradicate fistula epithelium. These procedures are primarily performed across the fistula terrain blindly although recently, the video-assisted fistula treatment (VAAFT) has advocated a visual electrode-based fistula ablation technique. The initial excitement with some of these therapies (most notably, the fibrin glues) has been tempered by a recognition that the later success rates are in some series quite mediocre and that the procedure is not readily applicable to any degree of success to Crohn's related fistulae or rectovaginal fistulae.

Glues, plugs, regenerative adipose-derived stem cell therapies, filac, radial emitting laser probe therapy, the OTSC® fistula Nitinol® clip, and the VAAFT procedures are still under study with no long-term data or randomised trials.

Glues

These fibrin sealants have had some success in the management of enterocutaneous and bronchial fistulae. The glue is a tissue adhesive consisting of fibrinogen and a thrombin component that are injected simultaneously into the fistula tract to form a fibrin clot thought to promote fistula healing. The initial testing as described by Jose Cintron and his group from Cook County used autologous blood donation for elution of autologous fibrin, although commercially produced fibrin glue, which is now freely available, has been shown to bind up to 10 times more strongly *in vitro* than autologous fibrin glue. Nonetheless, there does not seem to be a clinical healing advantage between the two types of fibrin glue. The system for use has become standardised with commercially available Tissucol Fibrin Sealant (Baxter, Vienna, Austria) providing a kit with a flexible catheter which is introduced into the fistula using a double-channel injector system forming a bed of sealant at the level of the internal fistulous opening. These treatments usually have been used after preliminary seton drainage, where the available data is extensive suggesting that the treatment is safe and relatively painless with an ability to repeat injections and without disruption of the anatomy, preventing other later procedures should the sealant fail. As the use of plugs, the initial enthusiasm has waned where the long-term results have disappointed, making its early use highly debatable within the algorithm of fistula management.

Plugs

There are currently limited data concerning bioprosthetic plugs in fistula management, where most have focused on treated porcine submucosa (the Surgisys Cook TM, Bloomington IN, USA) material. The aim is focused on its use in trans-sphincteric fistulae with contraindications for use in acute sepsis, abscesses, simple fistulae, porcine allergy, or for use in short, stout tracts like the ano- or rectovaginal fistulae. The plugs need to be secured at the point of the internal opening while cutting off the excess protruding plug. This part of the procedure needs to be performed carefully to prevent early plug loss (dislodgement). The external wound needs to be left open to provide initial drainage.

Comparative studies have been made between the plug and mucosal advancement showing very disappointing results after short-term follow-up (4.5 months), where the advancement results were also poor (33% complete healing) as were the plug results (overall success 32%). Some evidence has suggested that fistula tract length predicts for a successful outcome with plug use, where longer tracts (>4 cm) are more likely to heal. The fistula length was measured by comparing the end plug length and the original plug length. The closure does not appear to correlate with gender, age, tract locale, duration of a prelim-inary seton, or length of follow-up. Ellis also analysed failure factors with fistula plugs on multivariate analysis suggesting that tobacco smoking, a posterior fistula, and prior bioprosthetic failure were the main negative predictive factors. Overall, the place of plugs is unclear with poor results in those patients with recurrent surgery and where the plug is used as second- or third-line therapy. The shorter fistula tract, the posterior fistula and non-trans-sphincteric fistulae tend to do poorly with this approach as do rectovaginal fistulae. Overall, initial enthusiasm for the plug has waned with medium to longer-term results being relatively poor. The recent combination of a LIFT proce-dure with a small supplementary plug reported by a Chinese group showed a 95% success rate in 20 patients over a 14-month follow-up suggesting that hybrid procedures require further evaluation.

Stem Cells and Autologous Expanded Adipose-derived Cells

This technique has been recently introduced by Garcia-Olmo and col-leagues of Spain using *in vitro* cultured adipose tissue-derived mesen-chymal stem cells, initially achieving success in 70% of cases where it was tried on enterocutaneous fistulae secondary to Crohn's disease. The technique used lipoaspiration with cell concentration and cellular elution to release the stromal fraction of the lipoaspirate. In this setting, the adipose-derived stem cells (ADSCs) can be isolated and cultured *in vitro* with a wide variety of cellular elements including connective tissue, endothelial, and scar tissue cells and where even non-cultured cells contain an abundant proportion of endothelial progenitor cells and tissue macrophages. There is a debate in some series concerning the need for two procedures (harvest and installation) as well as the personalised expense, the problem of cell contamination and overall cellular viability. The latest data suggests in a multicentre study com-prising a clinical trial in 200 cases derived from 19 centres with fistula healing defined by re-epithelialisation of the external opening and MR imaging that there were healing rates of between 39% and 43% overall although these increased to 57% at one year. There seemed to be no advantage to fibrin glue addition in a randomised study that also discussed its use in scattered Crohn's cases. This approach has also utilised autologous fibroblasts and platelet-derived growth factors although data is in a nascent stage.

Visual and Non-visual Fistula Ablative Technologies

A series of potentially exciting ablative technologies using different instruments have been devised for fistula ablation. These include video-assisted anal fistula treatment (VAAFT), the FiLac™ radial emitting laser probe and the use of the OTSC® fistula Nitinol® clip. The best of these appears to be one performed under direct visual fistulosocopy, the VAAFT procedure, whereby a small angle fistulosocope traverses and straightens the fistula with glycine mannitol irrigation without any sphincteric approach and which then destroys the fistula epithelium using an electrode. This technique is supplemented by cyanoacrylate support of the internal aspect of the fistula and stapled or hand-sewn closure of the internal opening.

If the external opening is absent, as sometimes happens with chronic fistulae, the VAAFT cannot be used. Similarly, it may well be possible some circuitous, and iatrogenic fistulae will not allow the passage of a straight video scope, the inter-sphincteric route of the fistula tract, which is somewhat poorly delineated even on advanced imaging, still needs to be accurately defined by the operator to excise the internal opening site. It is thus clear that the technique of the LIFT and the VAAFT will be acknowledged only if their long-term outcomes prove to be advantageous. The good thing is that they both are unlikely to substantially compromise further attempts of definitive repair because they preserve sphincter muscle and function.

The FiLac™ (Biolitec, Germany) is a laser radial emitting probe and has encouraging initial results. However, the best laser type and wavelength are poorly defined, and the technique is, of course, performed blindly. Whether it should be covered with an advancement anoplasty is also unclear.

Recently, a shape memory Nitinol® alloy OTSC® clip (Ovesco AG, Tubingen, Germany) has been deployed at the site of the internal opening of a complex fistula in a porcine model of anal fistula. It was associated with complete closure in the few animals where it was tried with an intense inflammatory response and an excessive collagen response. The potential weakness of this approach is that the clip applicator is inserted blindly. This technique has been seen as an extension of clip use in other gastrointestinal fistulae.

Follow-up

The follow-up is simple with the use of sitz baths, analgesics, and stool softeners. Frequent office visits within the first few weeks help keep an eye on proper healing and wound care. One must ensure that the internal wound does not close prematurely, causing a recurrent fistula. Digital examination findings can help distinguish early fibrosis.

Complications

Early post-operative include urinary retention, bleeding, faecal impaction, and occasionally thrombosis in the haemorrhoids.

Delayed post-operative complications include recurrence, incontinence, anal stenosis, and delayed wound healing.

Outcome and Prognosis

Following standard fistulotomy, the reported rate of recurrence is 0–18%, and the rate of stool incontinence is 3–7%. Following seton use, the reported rate of recurrence is 0–17%, and the rate of any incontinence of stool is 0–17%. Following mucosal advancement flap, the reported rate of recurrence is 1–10%, and the rate of anal incontinence for stool is 6–8%.

CLINICAL PEARLS

- Perianal abscesses are caused by cryptoglandular infections at the dentate line between the anal sphincters.
- Cryptoglandular anal fistulae are the most frequently occurring form of perianal sepsis.
- Characteristically they have an endoanal primary opening, a fistula tract, and an abscess and/or an external purulent opening. Antibiotic therapy is not of use in initial management except in special cases.
- Treatment of an abscess, if present, is required urgently and when possible, consists of its incision under local anaesthesia. Treating the fistula tract occurs afterwards and aims to dry up the purulent discharge and avoid recurrence of the abscess using surgical fistulotomy.
- The challenge in the therapy of perianal fistulas balances between the best possible cure and the preservation of continence.
- Low perianal fistulas are defined as fistulas of which the fistula tract is located in the lower third of the external anal sphincter. High fistulas are fistulas in, which the fistula tract runs through the upper two-thirds of the external sphincter muscle.
- Lower, inter-sphincteric fistulas can be treated by fistulotomy without risking a substantial loss in continence, but higher, supra-sphincteric, or complex fistula systems might be treated as a first step with a seton, followed by surgery as a second step. Internal opening identification is also essential for obtaining good results.
- Excision of the external fistula tract, closure of the internal opening, and a local advancement flap are now competing with fistulotomy, curettage, and immediate reconstruction.
- Endorectal ultrasound with H_2O_2 was the most accurate diagnostic modality in the pre-operative assessment of the fistula-in-ano.
- Most techniques are very effective regarding eradication of the problem, but there is sometimes a risk of anal incontinence. This explains the increasing interest in sphincter-preserving techniques using the advancement of a covering flap of rectal mucosa and the injection of fibrin glue. LIFT technique is another sphincter saving approach.
- Initial results with glues and fistula 'plugs' were promising but with increasing follow-up, the enthusiasm has been tempered because of disappointing results.
- A series of potentially exciting ablative technologies using different instruments have been devised for fistula ablation. These include VAAFT, the Filac™ radial emitting laser probe, and the use of the OTSC® fistula Nitinol® clip.

SUGGESTED READINGS

Davies M, Harris D, Lohana P, et al. The surgical management of fistula-in-ano in a specialist colorectal unit. *Int J Colorect Dis*. 2008;23: 833–88.

Eisenhammer S. The internal anal sphincter and anorectal abscess. *Surg Gynecol Obstet*. 1956;103: 501–06.

Eitan A, Koliada M, Bickel A. The use of the loose seton technique as a definitive treatment for recurrent and persistent high trans-sphincteric anal fistulas: a long-term outcome. *J Gastrointest Surg*. 2009;13:1116–19.

Ferguson EF Jr., Houston CH. Iatrogenic supralevator fistula. *South Med J*. 1978;71: 490–95.

Garcia-Olmo D, García-Arranz M, Herreros D, Pascual I, Peiro C, Rodríguez-Montes JA. A phase I clinical trials of the treatment of Crohn's fistula by adipose mesenchymal stem cell transplantation. *Dis Colon Rectum*. 2005;48:1416–23.

Garcia-Olmo D, Herreros D, Pascual I, et al. Expanded adipose-derived stem cells for the treatment of complex perianal fistula: a phase II clinical trial. *Dis Colon Rectum*. 2009;52:79–86.

Giamundo P, Geraci M, Tibaldi L, Valente M. Closure of fistula-in-ano with laser—FiLaC™: an effective novel sphincter-saving procedure for complex disease. *Colorectal Dis*. 2014;16:110–15.

Goligher JC, Ellis M, Pissidis AG. A critique of anal glandular infection in the aetiology and treatment of idiopathic anorectal abscesses and fistulas. *Br J Surg*. 1967;54:977–83.

Goodsall DH, Miles WE. Ano-rectal fistula. In Goodsall DH, Miles WE (eds). Diseases of the anus and rectum. Longmans, Green & Co., London 1900;92–137.

Ho KS, Tsang C, Seow-Choen F, et al. Prospective randomised trial comparing ayurvedic cutting seton and fistulotomy for low fistula-in-ano. *Tech Coloproctol*. 2001 Dec;5(3):137–41.

Kelly ME, Heneghan HM, McDermott FD, et al. The role of loose seton in the management of anal fistula: a multicenter study of 200 patients. *Tech Coloproctol*. 2014;18:915–19.

Lohsiriwat V, Yodying H, Lohsiriwat D. Incidence and factors influencing the development of fistula-in-ano after incision and drainage of perianal abscesses. *J Med Assoc Thai*. 2010;93: 61–65.

Malouf AJ, Buchanan GN, Carapeti EA, et al. A prospective audit of fistula-in-ano at St. Mark's hospital. *Colorectal Dis*. 2002;4:13–19.

McCourtney JS, Finlay IG. Setons in the surgical management of fistula in ano. *Br J Surg*. 1995;82:448–52.

Mitalas LE, van Onkelen RS, Monkhorst K, Zimmerman DD,Gosselink MP, Schouten WR. Identification of epithelialization in high transsphincteric fistulas. *Tech Coloproctol*. 2012;16:113–17.

Meinero P, Mori L. Video-assisted anal fistula treatment (VAAFT): a novel sphincter-saving procedure for treating complex anal fistulas. *Tech Coloproctol*. 2011;15:417–22.

Nomikos IN. Anorectal abscesses: need for accurate anatomical localization of the disease. *Clin Anat*. 1997;10: 239–44.

Nwaejike N, Gilliland R. Surgery for fistula-in-ano: an audit of practice of colorectal and general surgeons. *Colorectal Dis*. 2007;9:749–53.

Oztürk E, Gülcü B. Laser ablation of fistula tract: a sphincter-preserving method for treating fistula-in-ano. *Dis Colon Rectum*. 2014;57:360–64.

Parks AG. The pathogenesis and treatment of fistula-in-ano. *Br Med J*. 1961;i: 463–69.

Parks AG, Gordon PH, Hardcastle JD. A classification of fistula in-ano. *Br J Surg*. 1976;63: 1–12.

Prasad ML, Read DR, Abcarian H. Supralevator abscess: diagnosis and treatment. *Dis Colon Rectum*. 1981;24: 456–61.

Shawki S, Wexner SD. Idiopathic fistula-in-ano. *World J Gastroenterol*. 2011;17:3277–85.

van Koperen PJ, ten Kate FJ, Bemelman WA, Slors JF. Histological identification of epithelium in perianal fistulae: a prospective study. *Colorectal Dis*. 2010;12:891–95

Wilhelm A. A new technique for sphincter-preserving anal fistula repair using a novel radial emitting laser probe. *Tech Coloproctol*. 2011;15:445–49.

Chapter 9

Pruritus ani or anal itch

Pruritus ani is characterised by intolerable itching around the anus. It is an irritating situation for both sufferers and clinicians as many patients suffer persistent and intractable symptoms and medication is probably unsuccessful. A proctologist, a dermatologist, or a physician may treat irritation or itching of the perianal skin. Pruritus ani affects 1–5% of the population and is four times more prevalent in men than in women. It most commonly presents in the 4–6th decades of life. Pruritus ani is categorised as either primary (idiopathic) or secondary. In this regard, there are nearly 100 different listed causes for pruritus ani making the differential diagnoses and treatment options extensive.

INTRODUCTION

Pruritus ani is characterised by an unpleasant itchy or burning sensation in the perianal region. There are many definable perianal dermatologic conditions which lead to pruritus ani such as lichen sclerosus et atrophicus, or psoriasis but most cases are idiopathic; some contributing factors like vigorous perianal hygiene, prolapsing haemorrhoids, loose stools, and repeated use of ointments and creams result in gross perianal wetness with maceration of the perianal skin. Patients develop a minor itch, which may progress to severe pruritus over the entire perineum. Frequent scratching causes damaging excoriations, which may bleed. A vicious circle of itching and scratching develops which is hard to break and induces a state of nervous exhaustion.

An accurate understanding of dermatologic terms aids in the assessment of comparative treatment regimes. Plaques are well-circumscribed, elevated, and solid lesions; whereas, papules are well-circumscribed, elevated, and dome-shaped lesions. Pustules are circumscribed superficial elevations of the skin filled with purulent material; whereas, ulcers are superficial skin breaks resulting from trauma, and that include ruptured vesicles and secondary infections. Itch is an unpleasant sensation leading to a desire to scratch and can be categorised into the following main diagnostic groups—cutaneous, neuropathic, neurogenic, and psychogenic. While cutaneous or perceptive itch is caused by inflammation of the skin, the neuropathic itch occurs because of the damage to the peripheral nervous system that may be present anywhere along the afferent nerve pathway. It is centrally induced. Psychogenic itch may be associated with organic causes but is exacerbated by habitual activity and psychogenic or frankly psychiatric overlay.

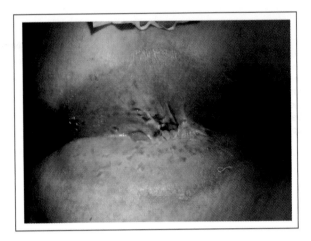

Figure 9.1 Perianal excoriations.

Courtesy: Pravin Jaiprakash Gupta.

AETIOLOGY

Certain foods like coffee, spicy foods, dairy products, citrus fruits, and alcoholic beverages, especially beer and wine, have been found to be associated with pruritus; in addition, milk or milk products like chocolates and cheese, and nuts may aggravate the condition. The moistness caused by anal fissures, fistulas, or mucosal prolapse, and the successive attempts to deal with such fluid may contribute towards pruritus. Neoplasms such as Bowen's disease, Paget's disease, and cloacogenic carcinoma can also cause pruritus. Fungal or bacterial infections, or parasites like the pinworms, are occasional causes. Several dermatologic conditions can also affect the perianal region. Contact dermatitis (Figure 9.1) could be due to the application of topical anaesthetics, neosporin, lanolin, or even overuse of topical steroids. Similarly, conditions such as psoriasis, seborrhoea, lichen planus, and hormonal deficiency in menopausal women are also uncommon yet specific causes of pruritus ani.

Usually, pruritus gets aggravated by over-cleansing with irritating soaps, excessive use of ointments, creams, or continuous scratching, which further irritates the skin to increase the inflammation and symptoms.

TRANSMITTED DISEASES

The list of secondary causes of pruritus is unending and includes psoriasis, pilonidal disease, gonorrhoea, atopic dermatitis, hidradenitis suppurativa, syphilis, contact dermatitis, Crohn's disease, chancroid, seborrhoeic dermatitis, tinea cruris, granuloma iguinale, scleroderma, herpes zoster, molluscum contagiosum, erythema multiforme, trichomoniasis, herpes simplex, pemphigus vulgaris, bilharziasis, condyloma acuminata, dermatitis, herpetiformis, oxyuriasis (pinworm), chlamydia, lichen planus, larva currens, lichen sclerosis et atrophicus, cimicosis (bed bugs), radiation dermatitis, pediculosis (lice), Darier's disease, scabies, diabetes mellitus, haemorrhoids, acanthosis nigricans leukaemia and lymphoma anal creases, leukoplakia, hepatic diseases, fistula-in-ano, mycosis fungoids, thyroid disorders, fissures, leukaemia cutis, renal failure, rectal prolapse, squamous cell carcinoma, iron deficiency anaemia, basal cell carcinoma, vitamin A and D deficiencies, Bowen's disease, aplastic anaemia, melanoma, dysplastic nevus, Paget's disease, etc.

Men are more commonly affected than women are. Faecal contamination of the perineum with the lack of gross soiling, allergies to locally applied agents or components of the diet, and irritant chemicals in the faeces have been implicated but not conclusively proved to be of relevance. A psychosomatic aetiology has been suggested; in its most severe forms, the condition undoubtedly provokes great anxiety. This condition is worse during the summer when sweating is the most.

Small particles of faeces may accumulate in perianal region and cause irritation if the patient finds it difficult to wipe off due to any existing condition like anal fissures, anal fistulas, papillomas, skin tags, prolapsing haemorrhoids, or rectal prolapse. Excessive sweating exacerbated by poorly fitting undergarments along with poor personal hygiene is also implicated. Threadworms, scabies, pediculosis pubis, and fungal infections are easily treatable but they are easily overlooked causes of pruritus ani. Usually, the symptoms get worse at nights as they are the only focus of attention then.

PATHOPHYSIOLOGY

The sensation of itch can be brought on by various stimulus modalities including thermal, electrical, mechanical (heat, xerosis, etc.), and chemical stimuli. In this respect, histamine has been studied extensively as a potential neuronal mechanism of itch; however, it is not the only substance that produces itching. Kallikrein, bradykinin, papain, and trypsin are all itch-mediating substances that are nonresponsive to blockade with classical histamine antagonists such as diphenhydramine. Consequently, antihistamines have proven ineffective in treating pruritus in many instances. Neurologically, an itch is a surface phenomenon initiated by the stimulation of C-fibres located in the epidermis and sub-epidermis. These C-fibres are slow conduction velocity unmyelinated fibres with extensive terminal branches that transmit messages centrally. Itch receptors may be located more superficially than pain receptors and are stimulated by minor mechanical stimuli so that pruritus is believed to represent a sub-threshold response of pain. In this sense, scratching of the affected skin provides inadequate feedback to inhibit itching so that prolonged itching can lead to damaging excoriations and infections, which themselves provide additional itching stimuli. The effect is the creation of a vicious cycle resulting in clinical skin damage, a secondary infection that prolongs the process and secondary psychological overlay.

Pruritus ani is considered primary or idiopathic when no other demonstrable cause can be found. The Washington Hospital Center devised a useful classification system for pruritus ani based upon the physical features of the skin where—stage 0 is normal skin; stage 1 is erythematous and inflamed skin; stage 2 is lichenified skin; and stage 3 is lichenified, coarse skin often with associated ulceration(s). The likely cause of these cases is faecal contamination as shown by Caplan's faecal patch test study. For this purpose, by applying autologous faeces patch tests to males on both the inner arm and the perianal region, Caplan was able to show that the perianal skin reacts differently to skin elsewhere on the body. In this study, anal symptoms were present in one-third of men with pruritus ani and 53% of asymptomatic males. These effects were seen within hours and alleviated by washing, suggesting a local irritation rather than any particular allergy. Symptoms ceased when the area was washed and did not show any allergic reaction. Any factor that leads the perianal area to become moist, soiled, or irritated also has the potential to result in pruritus ani symptoms.

Numerous studies have shown that patients with pruritus ani are more likely to have loose stools, drink more water, and have weekly faecal soiling than patients without this condition. Exaggerated recto-anal inhibitory reflexes and earlier incontinence were also found in patients presenting with pruritus ani. The recto-anal inhibitory is the natural relaxation of the internal anal sphincter in response to rectal distension. Such exaggerated reflex and leakage are concomitantly seen with an infusion of smaller volumes of a saline distention test in patients with idiopathic pruritus ani providing some explanation for the role of soiling as the principal cause of idiopathic or primary pruritus ani.

EXAMINATION

A patient who presents with pruritus ani should initially undergo a detailed history and physical assessment with attention to the afore-mentioned potential aetiologies. Some patients with severe pruritus ani have an entirely normal-looking perineum and anus; others have pronounced perianal skin creases and folds. The skin may have a moist white appearance or be various shades of red with excoriations from scratching. In its most severe form, the perineum is red, raw, and bleeding. Assessment of the patient includes questioning the overzealous use of perianal hygiene, stool consistency, the amount of fluid in the diet, or stool leakage. Threadworms appear as thin white threads about 6 mm in length and seen around the anal orifice. They can also be located in the effluent of a diagnostic saline enema. If the reddened skin has a clearly demarcated margin, fungal infection should be strongly suspected. The diagnosis is confirmed by micro-scopic examination of skin scrapings.

A thorough anorectal examination helps to identify potentially treatable causes of pruritus ani. Haemorrhoids and tags should be treated surgically with the aim of achieving a smooth anus to avoid faecal accumulation due to inability to wipe it off clear (Figure 9.2).

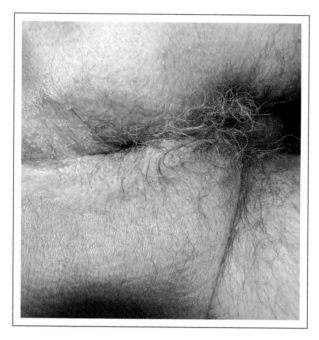

Figure 9.2 Perianal soiling and pruritus.
Courtesy: Pravin Jaiprakash Gupta.

A gynaecological examination should be carried out in women to look for any underlying disease process, like vaginitis. Investigations should be conducted to determine if pruritus ani is the result of a systemic disorder or from local causes. Tests should include blood glucose levels, blood nitrogen levels, erythrocyte sedimentation rate (ESR), haemachrome, liver (hepatic) functions, analysis of faeces, and a skin biopsy.

Pathology

Histological abnormalities are observed in skin biopsy samples though these are rarely accurate. Hydrops of the epidermis, an irregular proliferation of the stratum mucosum, and oedema of the dermis are commonly observed. A rectosigmoidoscopic examination should also be undertaken.

Treatment

Although potential causative conditions should be treated appropriately, the patient with idiopathic pruritus ani needs a detailed discussion on optimal anal hygiene and reassurance.

Once a diagnosis of primary pruritus ani has been made, treatment is directed towards proper anal hygiene, avoiding moisture in the anal area, removing offending agents, altering the diet accordingly directed to identifiable initiating targets, and protecting the skin. Patients are also encouraged to view therapy as control of chronic symptoms with the institution of new anal hygiene habits rather than as a once only treatment. All patients, wherever possible, receive a patient education handout for reference at home and will often benefit from ancillary education sessions with a colorectal practice nurse. Optimal anal hygiene includes avoidance of over-wiping of the anus, alcohol-based wipes, perfumes, dyes, and witch hazel products. Patients should only use plain, white, unscented, toilet paper for wiping the anal area that may be coated in Sorbolene.

In severe circumstances, patients must be inspired to take a shower after a bowel motion and cleanse the area with a detachable shower head. The use of bidet is advisable if it is easily available although it is less in the tradition of Americans and Anglo-Saxon (as opposed to European) households. The anal area is then pat dried with a towel or dried with a hair dryer on its cool setting. Any kind of seepage or leakage should be checked with either using fibres or anti-diarrhoeal which will not only eliminate offending agents, but will also make anal hygiene simpler.

The ideal consistency of stool must be soft and bulky so as to be easy to scrub with a single wipe. After cleaning the anal area, the skin should be protected with zinc oxide-based barrier ointment. Recommended dietary changes include the avoidance of some of the 'C's—coffee (and tea), cola, chocolate, citrus (tomatoes), and calcium (dairy products).

Tight fitting clothing will also promote moisture in the anal area and should be avoided. Replace synthetic underwear with cotton ones. Athlete's foot powder instead of a barrier cream may also be used in patients who have significant perspiration in both the anal and crural (groin) regions. This may be fortified by using topical antifungals as a preliminary trial in resistant cases. Topical steroids used in low dose for short periods are often effective in breaking the itch-injury cycle and may be necessary to provide symptomatic relief when starting therapy. The adverse effects of steroids should be discussed with the patient and include skin atrophy, ulceration, rebound symptoms after withdrawal, striae, and spontaneous bleeding that may themselves on occasion be a cause of itching.

When initiating therapy, 1% hydrocortisone for a limited period and then change over to a barrier ointment is a safe strategy. If prolonged and potent steroids have been in prescription, they should be tapered down slowly. It is advisable to have a tailored preparation of steroids for each patient for differential use. In general, ointments are less prone to skin atrophy when compared with creams constructed from the same constituents. Lately, there has been an interest in the local application of capsaicin, which although it causes an initial stinging sensation, appears in some studies to be effective. In one randomised, cross-over trial using a 0.006% capsaicin cream applied three times a day, 70% response was reported within three days while many of them responded on the first day itself.

Finally, anal tattooing has been advocated as a therapy for patients who have failed many other regimens. The technique involves the intradermal injection of a solution of 1% methylene blue, bupivacaine, and lidocaine. However, when used as a last resort, it should be noted that skin necrosis is a recognised complication of the technique. Modification of this method uses an intradermal and subcutaneous injection of 1% methylene blue (10 mL), 5 mL of normal saline, and 7.5 mL of 0.5% lignocaine with adrenaline into the perianal skin. The patients may experience some perianal hypoesthesia for this injection although this will recover over a period, as local nerve endings are eliminated due to this procedure. When effective, the tattoo should remain visible for 2–6 weeks; whereas, a less noticeable mark is suggestive of a too deeply placed solution.

It should always be remembered that psychological as well as sleep disorders can play a significant role in pruritus ani where it may be a manifestation of anxiety or depression. Patients may describe an intense desire to itch despite adequate empiric treatment of primary pruritus ani with no other secondary cause. In these cases, the use of central acting medications including doxepin, amitryptiline, nortriptyline, gabapentin, and cimetidine may be very useful as can the old trick of placing socks over the hands at night to prevent nocturnal scratching.

The anus must be kept clean and dry and should be gently blotted with non-scented toilet paper after bowel movements rather than vigorously rubbed. Patients should cleanse especially after activities that promote heavy sweating. An especially useful manoeuvre is the application of a wisp (not a ball) of cotton to the perianal area. The cotton wisp absorbs anal mucous discharge and is exchanged after bowel movements and baths. The perianal region may be dried regularly with a fan or a hair dryer after a bath but this may not be feasible on a regular basis. The patient must be encouraged to adapt the new approach and prevent excessive irritation of the area. Reassurance can help to alleviate focus and discomfort in the area. Nonetheless, any lesion that remains active despite treatment with a reasonable amount of time should undergo further investigation with biopsy and dermatologic consultation. If threadworms are discovered, patients and their families are treated with a course of mebendazole and strict measures of hygiene adopted to prevent reinfection. Pediculosis pubis and scabies are treated with topical lindane or malathion.

Antihistamines with a sedative effect may limit night time symptoms. In some patients, psychotropic agents are required to achieve adequate sedation. Anti-depressants may be necessary for patient's refractory to treatment or with underlying psychiatric disorders.

In spite of all this, there are few patients who do not have an identifiable lesion to treat and some might have undergone surgery for potentially suspicious anorectal conditions and will continue to have symptoms. If confirmed, treatment with a topical anti-fungal agent is given. Candida infection is treated with nystatin ointment.

Instructing the Patients

Certain advice given to the patient would help them get rid of this troublesome condition. These are:

- Avoid scratching the itchy area as much as possible. Scratching produces more damage, which in turn makes the itching worse.
- Cleanse meticulously, thoroughly, and gently after bowel movements.
- Wash the anal area using a tub full of lukewarm water or a bidet. Wet tissues or soft toilet paper is the next best option. Use mineral oil, aqueous cream, or another soap-free cleanser. Avoid customary soaps and harsh toilet paper.
- Gently apply the prescribed ointment, cream, or lotion as directed.
- It is prudent to avoid any over-the-counter cream, suppository, or medicine without medical advice as many of them can cause allergic contact dermatitis.
- Constipation should be avoided; so, have plenty of high-fibre foods. Similarly, exerting at stool causes fissures in the anus, which are irritable and invite organisms to harbour.
- Avoid loose and irritating motions. Consumption of spicy food should be minimal. So also prunes, figs, orange juice, coffee, or beer.

Pruritus ani is a condition with multiple causes and, therefore, effective therapy may be elusive at first. Primary causes are thought to be due to faecal soiling or food irritants. Secondary causes include malignancy, infections such as sexually transmitted diseases, benign anorectal diseases, systemic diseases, and inflammatory conditions. Therapy is directed at the underlying cause when identified. The list of differential diagnosis is always vast and huge, and reassessment of therapy is paramount. Although the proctologist needs to treat associated anorectal disorders, anal surgery is often not indicated and will not benefit the majority of patients. When there is no apparent secondary cause, an empiric treatment is directed at improving anal hygiene, removal of common irritants, and protection of the anal skin.

CLINICAL PEARLS

- Pruritus ani, or perianal itching, affects 1–5% of the population and is the second most common anorectal condition after haemorrhoids. Almost all the patients had indulged in self-treatment for a year before consulting a physician.
- Pinworm infection is prevalent among young children and institutionalised adults. A self-propagating itch-scratch cycle results irrespective of the cause.
- The scratching precipitated inflammation leading to an irresistible urge to scratch further. Chronicity of the disease can well be demonstrated by lichenification of the perianal skin.

(Cont'd)

- When treatment matches the cause of itching, then only it becomes effective and successful.
- Parasites or bacterial infections are treated appropriately using anti-infestive and antibiotics. Underlying disease processes like diabetes mellitus need treatment.
- Injuries, fistulas, and haemorrhoids should be appropriately addressed. A mere change of soaps or detergents can check allergic reactions.
- While it is important that poor anal hygiene needs to be corrected, overzealous or vigorous cleaning should also be avoided as it can precipitate the itching further.
- Use of a blow dryer on the perineum may be effective. Water alone may be adequate hygiene for the over-sensitive skin.
- For cases where the cause is never determined, injection of methylene blue under the skin of the affected area may be curative. Individual should be re-examined again in 2–3 weeks to evaluate the effectiveness of treatment.
- Patient must always be kept in confidence and an honest opinion must be shared even if the precise cause for their condition cannot be identified. They must be reassured that with proper personal hygiene their symptoms can be minimised.
- Dermatological opinion is valuable in chronic cases as it might be able to rule out dermatological causative factors like psoriasis.

SUGGESTED READINGS

Alexander S. Dermatological aspects of anorectal disease. *Clin Gastroenterol*. 1975;4:651–7.

Al-Ghnaniem R, Short K, Pullen A, Fuller LC, Rennie JA, Leather AJ. 1% hydrocortisone ointment is an effective treatment of pruritus ani: a pilot randomized controlled crossover trial. *Int J Colorectal Dis*. 2007;22:1463–7.

Chaudhry V, Bastawrous A. Idiopathic pruritus ani. *Semin Colon Rectal Surg*. 2003;14:196–202.

Daniel GL, Longo WE, Vernava AM., 3rd Pruritus ani. Causes and concerns. *Dis Colon Rectum*.1994;37:670–4.

Eyers AA, Thomson JP. Pruritus ani: is anal sphincter dysfunction important in aetiology? *Br Med J*. 1979;2:1549–51.

Friend WG. The cause and treatment of idiopathic pruritus ani. *Dis Colon Rectum*. 1977;20:40–2.

Hanno R, Murphy P. Pruritus ani. Classification and management. *Dermatol Clin*. 1987;5:811–6.

Laurent A, Boucharlat J, Bosson JL, Derry A, Imbert R. Psychological assessment of patients with idiopathic pruritus ani. *Psychother Psychosom*. 1997;66:163–6.

Lysy J, Sistiery-Ittah M, Israelit Y, Shmueli A, Strauss-Liviatan N, Mindrul V, et al. Topical capsaicin—a novel and effective treatment for idiopathic intractable pruritus ani: a randomised, placebo controlled, crossover study. *Gut*. 2003;52:1323–6.

Robinson N, Singri P, Gordon KB. Safety of the new macrolide immuno-modulators. *Semin Cutan Med Surg*. 2001;20:242–9.

Sauer T. The role of the bidet in pruritus ani. *Aust Fam Physician*. 2010;39:715.

Smith LE, Henrichs D, McCullah RD. Prospective studies on the etiology and treatment of pruritus ani. *Dis Colon Rectum*. 1982;25:358–63.

Sullivan ES, Garnjobst WM. Symposium on colon and anorectal surgery. Pruritus ani: a practical approach. *Surg Clin North Am*. 1978;58:505–12.

Chapter 10

Rectal prolapse

Prolapse of the rectum completely, or in part, is a lifestyle altering disability that commonly affects older people. This prolapse occurs when a mucosal or full-thickness layer of rectal tissue slides through the anal orifice. A full-thickness prolapse of the rectum causes variable and annoying discomfort because of the sensation of the prolapse itself and the mucous that it secretes, and as it tends to stretch the anal sphincters, it could lead to incontinence. Rectal prolapse is defined as the protrusion of one or more layers of rectum through the anal sphincter. If mucosa alone is involved, the prolapse is called incomplete; if all layers of the rectal wall protrude, it is termed as complete (Figure 10.1).

There is a frequent coexistence of rectal prolapse with other pelvic floor abnormalities. Patients having symptoms associated with combined rectal and genital prolapse is not uncommon. The list of surgical methods proposed to correct the underlying pelvic floor defects in a complete rectal prolapse is in itself a proof that there is no agreement about the choice of the best option.

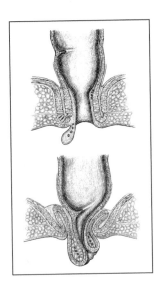

Figure 10.1   Incomplete and complete rectal prolapse.

Illustration: James Oinam.

The terminology implies that incomplete rectal prolapse has the same causes and is merely an earlier stage of complete prolapse, but there are many reasons to doubt this assumption. Moschowitz stated that complete rectal prolapse is a true 'hernia-en-glissade' of rectum and distal colon through the pelvic diaphragm, and this can clearly occur without antecedent mucosal protrusion. Mucosal (incomplete) prolapse can be treated by surgical manoeuvres directed at the mucosa (and its local supporting structures) but complete rectal prolapse can be cured only by operations which include retethering the rectum within the pelvic cavity.

Although complete rectal prolapse was described in the *Ebers Papyrus* of 1500 BC, until recently it was regarded as untreatable since there was no practical method for permanently replacing the prolapsed rectum. Operations were devised in the nineteenth century that amputated the excessive tissue protruding from the anus, but insofar as these did not affect the origin of the prolapse at the pelvic diaphragm they were usually unsuccessful and in the course of time further lengths of bowel inevitably descended through the weakened pelvic floor.

PRESENTATION

Rectal prolapse is commonest in children below the age of three and in elderly women. In both age groups, straining at defaecation and pelvic floor weakness are common.

It may present with constipation or incontinence, and patients may have bleeding, mucous discharge, or tenesmus. In the earlier disease process, prolapse takes place only during bowel movements or while straining, and gradually progresses as tissues become laxer over time.

In adults, females predominate in the proportion of 6:1 and most of them are thin elderly women. In men, the peak incidence falls off after the age of 40; whereas, in women it climbs steadily to reach its maximum incidence in the seventh decade. The previous pregnancy and labour are important aetiological factors. Kupfer and Goligher (1970) investigated this and found that the incidence of complete prolapse was, in fact, higher in those female patients who were nulliparous. More than half the adult cases give a clear history of straining associated with intractable constipation and this probably provides the abdominal squeeze that produces the prolapse.

Weakness of the pelvic floor is clearly an important aetiological factor. Neurological disorders affecting the cauda equina and the pelvic nerves (for example, multiple sclerosis, tabes dorsalis, neoplasms, or trauma) have a definite incidence of complete rectal prolapse, but overall only account for 1.5% of cases.

PHYSICAL EXAMINATION

The continence of the patients can be most accurately judged from the history when they are prepared to divulge all the facts. If the anal sphincters are markedly patulous, this constitutes a subsidiary problem that may require treatment in addition to that aimed at the prolapse itself.

A confident diagnosis is made when a circumferential or segmental mass is visualised protruding from the anus (Figure 10.2). Before embarking on treatment, a thorough appraisal of each case is necessary. There are three equally important facets to this clinical assessment, viz.—the degree of prolapse, the state of continence, and the fitness of the patient.

In order to determine whether a prolapse is complete or not, it is essential that the full extent of the rectal protrusion should be produced to the examining surgeon. This can usually be brought about by asking an adult patient to strain, but can be almost impossible to achieve in children. In such cases of difficulty or doubt, the answer can often be obtained by examining the patient immediately after an attempt at defaecation produced by a glycerine suppository. If the prolapse is small, visual examination may not be enough to decide if full rectal wall descent is present, but in complete prolapse while rolling the prolapse between the finger and thumb, the surgeon will be able to feel the characteristic thickening present near the anal verge where the bowel wall doubles back on itself. Other aids to diagnosis include the observation that in complete prolapse, concentric circular folds of mucosa are usually seen, and on sigmoidoscopy the mucosa of the rectum may be boggy, oedematous, and friable, testifying that it has been prolapsing in the recent past.

The upper limit of such mucosal changes provides an exact guide to the extent of prolapse that is present. Very rarely, the anterior hernial (rectovaginal) sac that is invariably found at operation in cases of complete prolapse may be seen or felt prior to surgery, and even when the prolapse cannot be extruded by the patient, small bowel in the sac may be felt with the finger between the rectum and the back of the vagina and uterus. Complete prolapse begins by descent of

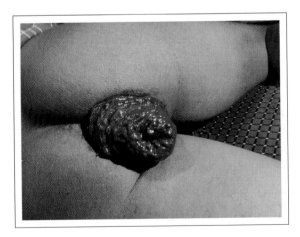

Figure 10.2 Complete rectal prolapse.
Courtesy: Pravin Jaiprakash Gupta.

the anterior rectal wall and its accompanying peritoneal pouch, which causes the anterior wall to be characteristically more bulky than the posterior, and the lumen of the bowel to be directed posteriorly. If a markedly patulous anus is present, the case is likely to be one of complete prolapse.

PATHOLOGICAL CHANGES

Defaecation is a delicately synchronised response in which relaxation and contraction of the large bowel, pelvic floor, and abdominal muscles are completely co-ordinated. Prolonged straining abolishes anal sphincter tone and if the puborectalis is weak or damaged by the factors already discussed, then the whole pelvic floor sags. With this downward descent, there is a degree of invagination of the rectal wall which causes it to turn itself inside out as it emerges from the anal canal. Cineradiographic studies have shown that in many cases the prolapse starts as an internal intussusception of the rectum in the region of the middle to upper two-thirds. Once the leading edge of the prolapse reaches the anal canal, it itself causes further reflex anal inhibition with the development of the typical gaping patulous anus which accompanies the condition. The prolapsed rectum becomes traumatised and the mucosa ulcerated with histological changes identical to those of a solitary ulcer syndrome. There is now considerable evidence that pelvic floor weakness may be associated with a traction neuropathy of the pudendal nerve as a result of downward displacement of the pelvic floor; for example, during straining or childbirth. This may be responsible in many cases not only for the prolapse, but also for the incontinence that frequently accompanies it.

LABORATORY STUDIES

* Rectal prolapse is merely a symptom, and evaluation should focus on the discovery of an underlying disorder.
* It is wise to perform a sweat chloride test for paediatric patients as more than 10% of children with rectal prolapse do have cystic fibrosis.
* Consider a stool examination and culture for infectious agents, particularly in paediatric patients.

IMAGING STUDIES

* A barium enema can assess for concurrent colonic diseases or tumours.
* Defecography may reveal intussusception of the proximal colon or pelvic outlet obstruction.

OTHER TESTS

* Colonic transit study.
* Proctosigmoidoscopy can be a valuable tool to examine rectal mucosa for ulceration, inflammation, or other contributing colonic disease.
* Anal sphincter manometry (aids in determining the degree of anal sphincter damage).

- Pudendal nerve terminal motor latency (assesses for neurological injury or dysfunction).
- Ultrasonography.

TREATMENT

Figure 10.3 shows an emergency treatment in case of irreducible or incarcerated prolapse. Its features are as follows:

- A prolapsed rectum can be reduced with gentle digital pressure. Sedation and local perianal anaesthesia may aid in the reduction.
- Significant bowel oedema may make manual reduction difficult. The topical application of granulated sucrose to the mucosal surface may reduce bowel oedema and allow a reduction.
- Precipitating factors, such as constipation or diarrhoea, should be treated on priority.
- Additional care may be required particularly in the presence of an irreducible prolapse and with gangrene or rupture of the rectal mucosa.

Differential Diagnosis

In both children and adults, mucosal prolapse must be distinguished from a prolapsing anal or third-degree haemorrhoids. The smooth glistening mucosa covering a juvenile polyp is easily differentiated from the rugose mucosa of prolapse, and the presence of haemorrhoids is obvious once they are looked for.

In every case of prolapse, the presence of other diseases of the colon or rectum must be excluded. Proctoscopy and sigmoidoscopy are mandatory in every case to exclude polyps or carcinoma of the

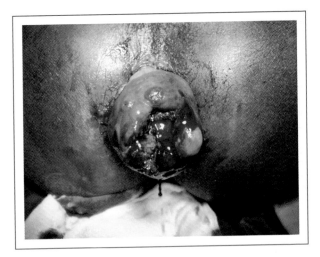

Figure 10.3   Irreducible, incarcerated rectal prolapse.

Courtesy: Pravin Jaiprakash Gupta.

rectum and lower-sigmoid colon. In adults, a radiographic appraisal of the whole colon should be made to exclude a carcinoma or severe diverticular disease, because in both instances treatment for the prolapse may have to be modified. Very occasionally, a carcinoma presents as an ulcer on the prolapsing bowel, and any suspicious lesion should be biopsied.

Definitive Treatment

In adults, the only way to control complete rectal prolapse is by operation. This is rarely the case in children where the condition usually resolves spontaneously on regulation of the bowel habit.

The general fitness of the patient to withstand an operation must be taken into account as many of them are elderly and enfeebled. However, in spite of this, surgery is remarkably well tolerated, so that the clinician can afford to err generously on the side of giving the patient the chance of cure. Bowel preparation is important and the operation should be covered by antibiotic prophylaxis. Pre-operative anti-coagulation is not advisable since a pelvic haematoma might lead to the possibility of infection in an area which may contain unabsorbable foreign material.

There are two principal types of procedures—abdominal and perineal. The major abdominal repair operations provide excellent anatomical restoration with the fewest recurrences but may produce urinary or sexual dysfunction. The more minor perineal approaches, on the other hand, provide only a moderately good anatomical reconstruction with a considerable chance of recurrence, but a lower risk of pelvic nerve damage. In the elderly, anatomical restoration is usually the overriding concern of the surgeon, and should be treated almost exclusively by major anatomical repair, whilst in the young adult a more conservative approach may be advisable.

It can also be performed laparoscopically with equally low rates of recurrence.

Abdominal Approach

There are many operations described aimed at fixing the rectum, removing redundant large intestine, or repairing the pelvic floor from above. This is not the place for a detailed exposition of surgical technique. Ripstein's Teflon sling procedure is safe and gives good results, but serious complications have been reported. Anterior resection is a more major operation, and the risk to life is much greater than with those alternative abdominal operations which do not involve opening the bowel and performing an anastomosis. Excision of the rectum and a permanent colostomy is reserved for those cases whose rectal function is beyond salvage.

The technique of the extended Ivalon sponge rectopexy is summarised as follows. The rectum is mobilised posteriorly down to the level of the coccyx and the anterior peritoneal pouch is excised. The lateral ligaments of the rectum are then mobilised and divided near the pelvic wall. The Ivalon sponge is not attached to the presacral fascia but instead is wrapped around the rectum to cover its posterior and lateral aspects; this avoids any danger of pricking the presacral veins, but nevertheless, many surgeons do in fact, attach the sponge to the presacral fascia. The edges of the sponge, which stiffens the rectal wall enough to prevent intus-susception, while promoting adhesions between the rectum and surrounding tissues, are stitched to the rectal wall and the stumps of the lateral ligaments are sutured to the sacral promontory. This operation corrects all the major anatomical defects with the exception of the pelvic floor laxity. However, in approximately half the patients with pre-operative incontinence, satisfactory continence is restored.

Perineal Approach

The perineal approach allows a repair of the puborectalis portion of the levator ani. The rectum itself cannot be fully mobilised or returned to its normal position, so that the operations necessarily have the aspect of 'plugging back' the descending tissues rather than a total correction of the situation. With these reservations, it is true to say that with a young patient who will co-operate in avoiding straining on defaecation post-operatively, a successful repair can be done through the perineum, with negligible risk to the pelvic nerves.

The operation of choice involves a posterior approach through the inter-sphincteric space. When the level of the puborectalis sling is reached, the rectum is pushed upwards into the pelvis and the puborectalis muscles are then drawn together behind the rectum using a darn of stout monofilament nylon. If the operation is carried out satisfactorily, the gap in the pelvic floor is closed, the puborectalis sling made taut, and the anorectal angle restored. At the same operation, the patulous external anal sphincter muscle may be tightened. Recurrences with this technique seem more likely than with any of the abdominal operations.

The Thiersch operation is simple, but has very poor long-term results. It often increases the problem of constipation (by narrowing the anal orifice too much) or the wire fractures with immediate recurrence. The results are slightly better with new more plaint materials for the encircling stitch (nylon or Mersilene® mesh). Rectosigmoidectomy has such a high recurrence rate that it has been virtually abandoned.

Complications

- Mucosal ulceration.
- Necrosis of rectal wall.
- Post-operative mortality is low, but recurrence rate can be as high as 15%, regardless of the operative procedure.
- The most common post-operative complications include bleeding and dehiscence at the anastomosis.
- Untreated rectal prolapse can lead to incarceration and rarely strangulation.
- More commonly, increasing incidences of rectal bleeding (usually minor), ulceration, and incontinence may occur.

RECTAL PROLAPSE IN CHILDREN

Background

In the paediatric population, rectal prolapse is most commonly a self-limited and benign condition.

In children, an obsessional mother is often the cause of the straining, and pelvic weakness may be present as a result of malnutrition and absence of ischiorectal fat; whooping cough, measles, and tuberculosis may also cause wasting and laxity of the levator muscles and may be associated with a chronic cough causing bursts of raised intra-abdominal pressure to stretch the tissues still further. Chronic urinary obstruction can also substitute for constipation as a cause for prolonged straining, and the shallow sacral curve of the infant has also been suspected as aggravating the tendency to pelvic floor deficiency. It is clear that most of these factors are reversible, and the great majority of childhood prolapses recover on conservative management; 10% of cases persist, an in these children some permanent abnormality of the pelvic floor or mental defectiveness is often present. In these instances, careful search for spinal defects and paralysis of the pelvic diaphragm must be made by suitable radiographic studies, including myelography and electromyography. Cystic fibrosis is another cause.

Pathophysiology

Prolapse of the rectum may involve only the mucosa, which is the innocuous form and the most common in the paediatric population; in the severe form, it includes all layers of the rectum protruding through the anus (Figure 10.4).

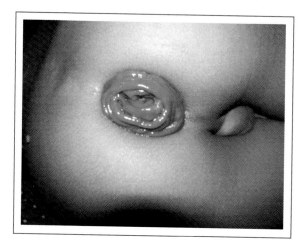

Figure 10.4   Rectal prolapse in a child.
Courtesy: Pravin Jaiprakash Gupta.

While cystic fibrosis is not a likely diagnosis in patients who come with a rectal prolapse, a sweat test should be performed in all patients who present without an underlying anatomic abnormality.

Physical Examination

Because most prolapses spontaneously reduce before arrival for evaluation, a brief examination of the patient in a squatting position and observation for recurrence of prolapse is recommended. Parents often provide a history of protrusion of a dark or bright red mass from the child's anus, but the child appears to be pain-free or in minimal discomfort.

In children, complete rectal prolapse may have to be distinguished from an intussusception. This is usually very obvious from the history, but in any case of difficulty the finger should be inserted into the anal sulcus; if the finger passes freely into the rectal ampulla, the case is one of sigmoido-rectal intussusception and not rectal prolapse.

Treatment

Medical care

Patients landing with a prolapsed rectum should undergo manual reduction at the earliest. They should be provided with gloves and lubricant and taught how to reduce the prolapse. However, prolapse often spontaneously reduces without the need of any reduction techniques.

Conservative management is started in children younger than four years and in children older than four years who have non-complicated, non-recurrent rectal prolapse. This management is aimed at treating the cause and reducing straining.

Constipation should be treated with dietary modification (total dose per day is 5 g of fibre with an additional gram for each year of age; dose for adults is 20 g once or twice daily) and stool softeners to reduce straining. Infectious diarrhoea or parasitic infestation should be appropriately treated.

Surgical care

Circumferential injection procedures: Injection methods use either phenol in oil, D50, isotonic sodium chloride, or ethyl alcohol as a sclerosant to induce fibrosis and adhesion formation, which stabilises the rectum. Possible complications include injury to nerves, injury to surrounding tissue, and possible damage from sclerosing agents that may be carcinogenic.

Cauterisation: In this approach, the prolapsed rectum is cauterised in a linear fashion extending to the submucosa divided into four quadrants. This induces perirectal inflammation and scarring that prevents prolapse.

Abdominal rectopexy: Endoscopic or open approach is possible. The perirectal tissues are fixed to the presacral area to assure correct anatomical positioning and tissue adherence.

Ekehorn's rectopexy: A suture is placed in the rectal ampulla through the lowest part of the sacrum to induce inflammation and adhesions. This produces adhesions between the rectal wall and peri-rectal wall to perform a sacrorectopexy that fixes the prolapse.

Prognosis

- Ten per cent of patients who had experienced rectal prolapse as a child continue to experience it in their adult lives.
- Approximately 90% of children aged from nine months to 3 years who experience rectal prolapse respond to conservative management up to six years of age.
- Spontaneous resolution is much less likely in children who first experience prolapse when they are older than four years.

RECTAL MUCOSAL PROLAPSE

External rectal mucosal prolapse is defined as a circumferential descent of anorectal mucosa through the anus (Figure 10.5). Similarly, mucosal prolapse can result from a wide variety of causes of distortion of the tubular structure of the anal canal associated with laxity of the submucosa (such as third-degree haemorrhoids, pronounced rectocele, perineal descent, anal sphincter weakness, and after operations for fistula-in-ano) without any evidence of pelvic floor hernia and with little or no tendency to progress to a complete rectal prolapse. However, while there is considerable reason to doubt that the two types of rectal prolapses are of similar aetiology; they often coexist and the terms complete and incomplete which have been hallowed by long clinical use serve to emphasise the major difference between them.

The symptoms related to partial rectal mucosal prolapse are quite similar to the symptoms of the advanced haemorrhoidal disease that

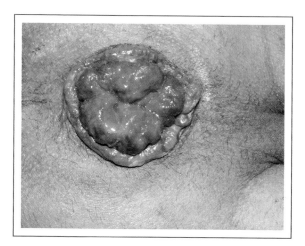

Figure 10.5   Rectal mucosal prolapse.
Courtesy: Pravin Jaiprakash Gupta.

include pain, bleeding, mucous discharge, and pruritus. The pathology is usually self-limiting in children and responds well to appropriate toilet training, use of laxatives, and in exceptional cases with the submucosal injection of sclerosant solution. Nevertheless, in adults, it needs a more complex treatment to contain the prolapse and associated symptoms. This would either need the traditional extended haemorrhoidectomy with ligature and excision of the prolapsing mucosa or the stapled transanal excision of the prolapse using the Longo's technique.

CLINICAL PEARLS

- Rectal prolapse is an uncommon, disabling condition that has long fascinated surgeons. Very few clinical disorders have generated such a large number of surgical procedures, with varying degree of successful outcome.
- Confusing terminology is a major problem in the study of rectal prolapse. The terms that must be distinguished are mucosal prolapse, internal intussusception (occult rectal prolapse), and complete rectal prolapse (procedentia).
- Mucosal prolapse is caused by a looseness or breaking down of the connective tissue between the submucosa of the rectum and anal canal and the underlying muscle. This usually starts in the anal canal and, in its earliest form, is represented by prolapsing haemorrhoids.
- The goal of surgery for rectal prolapse is to correct the prolapse, avoid faecal incontinence, and constipation, and to do so with little or no mortality and morbidity.
- Great care should be undertaken in selecting the right operation for patients with rectal prolapse. This is one operation where the surgical procedure must be tailored to physiologic needs; thus, the evaluation of pudendal nerve latency, anorectal sensation, rectal emptying, perineal descent, and colonic transit is essential.
- Patients too frail for surgery should be given bulk laxatives and taught how to reduce the prolapse. Urgent treatment required if the prolapse is irreducible or ischaemic.

SUGGESTED READINGS

Boccasanta P, Rosati R, Venturi M, et al. Comparison of laparoscopic rectopexy with open technique in the treatment of complete rectal prolapse: clinical and functional results. *Surg Laparosc Endosc*. 1998; 8:460–5.

Frykman HM, Goldberg SM. The surgical treatment of rectal procidentia. *Surg Gynecol Obstet*. 1969;129:1225–30.

Frykman HM. Abdominal proctopexy and primary sigmoid resection for rectal procidentia. *Am J Surg*. 1955;90:780–9.

Gordon PH, Hoexter B. Complications of the Ripstein procedure. *Dis Colon Rectum*. 1978;21:277–80.

Jacobs LK, Lin YJ, Orkin BA. The best operation for rectal prolapse. *Surg Clin North Am*. 1997;77:49–70.

Kuijpers HC. Treatment of complete rectal prolapse: to narrow, to wrap, to suspend, to fix, to encircle, to plicate or to resect? *World J Surg*. 1992;16:826–30.

Madden MV, Kamm MA, Nicholls RJ, Santhanam AN, Cabot R, Speakman CT. Abdominal rectopexy for complete prolapse: prospective study evaluating changes in symptoms and anorectal function. *Dis Colon Rectum*. 1992;35:48–55.

Madiba TE, Baig MK, Wexner SD. Surgical management of rectal prolapse. *Arch Surg*. 2005;140:63–73.

Munro W, Avramovic J, Roney W. Laparoscopic rectopexy. *J Laparoendosc Surg*. 1993;3:55–8.

Novell JR, Osborne MJ, Winslet MC, Lewis AAM. Prospective randomized trial of Ivalon sponge versus sutured rectopexy for full-thickness rectal prolapse. *Br J Surg*. 1994;81:904–6.

Ramanujam PS, Venkatesh KS. Management of acute incarcerated rectal prolapse. *Dis Colon Rectum*. 1992;35:1154–6.

Solla JA, Rothenberger DA, Goldberg SM. Colonic resection in the treatment of complete rectal prolapse. *Neth J Surg*. 1989;41:132–5.

Solomon MJ, Young CJ, Eyers AA, Roberts RA. Randomized clinical trial of laparoscopic versus open abdominal rectopexy for rectal prolapse. *Br J Surg*. 2002;89:35–9.

Stevenson AR, Stitz RW, Lumley JW. Laparoscopic-assisted resection-rectopexy for rectal prolapse: early and medium follow-up. *Dis Colon Rectum*. 1998;41:46–54.

Chapter 11

Paediatric proctology

Problems related to the rectum and anus are frequent and bothersome in infants and children. Most of these are not associated with severe morbidity, but they can lead to a significant anxiety in patients and parents and frequent medical consultation until the problem is successfully treated. The approach to such disorders in children has been little studied. The region, however, is readily accessible for direct examination, and the predominant pathologies are the consequences of passing hard and voluminous stools that are often responsible for pain and bleeding. Few proctological problems, such as constipation and anal fissure, are seen in both children and adults. Congenital problems such as anorectal agenesis and Hirschsprung's disease present themselves in early infancy. Despite treatment in childhood, the sequel may require continuing management in adult life.

FISSURE-IN-ANO

Anal fissures present themselves as painful defecation and hematochezia, and are common in children and infants alike. The child presents with a history of pain on defecation with crying 'holding back'. There may be streaks of blood seen on toilet paper or the stool or a skin tag (sentinel pile) may indicate a fissure. It was noticed that toddlers and young children with chronic constipation and anal fissure had been found to consume larger amounts of cow's milk in comparison with children with a normal bowel habit. Additionally, shorter duration of breastfeeding and early bottle-feeding with cow's milk might be playing some role in the causation of hard stools and anal fissure in infants and young children. Rectal examination should not be attempted if the diagnosis is obvious.

Treatment includes toilet training, reassurance to the parents, dietary regulation, oral laxatives for constipation, and applying local anaesthetic cream to the area. Suppositories should preferably be avoided. Significant proportions are resistant to simple stool softening therapy, and no single surgical treatment has been described which is not fraught with the risk of compromising sphincteric function. Fissurectomy could be a successful treatment for anal fissures when combined with post-operative laxative therapy. As the internal anal sphincter division is not involved, the risk of iatrogenic faecal incontinence is obviated. Application of topical GTN ointment is found to be effective in healing chronic anal fissures in children.

At the beginning of GTN therapy, many formal trials comparing its use to placebo were reported. Some of these included only children in treatment where GTN showed an advantage over placebo although there was heterogeneity of placebo response rates in some studies that provided some conflicting data.

Anorectal injuries in children are uncommon, and those caused by sexual abuse are rarely reported. However, these can present with fissure-in-ano. While anal fissures are not rare in children, it might be necessary to exclude sexual assault and undertake appropriate evaluation and treatment. The child must be shielded from further abuse.

HAEMORRHOIDS

Haemorrhoids in children are not common (Figure 11.1). There is hardly any evidence of a presence of haemorrhoids in children who were examined for sex abuse or even in the postmortem perianal findings.

The most frequent cause of haemorrhoid in young children is portal hypertension. The extrahepatic disease is associated with a higher incidence of both haemorrhoids and anorectal varices. The occurrence and severity of haemorrhoids are related to the number of previous oesophagal sclerotherapy sessions. On few occasions, haemorrhoids may be found in association with colorectal malignancies, rectal mucosal prolapse, and as pseudo-haemorrhoidal vascular swellings.

A strong family history of such disease and history of constipation could be contributing factors to initiate this rarity. A high-calorie and low-roughage diet could be one factor that could be responsible for initiating this pathology. A structural weakness of the haemorrhoidal venous walls may be present congenitally to cause haemorrhoids or pseudo-haemorrhoidal vascular swellings.

Haemorrhoids at times may be confused with rectal prolapse or prolapse of a rectal polyp. The lesions may not be apparent when the child is anaesthetised because of the absence of straining. This will impair accurate diagnosis and impede identification of the lesion if surgery is being attempted. By inserting a 20 F Foley catheter with 30 mL balloon in the rectum and applying gentle traction to reproduce the raised venous pressure generated during straining, it is possible to demonstrate haemorrhoids. Haemorrhoids in children can be managed with sclerotherapy or banding.

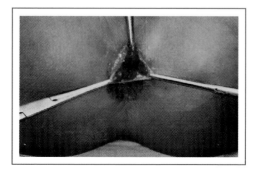

Figure 11.1   Prolapsing haemorrhoids.
Courtesy: Pravin Jaiprakash Gupta.

HIRSCHSPRUNG'S DISEASE

Any child who has had constipation since birth, irrespective of age, may have Hirschsprung's disease. The disease presents either in a neonate as large bowel obstruction or later as chronic dyschezia. The diagnosis should be considered and excluded in any child who does not pass meconium for 48 hours or who passes a meconium plug only after rectal examination or insertion of a thermometer. The diagnosis should be considered in all constipated children, especially if constipation starts from birth or with the delay in the passage of meconium. Soiling and faeces in the rectum may indicate that the disease is of short length. There is an absence of the ganglion cells in Auerbach's plexus for varying lengths of bowel proximal from the anus. Total lack of ganglion cells throughout the colon or even the small bowel can occur. At times, in some children, the affected segment is very short and the disease may remain silent until they are teenagers. Anorectal manometry may be helpful in making the diagnosis in these children.

TREATMENT

Colostomy is used as an initial treatment to deflate the bowels. It can either be in the right transverse colon, if the stoma is created blind, or at the junction of ganglionic and aganglionic bowel, if laparotomy has been necessary to confirm the diagnosis.

JUVENILE POLYP

Juvenile colorectal polyps are the most common cause of paediatric haematochezia and contribute to significant morbidity if not treated early. Most children presented with painless rectal bleeding associated with other symptoms, such as protrusion of mass through the anus (Figure 11.2), diarrhoea, anaemia, and recurrent abdominal pain.

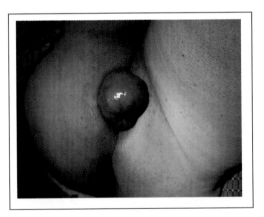

Figure 11.2 Juvenile rectal polyp.
Courtesy: Pravin Jaiprakash Gupta.

It is present in 3–4% of the population below 21 years of age and represents 90% of all polyps in childhood. Diagnosis can be clinched by digital rectal examination, proctosigmoidoscopy, and barium enema. Rectosigmoidoscopy and colonoscopy remain as the diagnosis and therapeutic methods in children with juvenile polyp (JP) as these polyps can be removed by proctosigmoidoscopy. Histological examination usually shows inflammatory changes. Recurrence is rare.

As the juvenile colorectal polyps can cause a substantial morbidity in children and do carry a minimal risk of developing dysplastic changes, they should be removed early. Colonoscopy is the investigation of choice in children with prolonged rectal bleeding.

FISTULA-IN-ANO

Anal fistula in children has its origin in a cryptitis which proceeds to a perianal abscess and subsequent fistula formation. They are usually encountered in otherwise healthy boys of less than a year. Multiple studies have indicated that an anal cryptitis seems to be the precipitating event that ends in the formation of a perianal abscess. It has been suggested that high amount of androgens or its imbalance with oestrogen levels during pregnancy can be the origin for the formation of abnormal and thick Morgagni crypts; the latter are often the centre of cryptitis and perianal abscesses.

Few available studies of perianal abscess and fistula-in-ano in children have shown a different natural history of the disease. It is under the age of two years that the disease occurs exclusively in males with a very low incidence of systemic signs of sepsis and a high rate of spontaneous resolution. A disease occurring in older children (>2 years of age) is particularly rare and has usually been reported on a background of immunocompromised, diabetes, or childhood Crohn's disease. A recent report showed that simple abscess aspiration resulted in good outcomes in most cases between the ages of 2–14 years with a rare need for subsequent fistula treatment.

The possible cause of development of fistulae in the child could be seen in the parental negligence of episodes of perianal abscesses in the child following cryptoglandular infection, which is allowed to burst open. The infective focus persists in the crypts and at the site of the lesion to give rise to recurrent suppuration and subsequent bursting of the abscess at different times and different locations around the primary lesion (Figure 11.3).

The other rare predisposing condition in the formation of anal fistula includes a recent rectal surgery (rectal dilatation or myotomy) for anal imperforation or Hirschsprung's disease, severe neutropenia (due to cytotoxic chemotherapy or of malignant or autoimmune origin), HIV infection, Crohn's disease, ulcerative colitis, diabetic ketoacidosis, severe combined immune deficiency, septic granulomatosis, and juvenile polyarthritis treated with high-dose corticosteroids.

In a developing country like India, tuberculosis is another significant cause of anal suppuration and subsequent fistula formation.

It is estimated that about 45% patients with a perianal abscess are destined to develop anal fistula, and the incidence could further

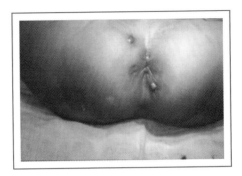

Figure 11.3 Multiple fistulae-in-ano.
Courtesy: Pravin Jaiprakash Gupta.

increase with the subsequent development of similar abscesses in
the surrounding region. Various modalities have been suggested in
the treatment of anal fistula in children including fistulectomy, use of
setons, and fibrin sealant. However, a simple lay open technique of
fistula tract (fistulotomy) is found to give satisfactory results with minimal complications like continence disorder, problems related to large
wounds, and possibility of a recurrence.

PERIANAL ABSCESS

A perianal abscess is not uncommonly found in neonates and children. Anal cryptitis seems to be the precipitating event that ends in
the formation of a perianal abscess (Figure 11.4). An abscess may
be associated with chronic fissure-in-ano or uncontrolled diabetes
mellitus in few patients. *Escherichia coli* and *Staphylococcus aureus*
are the commonly found organisms in the pus culture. Abscesses
are primarily saucerised, and fistulotomy and cryptotomy of the con-
fluent crypt are performed. Perianal abscess in infants is likely to be a
period-limited disorder and likely to resolve spontaneously over a period of one year. It is better to avoid or defer both fistulotomy and fistulectomy in infants. Drainage of the abscess by needle aspiration along
with antibiotics is effective in children younger than two years of age.

Thus, the primary treatment of perianal abscess in a child should
involve a careful search for a coexisting fistula and treatment of it
by fistulotomy. Treatment of perianal abscess by mere incision and
drainage is fraught with an unacceptably high recurrence rate, as
either fistula-in-ano or recurrence of abscess in older children.

It would appear that the transition to fistula after abscess formation
in children and infants, in particular, is low and, therefore, the need for
secondary surgery that places the sphincters at risk as well as seton
usage is less. In some of these patients, needle drainage and antibiotic
therapy alone may be sufficient, with secondary fistula surgery being
reserved for resistant cases. Others have suggested that a cut-off of
two years may define the fistula risk with actually a higher incidence of
fistulae in infants elder that two years of age, particularly in male children.

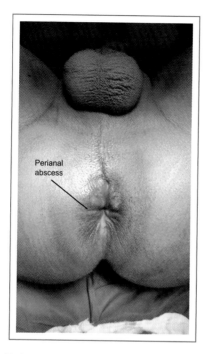

Figure 11.4 Perianal abscess.
Courtesy: Pravin Jaiprakash Gupta.

SINUSES AROUND ANUS

Though fistulae are the most common perianal discharging lesions in neonates and infants, blind sinuses are another cause in few of the patients. This blind sinus tract has a high bacterial yield of non-gut derived organisms on the culture of the pus or discharge. These perianal sinuses may be blind without an inner end or connection to the anal canal; few others have a different histological pattern. Complete surgical excision and primary closure of the wounds can cure these patients.

INFLAMMATORY BOWEL DISEASE

Ulcerative colitis and Crohn's disease are chronic intestinal inflammatory diseases that can present as bloody diarrhoea, abdominal pain, and malnutrition, and are capable of inducing disease-induced delays in linear growth or physical development. Twenty per cent of such patients present themselves during childhood or adolescence. The differences in drug dosage and the changes in social and cognitive development also occur as children move from the school-age years into adolescence and early adulthood.

Therefore, gastroenterologists caring for these children must plan an optimal regimen of pharmacologic therapies, psychological support, nutritional management, and properly timed surgery when necessary. This approach will also maintain disease remission, minimise disease-and-drug-induced adverse effects, and optimise growth and development.

For children, the presentation and natural history of perianal Crohn's disease (PACD) are different to that of adults, where the worldwide incidence is region-dependent ranging from 0.2–8.5 per 100,000 children, and where between 49% and 62% of children with known Crohn's disease will manifest significant PACD.

RECTAL BLEEDING OR HAEMATOCHEZIA

Rectal bleeding in children, though uncommon, is a significant complaint and an alarming event for the parents. Colorectal polyps should be considered as a first and commonest possible cause, but differential diagnosis is broad and includes allergic enteropathy, chronic inflammatory bowel disease, Meckel's diverticulum, intestinal obstruction (intussusception), anal fissure, trauma, infective enteritis, and congenital anomalies (duplication, malrotation). Intermittent but painless and fresh rectal bleeding is likely to be due to a polyp in the large bowel in a child who is well grown and not otherwise ill (Tables 11.1 and 11.2).

Fibreoptic colonoscopy and colonoscopic polypectomy are routinely practised in adults, and the introduction of these procedures in children now permits a similarly safe, efficient method to investigate the entire colon, with the possibility of immediate therapeutic polypectomy.

Table 11.1 Common causes of lower gastrointestinal bleeding in children

Age group	Causes
Neonates	Anal fissure (commonest) 40–70%
	Necrotizing enterocolitis
	Malrotation with volvulus
Infants aged one month to 1 year	Anal fissure (commonest) 60–77%
	Intussusception 10–35%
	Gangrenous bowel
	Milk protein allergy
Infants aged 1–2 years	Polyps (commonest) 60–70%
	Meckel diverticulum 22%
Children older than two years	Polyps (commonest) 65–77%
	Inflammatory bowel diseases 4–20%
	• CD
	• Ulcerative colitis
	• Indeterminate colitis
	• Infectious diarrhoea
	Vascular lesions
	• Haemangiomas
	• Arteriovenous malformations
	• Vasculitis
	Peutz–Jeghers syndrome
	Familial adenomatous polyposis (FAP)

Reproduced with permission from: PJ Gupta. Advanced grades of bleeding hemorrhoids in a young boy. *Eur Rev Med Pharmacol Sci*. 2007;11(2):129–32.

Table 11.2 Rare causes of lower gastrointestinal tract bleeding in children

- Haemorrhoids
- Lymphonodular hyperplasia
- Haemolytic uraemic syndrome
- Henoch-Schönlein purpura
- Cytomegalovirus (CMV) in HIV-infected child
- Solitary rectal ulcer
- Enteric fever
- Intestinal tuberculosis
- Amoebic ulcers

Reproduced with permission from: PJ Gupta. Advanced grades of bleeding hemorrhoids in a young boy. *Eur Rev Med Pharmacol Sci.* 2007;11(2):129–32.

The polyp can be located and removed safely and painlessly by colonoscopic polypectomy in an appropriately sedated child during the first, diagnostic examination.

DOCTOR'S ADVICE TO PARENTS

Perfect personal hygiene is obligatory. Always wash the rectal area after a bowel movement and dry it gently with a soft cotton towel. Vaseline® can be applied to the subject area to relieve the symptoms to some extent. If the symptoms are painful, you can use topical analgesics for temporary relief from the pain.

There are no safe and useful haemorrhoidal creams or ointments specific to children that are available. However, paediatric preparation of Ibuprofen is available over the counter and may help for both pain and inflammation. Leaving medication aside, warm sitz baths, given for 10 minutes at a time three times a day often bring great relief. The oatmeal powder can be added to the sitz bath for more soothing effects. If there is a perianal itch, plain cornstarch can be dusted over the area and into the child's diaper or underwear. Sitting on a towel-wrapped icepack for a few minutes can also help with the pain.

It is important to ensure that the child does not have any sensitivity or allergy to the current laundry soap or softeners being used. If unsure, use of hypoallergenic laundry detergent and softener is recommended. Exercise can be very beneficial; for a child, this means physical activity including playing.

CLINICAL PEARLS

- Children, simply as adults, have almost customary anorectal problems that can be fairly bothersome.

(Cont'd)

- The presentation of these problem could also be unique to their ages.
- Abscesses, fistulas, and fissures show up more regularly in infants and small children, whereas haemorrhoids and pilonidal diseases are prevalent in teens and young adults.
- Most of the fissures can be dealt with conservative therapy and very rarely require surgical intervention.
- Abscesses and fistulas are common in the young ones, especially, toddlers who have breastfed. About two-thirds of them can be managed with conservation, and anal fistulotomy is indicated in case of failure of medical treatment.
- Haemorrhoids are infrequent in young children; however, they could be an issue in the teens. Acute symptomatic lesions may just require excision if local measures cannot manage the symptoms.
- The role of weight loss plan, toileting habits, routine exercises, personal hygiene, and religious follow-up with the treating clinician can achieve the goal.

SUGGESTED READINGS

Burt R, Neklason DW. Genetic testing for inherited colon cancer. *Gastroenterology*. 2005;128:1696–716.

Corredor J, Wambach J, Barnard J. Gastrointestinal polyps in children: Advances advances in molecular genetics, diagnosis, and management. *J Pediatr*. 2001;138:621–8.

Doig CM. ABC of colorectal diseases. Paediatric problems–I. *Brit J Med*. 1992;305(6851):462–4.

Evans DA. Lateral subcutaneous sphincterotomy for treatment of anal fissure in children. *Br J Surg*. 1996;83(4):571.

Giardiello FM, Hamilton SR, Kern SE, et al. Colorectal neoplasia in juvenile polyposis or juvenile polyps. *Arch Dis Child*. 1991;66:971–5.

Gourgiotis S, Baratsis S. Rectal prolapse. *Int J Colorectal Dis*. 2007;22(3): 231–43.

Gupta PJ. Advanced grades of bleeding hemorrhoids in a young boy. *Eur Rev Med Pharmacol Sci*. 2007;11(2):129–32.

Jass JR, Williams CB, Bussey HJ, Morson BC. Juvenile polyposis—a prepre-cancerous condition. *Histopathology*. 1988;13:619–30.

Lambe GF, Driver CP, Morton S, Turnock RR. Fissurectomy as a treatment for anal fissures in children. *Ann R Coll Surg Engl*. 2000;82(4):254–7.

Nugent KP, Talbot IC, Hodgson SV, Phillips RK. Solitary juvenile polyps: Not not a marker for subsequent malignancy. *Gastroenterology*. 1993; 105:698–700.

O'Connor JJ. Pediatric proctology. *Dis Colon Rectum*. 1975;18(2): 126–127.

Schreibman IR, Baker M, Amos C, McGarrity TJ. The hamartomatous polyposis syndromes: A a clinical and molecular review. *Am J Gastroenterol*. 2005;100:476–90.

Wu JS. Rectal prolapse: a historical perspective. *Curr Probl Surg*. 2009; 46(8):602–716.

Chapter 12

Proctology in ante- and postpartum period

Women often experience different anorectal symptoms during their pregnancy, or immediately after the delivery. The common problems include haemorrhoidal disease, anal fissure, and dyschezia. Inflammatory diseases and abscess formation are relatively rare during pregnancy. Consequent pregnancies have a tendency to aggravate the previous anorectal ailment and expand the incapacity and bleakness for the mother. These patients are also susceptible to anal thrombosis, strangulation, and ulceration.

There is no unanimity among obstetricians, proctologists, and others about the most efficient management of these anorectal complications affecting the normal course of pregnancy. It is, in any case, shrewd that a more extensive methodology ought to be received to handle these lesions, as the agony from these anorectal conditions is regularly far more prominent than the inconvenience of the pregnancy itself.

HORMONAL, ANATOMICAL, AND PHYSIOLOGICAL PELVIC CHANGES

It is now established that during pregnancy and in the postpartum period, few anatomical, hormonal, and physiological changes take place in the pelvis. The shifts in the levels of oestrogen, progesterone, gonadotropins, corticosteroids, thyroid function, and proteins are quite remarkable.

Pregnancy and vaginal delivery predispose women to develop haemorrhoids relatable to these hormonal changes and due to increase in intra-abdominal pressure. It has been evaluated that around 25–35% of pregnant ladies are influenced by this condition. There is anorectal vascular dilatation and enlargement along with the laxity of the peri-anorectal structures. Similarly, the increases in the intra-pelvic pressure during labour is also an important secondary factor in the causation of haemorrhoids before and during childbirth, while these effects being most prominent during the final trimester. Mucosal piles, often seen associated with pregnancy and with older people, appear to consist mainly of thickened mucous membrane only.

The precipitating factors include an irregular diet, lack of exercise, pushing off the bowel to the periphery by the enlarged uterus, and release of the hormone 'relaxin'. All these contribute to constipation and straining during or after pregnancy. Third-trimester symptomatology is commonest when venous engorgement is greatest in the pelvis and when dehydration may lead to relative constipation with most of the symptoms alleviating after delivery.

Besides these anatomical and physiological changes in the pelvis during gestation, there is an increase in the elasticity of the perianal, anorectal, and recto-pelvic structures; hypertrophy of the sphincters and pelvic muscles is present, and the blood vessels become dilated and hypertrophied; the vascular structure is enlarged and congested. The blood volume goes up to 25% above its average level and it remains at the higher level until childbirth, decreasing rapidly to near normal towards the tenth day after labour. If these changes were not present, the anorectal tissues would have been significantly damaged during delivery.

The anorectal vascular dilatation and enlargement and the laxity of the peri-anorectal structures, as well as the increased intra-pelvic pressure during labour, are important secondary factors in the causation of various anal lesions before and during childbirth.

SYMPTOMATOLOGY OF ANORECTAL LESIONS DURING ACTIVE MOTHERHOOD

Anorectal symptoms are reported in both antepartum and post-partum periods. Straining to defecate, hard or lumpy stools, incomplete emptying, uncontrolled loss of gas or stool from the rectum, unpreventable soilage of underwear, and pain and bleeding from the anus are the most common complaints. Haemorrhoids become symptomatic when the external haemorrhoidal veins become varicose, which causes itching, burning, painful swellings at the anus, dyschezia, and bleeding. Many women recall postpartum haemorrhoidal symptoms as their worst nightmare. However, symptoms in most of them are mild and transient and include intermittent bleeding per rectum and pain. Depending on the intensity of pain, quality of life could be affected, varying from mild discomfort to real difficulty in dealing with the day-to-day activities. Pain during defecation and haematochezia are often the first signs of haemorrhoids.

Dyschezic symptoms are most frequently reported in the first trimester and anal incontinence most often in the third quarter while the loss of gas or stool is more in the postpartum period. Anal incontinence is more frequent in women who delivered by forceps.

HAEMORRHOIDS

Pregnancy and the puerperium predispose to symptomatic haemorrhoids being the most common anorectal disease at these times. Symptoms are often mild and transient and include intermittent bleeding from the anus along with pain. Most of the haemorrhoidal diseases in pregnancy are underestimated by obstetricians, often precluding patient access to possible medical and surgical or rehabilitative treatments designed to relieve eventual dysfunction related to the delivery. In this regard, it has been noticed that haemorrhoids affect about 25–35% of pregnant women with symptoms presenting most commonly in the second and third trimesters. The worst symptoms are usually noticed in the third trimester, which is the period of greatest pelvic pressure with associated periods of constipation and dehydration. Acute haemorrhoidal crisis can also occur with irreducible prolapse, thrombosis, and protracted pain along with external haemorrhoidal thrombosis.

Treatment during pregnancy is mainly directed at the relief of symptoms, especially pain control. Laxative treatment for patients with dyschezia during childbirth and the postpartum period significantly decreases the occurrence of anal lesions in the postpartum period. The conservative management comprises of dietary modifications, stimulants, or depressants of the bowel transit, local treatment, and phlebotonics. For most of the women, symptoms will resolve spontaneously immediately after the childbirth and so any corrective treatment is usually deferred although literature has reported a successful haemorrhoidectomy during pregnancy. Most forms of the haemorrhoids can be successfully treated by increasing the fibre content, administering stool softeners, increasing liquid intake, anti-haemorrhoidal medications, analgesics, and training in toilet habits.

The ideal approach is a cold sitz bath or mopping with cotton-wool pledgets and reduction of the prolapsed haemorrhoids in case it happens. Some women prefer natural and herbal approaches where relief may be obtained with oral rutosides, disodium flavodate, French maritime pine bark extract, hidrosmine, *Centella asiatica*, or grape seed extract, each of which can decrease capillary fragility and improve the micro-circulation in venous insufficiency disorders.

Although the treatment with oral flavonoids looks promising for symptom relief in first- and second-degree haemorrhoids, its blind usage cannot be recommended until new evidence reassures women and their clinicians about their safety. More aggressive therapies used in other haemorrhoidal disease are reserved for patients who have persistent symptoms after one month of conservative treatment either during pregnancy or in the postpartum period, although in the latter situation, it should be delayed for at least three months if possible. Once the real haemorrhoidal disease develops, correction should be performed before a subsequent pregnancy.

The acute haemorrhoidal crisis should have a short period of conservatism in pregnancy before a decision to operate is taken in case of persistence or development of a complication. The surgery has a septic risk, and the aim should be directed at removing only the symptomatic, complicated, or gangrenous area. Nonetheless, it is important to note that haemorrhoids are not the only cause of rectal bleeding in pregnancy and that the physician should accurately confirm the diagnosis and exclude other colonic causes where appropriate before initiating any treatment.

The thrombosed external haemorrhoids during pregnancy should be treated as for the non-pregnant population. Risk factors such as traumatic and late delivery, delivery of a large baby, and a prolonged first stage of labour are quite common during and immediately after the pregnancy; these always result in disabling situations and are many times accompanied by complications that may require surgical intervention.

More aggressive approaches like sclerotherapy, rubber banding, and infrared photocoagulation are saved for those subjects who have persistent symptoms after one month of conservative treatment. A few recent studies have shown the efficacy of botulinum toxin injections as a treatment for chronic anal fissure and haemorrhoids. However, due to its various mechanism of action, botulinum toxin is contraindicated during pregnancy and lactation.

Topical treatment with analgesics and anti-inflammatory medication does provide a short-term local relief from discomfort, pain, and bleeding. As used in small doses and with a limited systemic absorption, the pregnant women can use them with caution as the safety of any of them in pregnancy has not been adequately documented.

Most topical preparations for haemorrhoids are available over-the-counter. They often contain anaesthetics, anti-inflammatory, and corticosteroids in varying proportions. The majority of these products help to maintain personal hygiene and alleviate symptoms.

A real symptomatic haemorrhoidal disease, however, is relatively uncommon, but is more permanent and will need corrective treatment to prevent early complications and late aggravation. Advanced rectal and colonic problems demand endoscopic and other sophisticated investigation irrespective of the pregnancy. Clinical experience and studies have hinted that extreme conservatism in the treatment of severe complicated haemorrhoidal disease during pregnancy is unwarranted.

Once the real haemorrhoidal disease develops, correction should be done before a subsequent pregnancy to avoid later increased aggravation and morbidity. Lactation, strain, constipation, and diarrhoea merely act as trigger mechanisms to aggravate the pre-existing state. It is strongly advised that a prophylactic haemorrhoidectomy should be performed before a succeeding pregnancy whenever unresolved symptomatic disease had developed.

Extensive, symptomatic, unmanageable, and prolapsing internal haemorrhoids that have not responded to conservation and which are repeatedly interfering with a smooth course of pregnancy must be removed during the second trimester under necessary anaesthesia only after proctologic consultation and agreement of the parent couple. There is a possibility of thrombosis, strangulation, or ulceration in the third trimester or during parturition and corrective measures are required to be taken when these add to the morbidity to the mother. Profusely bleeding internal haemorrhoids can be treated during pregnancy by various sclerosing injections.

For thrombosed, prolapsed haemorrhoids (Figure 12.1), a semi-closed haemorrhoidectomy can be done. All the patients are instructed to exercise the anorectal sphincters and levator ani muscles after surgery to promote healing; these also help to prevent oedema and improve tonicity. Routine post-operative care is observed in these women.

It is imperative to note that haemorrhoids are not the only reason of haematochezia, and the physician should accurately confirm the diagnosis before the commencement of any treatment.

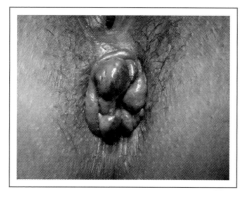

Figure 12.1 Prolapsed and thrombosed haemorrhoids.
Courtesy: Pravin Jaiprakash Gupta.

External Haemorrhoidal Thrombosis

External haemorrhoids usually develop over time and may result from straining with stools or childbirth. Traumatic delivery is known to be associated with thrombosed external haemorrhoids. External haemorrhoids represent distended vascular tissue in the anal canal distal to the dentate line. External haemorrhoids are covered by anoderm and skin that are richly innervated with somatic pain fibres. Lesions affecting the anal canal or the external haemorrhoidal vessels can be extremely painful.

External haemorrhoids can develop in pregnant women and may suddenly become thrombosed (Figure 12.2). Persons with thrombosed external haemorrhoids usually present with pain while standing, sitting, or defecating. The body slowly absorbs the thrombosis over several weeks. During resolution, the thrombus

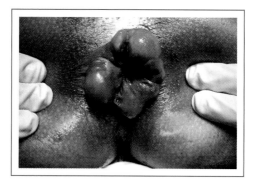

Figure 12.2 External haemorrhoidal thrombosis.
Courtesy: Pravin Jaiprakash Gupta.

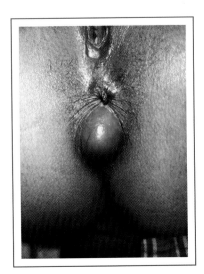

Figure 12.3 Perianal thrombosis or haematoma.

Courtesy: Pravin Jaiprakash Gupta.

may erode through the skin and can produce bleeding or may drain out slowly.

Acutely inflamed thrombosed external haemorrhoids can be surgically removed within the first 72 hours after onset. However, after that, the discomfort of the procedure is more than the relief provided by the procedure itself. Few patients still chose to undergo late surgery, although they should understand that even without surgery haemorrhoid would get fibrosed and resolve over a period of few days to weeks.

After making an elliptical incision over the thrombotic mass, the thrombus together with the complete offending haemorrhoidal plexus should be excised. It is wise to leave the site open; few physicians prefer to place 2–3 subcutaneous sutures aiming to limit postoperative pain and bleeding. Suturing in this area should better be avoided for the fear of complications since the rich vascularity in the anal tissues usually provides rapid healing.

A direct incision over a thrombus (Figure 12.3) under local anaesthesia just to squeeze out the clot has been fraught with a significant rate of rethrombosis. Experts now recommend excision of the entire thrombotic mass and the external haemorrhoidal vessels underneath. This process is more extensive than simple incision, but usually yields a better outcome.

ANAL FISSURE

One-third of females suffers from few symptoms of anal fissures in the antepartum and postpartum periods (Figure 12.4). The most important risk factor is dyschezia. The fissure can also occur due to precipitated labour, large foetus, episiotomy, and perineotomy. The

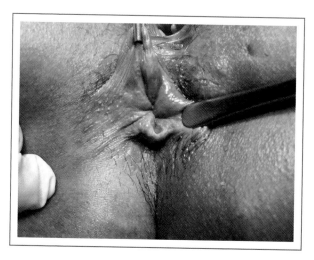

Figure 12.4 Anal fissure.
Courtesy: Pravin Jaiprakash Gupta.

conservative treatment of anal fissures can begin with local treatment by different means, which include the arrest of the pain syndrome by analgesics, local anaesthetic or diltiazem ointment, dietary regulation, and prevention of constipation. Long-term results are good. An anal sphincter hypertonia is commonly thought to be the source of anal fissure; however, in the anal fissure that is common after childbirth, the anal canal pressure is lower than normal. This paradox is not understood. Also, as puerperal anal fissures are associated with reduced anal canal pressures; thus, any surgical manipulation of the anal sphincter mechanism should be avoided.

OTHER ANORECTAL LESIONS IN PREGNANCY

Incontinence and difficult defecation are commonly reported among women and often ascribed to traumas sustained during childbirth; specifically, injuries to the anal sphincters and other structures that comprise the pelvic floor. These have been recognised as a significant contributor to the development of anal incontinence, or difficult defecation in later life. It is apparent that pregnancy forces changes, essentially through hormonal impacts, on colonic, anorectal, and pelvic floor physiology. Anorectal problems of vaginal delivery could be as anal fissure, anorectal abscess, sphincteric injury, and recto-vaginal fistula. Surgical correction of these complications results in a satisfactory outcome. Vaginal delivery and nulliparity are known risk factors for anal sphincter injury; especially, if vacuum or forceps are used.

Vaginal delivery is associated with reduced anal pressures and increased anal sphincter trauma; however, it has no effect on anal sensation. As there is an established association between sphincteric muscular damage and anal incontinence, all the patients should be informed about the risk of anal sphincter injury during operative vaginal delivery. It is prudent to follow such patients closely in the postpartum period to affirm any occurrence of potential anorectal complaints.

Different hormonal, physiologic, and anatomic changes, prone to create a relative increase in the haemorrhoidal pathophysiology, also decrease the incidence of inflammatory anorectal disease in the pregnant woman. Anal fissure, cryptitis, and papillitis are seen in the first trimester of pregnancy. Symptomatic care and improvement in bowel function are usually effective measures at this stage. The increase in vascular congestion and circulation prevents anorectal abscess and fistula formation during pregnancy. Still, if abscess should occur, incision and drainage should be done immediately. Subsequent formation of fistulas can be treated after the postpartum period.

Colorectal polyps, malignant neoplasia, and ulcerative colitis are rarely present during pregnancy. These conditions do not have any direct correlation with pregnancy and should always be treated on an individual basis. If a diagnostic problem exists concerning a severe rectal or colonic disease, a careful proctosigmoidoscopic study is safe and invariably be performed. Delay in diagnosing polypoid rectal disease or malignant growth could result in an incurable lesion.

It is imperative that obstetricians should pay due attention to the anorectal symptoms of their patients because the apparently insignificant lesions may result in complications and cause much physical and mental suffering.

CLINICAL PEARLS

- The commonly occurring pathologies during pregnancy include haemorrhoids, fissures, and thrombosed haemorrhoids.
- The management during pregnancy is usually limited to emergency care, consisting of palliation for symptomatic prolapsing internal haemorrhoids, evacuation, or excision of external anal thromboses and drainage of the perianal abscess.
- Haemorrhoids in pregnancy ought to be dealt with by expanding fibre content in the foods, softening the stools, enhancing fluid consumption, and toilet training.
- It is normal that these preservationist measures can ease the sufferings in many patients. If required, patients ought to get topical treatment.
- For numerous females, most of these symptoms will resolve on their own after parturition, and just a couple cases will require a surgical assessment amid pregnancy or in the postpartum period.
- The patient has to have a frank discussion with her physician about the pros and cons of operative and non-operative approaches, which can result in either therapeutic abortion or timely surgery versus preserving the foetus and taking on the unknown factor of whether the delay in treatment will cause an adverse outcome.

SUGGESTED READINGS

Abramowitz L, Batallan A. Epidemiology of anal lesions (fissure and thrombosed external hemorroid) during pregnancy and postpartum. *Gynecol Obstet Fertil*. 2003;31(6):546–9.

Abramowitz L, Benabderrhamane D, Philip J, Pospait D, Bonin N, Merrouche M. Hemorrhoidal disease in pregnancy. *Presse Med*. 2011; 40(10):955–9.

Abramowitz L, Sobhani I, Benifla JL, et al. Anal fissure and thrombosed external hemorrhoids before and after delivery. *Dis Colon Rectum*. 2002;45(5):650–5.

Abramowitz L, Sobhani I. Anal complications of pregnancy and delivery. *Gastroenterol Clin Biol*. 2003;27:77–83.

Avsar AF, Keskin HL. Haemorrhoids during pregnancy. *J Obstet Gynaecol*. 2010;30:231–7.

Medich DS, Fazio VW. Hemorrhoids, anal fissure, and carcinoma of the colon, rectum, and anus during pregnancy. *Surg Clin North Am*. 1995; 75:77–88.

Poskus T, Buzinskienė D, Drasutiene G, et al. Haemorrhoids and anal fissures during pregnancy and after childbirth: a prospective cohort study. *Br J Obstet Gynaecol*. 2014;121(13):1666–71.

Quigley EM. Impact of pregnancy and parturition on the anal sphincters and pelvic floor. *Best Pract Res Clin Gastroenterol*. 2007;21(5): 879–91.

Saleeby RG, Jr, Rosen L, Stasik JJ, et al. Acute anal fissures in puerperants. *Vestn Khir Im I I Grek*. 1999;158(4):80–3.

Saleeby RG Jr, Rosen L, Stasik JJ, et al. Hemorrhoidectomy during pregnancy: risk or relief? *Dis Colon Rectum*. 1991;34:260–1.

Wiseman OJ, Hombergh U, Koldewijn EL, et al. Sacral neuromodulation and pregnancy. *J Urol*. 2002;167:165–8.

Chapter 13

Anorectal problems in the elderly

Older people are at increased risk of colonic and anorectal problems, some of which occur in patients of all ages. Anorectal ailments like anal fissures, haemorrhoids, and anorectal abscesses are not unusual in the older population. These conditions, along with problems such as incontinence, rectal prolapse, and pruritus ani, cause tremendous morbidity and suffering. The key to diagnosis is primarily based on the patient history and confirmation via visible inspection and anoscopy. Expensive investigations are typically not required. The majority of those anorectal complaints can be easily controlled within the outpatient clinic by using dietary changes and comparatively minor and straightforward procedures. Patients having more advanced disease would require referral for surgical treatment. Although unusual, malignancies do arise in the anorectal region, and lesions that cannot be diagnosed by inspection have to be biopsied.

BOWEL COMPLAINTS

Bowel-related problems have a full-size effect on the quality of life in older people; in addition, these problems have many contributory reasons that are commonly amenable to treatment and control. Consequences of treatment, both conservative and surgical as appropriate, are convincing, leading to the alleviation of suffering and ability to enjoy a normal life. Most of the aged patients have a regular bowel activity, but their use of laxatives is accelerated.

CONSTIPATION

Dyschezia is the primary colorectal abnormality, mainly for people with mobility issues. Other contributory physiological problems in bowel dysfunction encompass reduced colonic propulsion, difficulty in defecating, and impaired rectal sensation. The entire gut-transit time does not appear to change with age; however, it has been observed to be extended (longer than 14 days) in immobile constipated patients.

The occurrence of constipation goes on increasing with growing age; specifically, after the age of 65 years. There are variable statistics on the age-related physiological modifications inside the colonic and anorectal characteristic; however, indeed, the anal sphincter pressures are reduced in old age even though the colonic transit time does not appear like altered.

Neurological illnesses, constipating drugs, bedridden conditions, and weak straining capacity are a few common causes of constipation. The amount of nutritional fibre within the weight loss programme is significantly reduced because of inadequate chewing potential. Parkinson's ailment is related to gradual colonic transit and impaired anal sphincter relaxation. Drug-induced constipation most possibly arises with anti-parkinsonism drugs (either anticholinergic or dopaminergic) and with tricyclic anti-depressants, iron, anticonvulsants, opiates, and aluminium- or calcium-containing antacids.

Constipation is often associated with 'faecal impaction' in aged people. The term 'faecal impaction' has historically indicated loading of the rectum with hard faeces. Many elderly patients have significant faecal loading with smooth or even liquid faeces, and they are much more likely to experience faecal soiling. Faecal incontinence is a distressing issue that is usually because of a combination of multiple factors in elderly people and is almost always related to urinary incontinence.

DIARRHOEA

Faecal incontinence can be the presenting characteristic of colorectal ailment causing diarrhoea; in particular, infective diarrhoea, colorectal carcinoma, inflammatory bowel disease, ischaemic colitis, diverticular disease, or the result of medicine (especially, long-term consumption of laxatives).

FAECAL INCONTINENCE

Numerous changes in anorectal function arise with growing age, which might also account for the increased risk of faecal incontinence in elderly people.

External Sphincter Weakness

The strength of contraction of the external anal sphincter muscle reduces with age. It can arise due to denervation, but does not appear to be caused by distal pudendal neuropathy. Though the age-related weakness and lack of the muscle's reflex act may additionally render sufferers liable to growing faecal incontinence, the latter does now appear to be associated with the degree of weakness. External sphincter pressures in lots of continent elderly persons are much like those recorded in younger incontinent patients. The resulting rectal distension results in relaxation of the internal sphincter and subsequent faecal soiling. The condition may be neglected though the right diagnosis is relatively easy, being made with a digital rectal examination.

Internal Sphincter Weakness

Anal resting pressure due to internal anal sphincter activity does not seem to alternate with age, but is appreciably reduced in patients with faecal incontinence regardless of age. Reduced anal resting pressure is one of the important factors leading to faecal incontinence in aged humans.

Anal Sensory Impairment

Anal sensation is decreased within the aged, with an extra degree of sensory loss amongst incontinent patients.

Faecal incontinence is a drastically unreported issue that has a devastating impact on the social and personal lifestyles of the sufferer in addition to their spouses and caretakers. There are the following three main categories of faecal incontinence in the elderly:

- Reservoir incontinence
- Overflow incontinence
- Rectosphincteric incontinence

The first two may be recognised by way of the patient's records and physical exam and the response to numerous nutritional and pharmacological interventions. The third one is assessed via a complete physical examination supplemented by diagnostic assessments directed towards the evaluation of anorectal continence function. The most crucial and easiest of most of these is anorectal manometry, which may be supported via anal ultrasonography or pelvic floor MRI and neuromuscular function just like the electromyogram.

A complete medical history and physical examination, information of the past clinical records, and evaluation of the situations in which symptoms of the intestinal disorder develop permit the intelligent direction of the scientific evaluation. Direct visualisation of the colorectal mucosa using fibre optic or video endoscopes frequently offers a prompt and accurate diagnosis and enables therapeutic intervention. Other ailments require radiological analysis and treatment or surgical intervention.

Treatment

The successful management of constipation in aged sufferers requires a know-how of colorectal characteristic, cautious evaluation of the affected person's grievance, and in few patients, a specialised research of colonic and anorectal function. The reasons for constipation in elderly are often multifactorial which comprise a state of reduced activity, melancholy and confusion, irrelevant diet, different medications, and neuromuscular diseases. The control of chronic constipation ought to be aimed towards the nature of the complaint and the pathophysiological mechanisms at work in each affected person. Treatment will rely upon one or more strategies along with dietary changes, laxatives, and in carefully described cases, surgical treatment.

When faecal incontinence is because of faecal impaction, the initial treatment is to empty the rectum and colon from below by way of the use of enemas or suppositories each day till the faecal mass is cleared. Laxatives or stool softeners have a tendency to be unsuccessful because many of those sufferers have impaction with even soft stools. Additional softening tends simplest to raise the frequency of incontinence.

At times, manual removal of faeces is required for patients impacted with very hardened faeces. Some patients with intense spinal cord lesions require manual evacuations twice weekly while all other treatments have failed. The rectum ought to be kept empty to prevent the recurrence of constipation. Numerous remedies, such as increased dietary fibre, are on trial. An affiliation has been shown, however, among high dietary fibre intake and colonic faecal loading in the bedridden elderly patients. It is therefore not useful to propose improved dietary fibre as a routine, as this will upload to faecal impaction and increase the possibility of faecal incontinence. If the stool is soft, laxatives need to be used (for instance, Senna). Osmotic laxatives (like lactulose) are used when the patients complain of hard stools. Once in a while, a mixed osmotic and stimulant laxative (for instance, co-danthrusate) is used.

A battery of therapeutic interventions is employed in patients with rectosphincteric incontinence; these include dietary, behavioural, pharmacological, and surgical interventions which might be based totally on the results of the diagnostic evaluation. For an isolated weakness of the internal anal sphincter, a cotton barrier in the anal canal is often pretty useful. Sphincter injury is treated with sphincteroplasty; however, those surgical approaches are of theoretical advantage. Peripheral neurogenic incontinence can be dealt with using anti-diarrhoeal medicines, bio-feedback techniques, and nutritional manipulations. Sacral spinal nerve stimulation is an emerging new method for few patients with neurogenic faecal incontinence and is presently being tested in different specialised centres. Significant modifications in the quality of life may be executed in most aged individuals with faecal incontinence.

LOWER GASTROINTESTINAL HAEMORRHAGE

Lower gastrointestinal bleeding is one of the common medical emergencies which can emerge as life-threatening in elderly sufferers. Internal haemorrhoids, diverticular bleeding, angiodysplasia, polyps, cancer, drug-induced (anti-coagulants, non-steroidal anti-inflammatory medications) lesions, ischaemic colitis, ulcerative colitis, solitary rectal ulcer, Crohn's disease, and colonic varices are the few causes to be cited. Increased prevalence of malignancy, polypharmacy, cerebro vascular and cardiovascular illnesses, and the use of nonsteroidal anti-inflammatory medications in aged sufferers adversely affect the outcome of bleeding.

Treatment

In a majority of instances, the bleeding stops spontaneously with resuscitation and supportive therapy. In those aged sufferers in whom bleeding is persistent, advantages of various endoscopic, angiographic, or surgical interventions should not be deferred simply because of their age. However, the timing of tests and the type of intervention should be custom tailored to the frail aged patient. The choice should depend completely on functional status, its impact on the final results, and the consent procedure.

COLORECTAL MALIGNANCY

It is important that a physician has to comprehend the gross modifications in the patterns of medical presentation of colonic or rectal neoplasia consisting of rectal bleeding, iron deficiency anaemia, alteration in bowel habit, and unexpected and unexplained weight reduction. Any affected person above 45 years of age coming with rectal bleeding needs to be evaluated with colonoscopy. In patients, while a colorectal neoplasm has been diagnosed, preoperative workup and counselling are of considerable importance. Primary treatment of colorectal cancers is resection and adjuvant chemotherapy. Patients with rectal tumours have a higher risk of complications of surgery and local recurrence than people with colonic tumours. Those with node-positive cancer are at enormous risk for recurrence, regardless of most efficient surgical treatment and elimination of the primary tumour. All such patients need to be provided with the benefits of early endoscopy and therapeutic interventions unless there are contraindications to the advance directives. Patient's advanced age should never be a deterrent to any of the diagnostic or therapeutic interventions.

CLINICAL PEARLS

- Diarrhoeal states tend to cause faecal incontinence in the elderly and constipation is commoner in immobile institutionalised elderly patients.
- The management of dyschezia incorporates the treatment of the basic cause and the clearing of the gut utilising bowel purges and suppositories given rectally and oral stool softening medicines.
- The neurological reasons for faecal incontinence might be local or all the more normally cortical. Conscious constipation and planned evacuation of the rectum may diminish the recurrence of faecal incontinence.
- Haemorrhoidal thrombosis, rectal mucosal prolapse, and pruritus should be dealt with a conservative approach or minimum possible surgical interventions.
- The potential risks of anaesthetic and surgical complications may be carefully weighed against the benefits of the surgical procedures.

SUGGESTED READINGS

Belsey J, Greenfield S, Candy D, et al. Systematic review: impact of constipation on quality of life in adults and children. *Aliment Pharmacol Ther*. 2010;31(9):938–49.

Camilleri M, Cowen T, Koch TR. Enteric neurodegeneration in ageing. *Neurogastroenterol Motil*. 2008;20(3):185–96.

Campion EW. The oldest old. *N Engl J Med*. 1994;330(25):1819–20.

Goode PS, Burgio KL, Halli AD, et al. Prevalence and correlates of faecal incontinence in community-dwelling older adults. *J Am Geriatr Soc*. 2005;53(4): 629–35.

Rao SS, Sadeghi P, Beaty J, et al. Ambulatory 24-h colonic manometry in healthy humans. *Am J Physiol Gastrointest Liver Physiol*. 2001; 280(4):G629–39.

Rao SS, Sadeghi P, Beaty J, et al. Ambulatory 24-hour colonic manometry in slow-transit constipation. *Am J Gastroenterol.* 2004;99(12):2405–16.

Rao SS. Diagnosis and management of fecal incontinence. American College of Gastroenterology Practice Parameters Committee. *Am J Gastroenterol.* 2004;99(8):1585–604.

Santos-Eggimann B, Cirilli NC, Monachon JJ. Frequency and determinants of urgent requests to home care agencies for community-dwelling elderly. *Home Health Care Serv Q.* 2003;22(1):39–53.

Schouten W, Gordon PH. Physiology. In: *Principles and Practice of Surgery for the Colon, Rectum, and Anus.* Gordon PH (ed.). New York, London: Informa Healthcare; 2007.

Schuster M, Mendeloff AJ. Characteristics of rectosigmoid motor function, Their relationship to continence, defecation, and disease. In: *Progress in Gastroenterology.* Glass C (ed.). New York: Grune & Stratton; 1970.

Chapter 14

Pilonidal sinus disease

Pilonidal disease is a disease of young adults, which can result in an abscess, draining sinus tracts, and moderate debility for some. It is a little mysterious why the management of the pilonidal disease has become the purview of the coloproctologist. The vast majority of the illness occurs in the natal cleft where its management has been somewhat controversial given the comparatively high rate of recurrence even with relatively radical procedures. Although quite rare after 45 years of age, most colorectal surgeons can recall seeing such patients in their practice. The exact incidence of the pilonidal sinus is unknown where data is limited. There is no racial predilection although it is intuitively more frequent in those with darker and stiffer hair and hirsute patients. It is rare in African-Americans and Africans and almost non-existent in Asian populations. It probably results from hair penetration beneath the skin, for reasons that are not very clear. Several surgical procedures have been proposed. However, no clear consensus as to the optimal treatment has been reported. Management has to be tailored according to the individual and depends on whether the disease is acute or chronic.

BACKGROUND

The pilonidal disease constitutes a group of entities spreading between asymptomatic hair containing cysts and sinuses to a large abscess most commonly located in the sacrococcygeal area. Although debated, the condition of the pilonidal sinus was most likely first described by Mayo in 1833 with Hodges coining the term 'Pilonidal' (where *pilus* in Latin means hair and *nidus* means nest) in 1880. In the intergluteal cleft, it is predominantly a disease of males (>80% of cases) with a peak incidence between the ages of 15–24 years and after that decreasing in incidence with increasing age.

PATHOPHYSIOLOGY

The debate concerning the aetiology and pathogenesis of the pilonidal sinus is something that can be found in most of the older colorectal textbooks. However, it is little addressed in the most recent literature that has focused more on novel surgical techniques.

The big debate in its etiopathogenesis is the 'congenital-acquired' argument, with most accepting that pilonidal sinus is an acquired disorder. Early on in the twentieth century, a lot of the literature focused on comparative anatomical dissections to explain an embryological origin. It was recognised relatively early on and in spite of a series of rather complex embryological theories that the high incidence of recurrence after wide soft-tissue excision along with the failure to demonstrate follicles and glands within cyst walls suggested that pilonidal sinus was probably an acquired condition. The original basic theory which is mostly adhered to some or other degree of an acquired condition was postulated by David H. Patey and R.W. Scarff, who proposed that hairs were sucked into the skin of the natal cleft similar to other sites (such as the hands of barbers). This resulted in a chronic foreign body granulomatous reaction. This process is the aetiology behind most of the disease with only rare elements arising from developmental anomalies of the lower spinal region. This would go along with the almost universal finding of the presence of coarse hairs in pilonidal sinuses and foreign-body style granulomata. The theory places no distinction between the origins of the hairs (which could be local or distant), but suggests that hair movement causes a drilling effect in the region of the natal cleft to form hair bundles that efficiently drill their way obliquely and cephalad through the skin. This is likely to be supplemented by a post-sacral suction mechanism particularly when sitting, which lifts the soft tissues off the sacrococcygeal fascia.

However, these hair follicles enter the subcutaneous tissues; mostly, the entry is in the midline where there is a dilatation of the orifices of the follicles particularly during adolescence and a stretching of the region due to powerful gluteal function. This is supplemented by an inflammatory reaction and exacerbated by friction with the clothes, desquamation of the epidermal cells, and maceration with faecal material. It had been postulated that the natural morphology of hairs propels them upwards and inwards and that hair tufts naturally lay laterally setting up lateral inflammatory sinuses where the small midline pits are no more than the distorted hair follicles. The high number of US Army personnel treated for pilonidal sinus during World War II resulted in the term 'jeep disease' as part of the acquired theory of prolonged sitting and jostling in vehicles as a potential cause.

These points paved the way for the modern-day acceptance of the acquired theory of pilonidal cysts. The acquired theory postulates that pilonidal disease is a result of hair and cellular debris finding a route of entry into the skin and hair follicles. The entering hair causes an inflammatory reaction and oedema. This reaction forms multiple micro abscesses that eventually migrate further into the subcutaneous tissue. A vacuum force created by the touting of skin when the patient bends over is believed to aid in the hair migration. Such abscesses eventually result in the creation of more sinus tracts and abscesses. At surgery, however, only 50–75% of all pilonidal cysts were found to contain hair in them (Figure 14.1).

Apart from the sacrococcygeal region, pilonidal sinus has been reported in the hands of hairdressers and barbers in the interdigital clefts as well as in sheep shearers, cow milkers, dog groomers, and even slaughterhouse workers. The disease has also been described not uncommonly in the umbilicus as well as in the chest wall, the anal canal itself, the ear, and the scalp. Other particularly unusual sites for the histological and clinical appearance of pilonidal sinus include the axilla, the perineum after abdominoperineal excision, the interdigital region of the foot, the penis, and old major amputation sites.

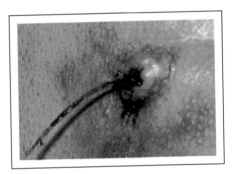

Figure 14.1   A tuft of hair protruding from pilonidal sinus.

Courtesy: Pravin Jaiprakash Gupta.

AETIOLOGY

The pilonidal disease involves loose hair and skin and perineal flora. Risk factors for the pilonidal disease include male gender, hirsute individuals, Caucasians, sitting occupations, presence of a deep natal cleft, and abundance of hair within the natal cleft. Family history is seen in 38% of patients with this disease. Obesity is another risk factor for the recurrent disease.

The pilonidal disease has a male preponderance in the general population. The ratio is three or four men per woman. In children, however, the ratio is the opposite, the disease occurring in four females for each male it afflicts. The pilonidal disease commonly affects adults in the second to the third decade of life. However, it is extremely uncommon after 40 years of age, the incidence gradually decreasing from the age of 25 years. The mean age of presentation is 21 years for men and 19 years for women.

PRESENTATION

The pilonidal disease has two major types of presentations.

- Completely asymptomatic sinus tracts that are noticed by the patient or primary care physician.
- Chronic disease: The average patient has two years of disease before seeking medical treatment. More than 80% of presentations of pilonidal disease are exacerbations of a chronic sinus tract.

The physical findings in the pilonidal disease depend on the stage of disease at presentation. In the early stages, the patient can notice a sinus tract or pit in the sacrococcygeal region (Figure 14.2). This can progress to midline oedema or abscess formation. As with any abscess, findings after the physical examination include tenderness to palpation, fluctuance, warmth, purulent discharge, and induration or cellulitis. Systemic signs of infection like fever or toxaemia are uncommon.

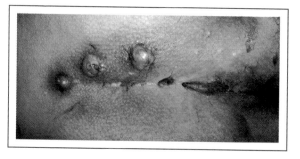

Figure 14.2 Multiple pilonidal sinuses.
Courtesy: Pravin Jaiprakash Gupta.

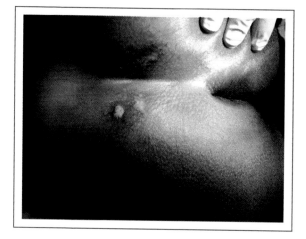

Figure 14.3 Multiple parasacral sinuses.
Courtesy: Pravin Jaiprakash Gupta.

Differential diagnosis includes anal fistula, hidradenitis suppuritiva, perirectal abscess, syphilis, tuberculosis, pyoderma gangrenosum, congenital abnormalities, pre-sacral sinus (Figure 14.3) or dimple, and implantation dermoid.

Pilonidal disease is a clinical diagnosis. The specific location is the easiest way to distinguish pilonidal disease from other disease entities.

TREATMENT

Some individuals with pilonidal sinus are clearly asymptomatic, with midline pits in the presacral area but without any secondary inflammation. It is debatable whether these pits ever become symptomatic where there is currently little available data to suggest any harm can come from a purely observational policy. The symptomatic disease most typically presents as an abscess or as purulent discharge. Clinical examination reveals an opening in the midline natal cleft and there may or may not be multiple sinus tracts and openings usually more predominantly off midline on one side only or where one side tends to dominate. Sinuses on both sides are often a feature of a recurrent disease or multiple operations in the past. There may be a cycle of the closure of an opening with acute infection and spontaneous drainage necessitating recurrent admissions. Loose hairs may often be seen projecting from the main orifice and secondary indurated tracts may be evident beneath the skin surface with brownish pyogenic granulation tissue.

There is surprisingly little data concerning specific conservative therapies for the definitive management of pilonidal sinus. Conservative approach may be considered for patients with minimal disease and minimal symptoms and may include the intermittent use of antibiotics and antiseptic creams along with local curettage including pit hair removal and cleaning in the office.

If the patients present with an abscess (Figure 14.4), incision and drainage should be performed in the office. The skin is infiltrated with local anaesthetic and incised lateral to the midline. All debris and hair should be removed. The wound should then be packed. No antibiotics are necessary for most instances unless surrounding cellulitis is present. Meticulous hygiene should be encouraged. Other alternatives include the use of neodymium-doped yttrium aluminium garnet (Nd:YAG) laser depilation that has found favour in young adolescents as a method to remove intergluteal hair as well as post-operative adjuvant treatment. Data would suggest a reduced recurrence rate where laser treatment is used as an adjunctive therapy to definitive surgery, where the treatment is commenced before and after definitive surgical treatment. The optimal type of specific laser

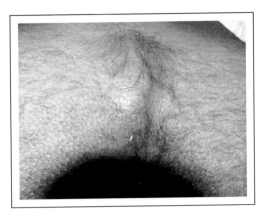

Figure 14.4 Acute pilonidal abscess.

Courtesy: Pravin Jaiprakash Gupta.

treatment is at present unclear where both Ruby and diode lasers have been employed.

Bacterial colonisation of these sinuses has categorically ranged from 50% to 70%, and typical isolates include *Staphylococcus aureus* and anaerobes such as bacteroides. Anaerobes can be isolated in 52% at initial presentation and 64% in recurrent conditions. The utility of antibiotics has been studied in three discrete situations: peri-operative prophylaxis, post-operative treatment, and topical use. However, few randomised trials have not been able to demonstrate any substantial improvement in wound healing with a course of antibiotics in an empirical form. Having previously shown an association between anaerobic infection and delay in healing of granulating wounds, studies have suggested that there is no role for empirical antibiotics in the conservative management and that antibiotics should be used in patients with clinical evidence of infection. Adjunctive use should be considered in the setting of severe cellulitis, underlying immunosuppression, or concomitant systemic illness. Non-surgical treatment for the active disease by careful perianal/postanal hygiene and shaving was introduced in 1947 because of prolonged disability amongst service personnel due to surgical treatment during World War II.

Conservative Experimental Treatment

These are considered for patients without severe symptoms. Looking at the diverse presentation of the disease, lack of unanimity towards a gold standard of treatment, and varied results of the conventional approaches within different institutions, few experimental procedures have emerged in the management of this disease complex. While they have been used with some success in the experienced hands, they have been a disappointment for others. However, a fair trial of such treatment options can be given as an attempt to prevent the need for surgery.

Phenol

This method was chosen to avoid excision of the sinuses, and it was based on the destruction of the pathologic epithelium of the sinus. Pioneers of the method thought that if the epithelium of the tract could be destroyed, any infection present sterilised, and if all the embedded hairs in the tracts are removed, then the sinus should heal.

Phenol injection can be given on an inpatient or an outpatient basis. Ideally, the injection should be done at a quiescent phase, and a pre-injection course of a broad-spectrum antibiotic may be useful in some cases. Most researchers advocating the use of phenol have reported a success rate of 59–95.1% in the first attempt and a recurrence rate of 6.3–17.1%. The median healing times was 6.2–8.7 weeks, while workdays lost were reported as 8.3–11.6 days.

The Procedure of Phenol Injection

The patient is placed in a prone jack-knife position. After shaving off the sacral area, the buttocks are held apart with 5–7 cm strapping to expose the sacral area and anal verge. The skin of the area is cleansed with an antiseptic solution and then dried and towelled up in the usual manner. The skin around the sinus is protected by liberal smearing of Vaseline® while protecting the anus with Vaseline® gauze. By a gentle probing, any loose hairs present are removed with forceps from the sinus and the side tracts. The main sinus tract is then injected with a solution of 80% phenol using a blunt-nosed needle, which can fit into the sinus opening snugly or by introducing an infant feeding tube in the tract. The solution is then injected into the tract gently and taking care to avoid phenol being transfused into the tissue surrounding the sinus and causing a local inflammatory reaction (Figure 14.5).

The injection is stopped when phenol is seen coming from any of the openings and any excess is quickly wiped away. The solution is made to remain in the tract for one minute, after which firm pressure is applied to the sinus tract to express the phenol and bring out loose hairs to the surface, which can be picked out. The whole procedure is repeated two times, each time allowing the phenol in place for one minute, thereby giving a total exposure time of three minutes. The whole tract is then washed out with saline and curetted. Vaseline® gauze and a light dressing are applied to the injected area. The patients are instructed to have frequent baths. Strict hygiene of the area is emphasised during the healing period. After the sinuses have healed, it is advisable to wash the natal cleft after defecation rather than using toilet paper. Particular care must be taken to dust off the loose hairs, particularly after a visit to the barber.

The commonly observed post-operative complications after phenol treatment are sterile abscesses and fat and skin necrosis which have been reported in about 7–16% of patients and is ascribed

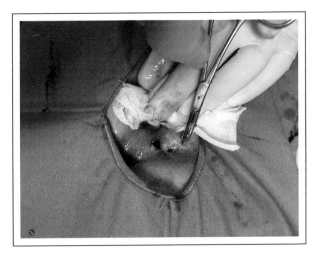

Figure 14.5 Phenolisation of the sinus tract.
Courtesy: Pravin Jaiprakash Gupta.

to leakage of phenol into the surrounding tissues either due to too much pressure at the time of injection, or due to opening up of a false tract during preliminary probing.

Gips et al. reported another minimal surgical treatment for the pilonidal disease. They used trephines for the excision of sinus tracts and bone curette and hydrogen peroxide for cleaning and debridement. Phenol application is less invasive than this method because there is no need for any tissue excision and cavity debridement with a curette, which is chemically done by crystallised phenol.

Use of Polyphenols

Humic substances or natural polyphenols are natural liquid biopolymers, which are the by-products of soil organic matter degradation and present in the environment. Humic substances have been in use in balneotherapy for a long time, and a similar hypothesis has been applied to use polyphenols in the treatment of pilonidal sinus disease.

Polyphenols are known to remove microorganisms located in the wound bed. They can cover and fill infected cavities, which in turn prevent atmospheric oxygen from reaching the microorganisms. Polyphenols can also prevent the microorganisms from using oxygen present in blood and neighbouring tissues produced due to their antioxidant actions.

Taking into consideration all the above factors, Sodium humate 25% was used as the source of polyphenol in one study. Three polyphenol product forms Pilonol® (solution, gel, and cream) were used altogether to achieve best results.

The study claimed a fair outcome of this conservative treatment for pilonidal sinus. The primary disadvantage of topical polyphenol treatment is the need for regular applications for a long time, which look to be cumbersome and unbearable to many of the patients. Few patients also experienced local reactions in the form of irritation, erythema, burning, and aching sensation.

Thread Dragging and Pad Pressure Therapy

This is one of the traditional Chinese medicine therapy used for complex fistulas and sinuses. In this procedure, the sinus tract is curetted free of all the debris and hairs. Ten threads are inserted from one end of the sinus tract to emerge from the other and tied. Each day, the part of the threads lying within the tract are pulled outside and cleaned with saline until the size of the wound is reduced and dragging of the thread becomes difficult. Five of the threads are then removed and remaining five are left behind until the wound is reduced further, and no more discharge is found. This is followed by the application of a pad over the wound with a pressure strapping to accelerate wound healing. This procedure was claimed to have a successful outcome.

Fibrin Glue

In the recent times, treatment of an epithelialised tract like the fistula-in-ano has been obliterated with a reasonable success using fibrin tissue glue. Fibrin glue has been proposed as an adjunct to reduce post-operative infection in primary wound closure after wide excision of the pilonidal sinus complex.

In one of the pilot studies, plugging the sinus tract with fibrin glue was performed as the sole treatment for pilonidal sinus. The pilonidal pits were identified under general anaesthesia, and all the debris were removed from the pits. The sinus tracts were thoroughly curetted or brushed through the midline pits with a small Volkmann spoon or cytology brush to remove the epithelium of the sinus. The pits were then injected with fibrin glue (Tisseel®, Baxter Healthcare Ltd, Newbury, UK). One to two millilitre of glue was injected into the sinus tracts to occlude as much of the sinus complex as possible (Figure 14.6). This was done as an outpatient treatment with a regular follow-up. Five of the six patients treated with this technique had their sinuses healed.

However, this procedure is suggested as the first-line treatment of patients who have no history of infection and having only one sinus.

Endoscopic Pilonidal Sinus Treatment

Recently, a new video-assisted minimally invasive technique using a fistuloscope has been proposed. The outer opening is excised, and the fistuloscope is introduced through the small hole. By directly visualising the anatomy of the tract, all the hair and debris can be removed, which is followed by ablation of the offending tissue under direct vision. No significant complications have been reported with the advantage of less pain and no recurrence in the first six months of therapy. The aesthetic results too were better than conventional procedures.

In a pilot project, the tract after ablation through fistuloscope was obliterated with a bioprosthetic plug to achieve better results. Four patients, who were analysed by this additional manoeuvre, were successfully treated achieving complete healing in all cases. There were no reports of infection or recurrence during a limited follow-up.

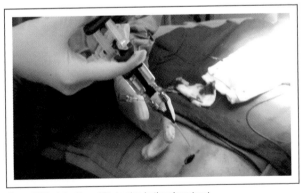

Figure 14.6   Injection of fibrin glue in the sinus tract.

Courtesy: Pravin Jaiprakash Gupta.

Minimalist Procedures: Less is More

The minimalist method is nowadays favoured except in complex recurrent disease or inpatients left with non-healing midline wounds, where Bascom found that 50% of the lateral wounds after a Bascom procedure were completely healed at three weeks, 99% by three months, and all wounds were healed by four months. Lately, there has been a return to much simpler procedures rather than the more complex flaps with their considerable wound morbidity. It is a practice to reserve Limberg flaps and other techniques now for complex bilateral disease and after perhaps a second failure of a trephine local excision procedure.

As far back as 1965, Lord and Millar postulated that midline pit excision should be successful if a pilonidal sinus were a foreign body sinus reaction so that hair removal and free drainage would result in healing. Bascom expanded upon this simple concept, removing the enlarged pathological follicles as an office procedure of pit-picking reporting his initial data in 1983 on 161 patients after a mean follow-up of 3.5 years (maximum 9 years). The healing rate was rapid (3 weeks on average) with, however, 16% reporting either the recurrence of disease or non-healing. The volume of tissue removed with each pit should be no greater than 'a grain of rice' so that the aim is to 'pick the pits' through small incisions and 'stay out of the ditch' of the natal cleft. The procedure of trephine excision is another attractive option. The technique simply uses a dermatological punch biopsy that is of variable size depending upon the size of the pits and which can be railroaded from one sinus point to another to simply core out the sinus. The majority of cases are performed under local anaesthesia. The data by Gips et al. showed that in a recent study of 1,358 cases, there was a 16.2% recurrence rate with a mean follow-up of nearly seven years and an average interval to recurrence of two years and seven months. This provided a disease-free probability of 86.5% at five years.

As mentioned above, controversy remains as to the best surgical approach for recurrent pilonidal disease. Initially, pilonidal disease was treated with wide excision and healing with secondary intention of the affected area. This method did not prevent recurrence of disease and was associated with extensive morbidity. Traditional wide excisional surgery, particularly with midline wounds, has a high incidence of debilitating wound problems that may be as high as 2–7%. The theory here would be that midline wounds are inherently more vulnerable to recurrent disease with secondary infection of the natal cleft particularly in those cases where the cleft is deep. In systematic reviews, although some studies have shown that midline healing can be faster, the overall recurrence rates are higher and were noticed in some series between 22% and 40% when compared with a non-randomised way to the lower recurrence rate of open non-excisional procedures.

The procedures presently advocated are as follows:

- Un-roofing and open secondary healing
- Incision and lying open

- Marsupialisation of the skin edges after excision
- Karydakis flap
- Bascom cleft lift (Bascom II)
- Rhomboid excision with Limberg/modified Limberg flap
- V-Y advancement flap
- S-plasty
- Gluteus maximus myocutaneous flap
- Complete excision with tension-free closure with fibrin glue application.

It is accepted that most recurrences after initial surgery present within five years, although it is known that some cases may recur decades after primary treatment. Non-healing of these small wounds in this series was acceptably low at 4.4%; whereas in three-quarters of these cases, a repeat trephine procedure was performed. Complete wound healing was achieved in this set in 82% over an average of three-and-a-half weeks. The relatively higher recurrence rates after simple excision of skin pits are tempered by the ease and success of a repeat procedure, which means that although one operation may cure less than 85% of patients, a second may finally cure more than 95% of all cases.

COMPLICATIONS

These include recurrence, systemic infection, abscess formation, and development of malignancy.

Prognosis

Although the pilonidal disease is associated with significant morbidity, the long-term prognosis is usually excellent.

Pilonidal sinus is still a troublesome disease entity because of the high morbidity of most treatment options. Management of chronic pilonidal sinuses is a far more controversial issue. The wide variety of surgical techniques described in the available literature reflects a lack of consensus as to an optimal surgical approach. Data suggests that both open and closed operative procedures are effective with no major differences in complication rates. Minimal approach with limited sinus excision is useful in patients with limited disease. If closed techniques are used, evidence supports placing the closure off the midline. Treatment must be tailored to the extent and severity of the disease. Diligent, long-term post-operative follow-up, and careful attention to wound care go a long way in managing the problem.

A deep and fatty natal cleft is a favourable environment for sweating, soddening, bacterial contamination, and hair piercing. So, for both treatment and prevention, these initiating factors must be eliminated as far as possible. An increased depth of the intergluteal sulcus leads to an anaerobic media and an increased chance of infection. Similarly, the vacuum effect created in such situations is thought to play an additional role in pilonidal disease development. The anaerobic bacteria, hair, and debris are sucked into the subcutaneous fat tissue. Therefore, it is prudent to eliminate such factors responsible for the development of the disease, as they will play a pivotal role in the development of disease recurrence as well.

CLINICAL PEARLS

- Asymptomatic sinuses do not require treatment.
- Options for the treatment of acute abscess include aspiration, drainage without curettage, and drainage with curettage.
- The choice of a particular surgical approach depended on the surgeon's familiarity with the procedure and perceived result regarding low recurrence of sinus and a quick healing of resulting cavity or surgical wound.
- Conservative non-operative management, closed methods, lying of the tract, wide excision and open drainage, wide excision and primary closure, and limited excision are the methods currently used.
- Recurrence rates vary with the technique, operator, and length of follow-up.
- Primary closure with a lateral approach appears to give the best results.
- Local hygiene and weekly shaving of the sacrococcygeal area have been shown to decrease the rate of recurrence.
- The modified rhomboid flap for the recurrent disease has consistently shown positive results regarding complication rates and recurrence.
- Newer procedures like fibrin glue and endoscopic sinus tract ablation are yet to prove their efficacy in the long term.

SUGGESTED READINGS

Aksoy HM, Aksoy B, Egemen D. Effectiveness of topical use of natural polyphenons for the treatment of sacrococcygeal pilonidal sinus disease: a retrospective study including 192 patients. *Eur J Dermatol*. 2010;20:476–81.

Altinli E, Koksal N, Onur E, Celik A, Sumer A. Impact of fibrin sealant on Limberg flap technique: results of a randomized controlled trial. *Tech Coloproctol*. 2007;11:22–5.

Armstrong JH, Barcia PJ. Pilonidal sinus disease. The conservative approach. *Arch Surg*. 1994;129:914–17.

Bascom J. Pilonidal disease: origin from follicles of hairs and results of follicle removal as treatment. *Surgery*. 1980;87:567–72.

Chia CL, Tay VW, Mantoo SK. Endoscopic pilonidal sinus treatment in the asian population. *Surg Laparosc Endosc Percutan Tech*. 2015; 25(3):e95–7.

Da Silva JH. Pilonidal cyst: cause and treatment. *Dis Colon Rectum*. 2000; 43:1146–56.

Gips M, Melki Y, Salem L, Weil R, Sulkes J. Minimal surgery for pilonidal disease using trephines: description of a new technique and long-term outcomes in 1,358 patients. *Dis Colon Rectum*. 2008;51(11):1656–62.

Greenberg R, Kashtan H, Skornik Y, Werbin N. Treatment of pilonidal sinus disease using fibrin glue as a sealant. *Tech Coloproctol*. 2004;8:95–8.

Handmer M. Sticking to the facts: a systematic review of fibrin glue for pilonidal disease. *ANZ J Surg*. 2012;82:221–4.

Humphries AE, Duncan JE. Evaluation and management of pilonidal disease. *Surg Clin North Am*. 2010;90:113–24.

Karydakis GE. Easy and successful treatment of pilonidal sinus after explanation of its causative process. *Aust N Z J Surg*. 1992;62:385–9.

Lu JG, Wang C, Cao YQ, Yao YB. Thread dragging and pad pressure therapy in traditional Chinese medicine for treatment of pilonidal sinus: a case report. *Zhong Xi Yi Jie He Xue Bao*. 2011;9:36–7.

Lund JN, Leveson SH. Fibrin glue in the treatment of pilonidal sinus: results of a pilot study. *Dis Colon Rectum*. 2005;48:1094–6.

Mankad PS, Codispoti M. The role of fibrin sealants in hemostasis. *Am J Surg*. 2001;182:21–8.

Meinero P, Mori L, Gasloli G. Endoscopic pilonidal sinus treatment (E.P.Si.T.). *Tech Coloproctol*. 2014;18(4):389–92.

Milone M, Bianco P, Musella M, Milone F. A technical modification of video-assisted ablation for recurrent pilonidal sinus. *Colorectal Dis*. 2014; 16(11):O404–6.

Neola B, Capasso S, Caruso L, et al. Scarless outpatient ablation of pilo-nidal sinus: a pilot study of a new minimally invasive treatment. *Int Wound J*. 2016;13(5):705–8.

Patey DH, Scarff RW. Pathology of postanal pilonidal sinus: its bearing on treatment. *Lancet*. 1946;2:13–14.

Seleem MI, Al-Hashemy AM. Management of pilonidal sinus using fibrin glue: a new concept and preliminary experience. *Colorectal Dis*. 2005; 7:319–22.

Vitale A, Barberis G, Maida P, Salzano A. Use of biological glue in the surgical treatment of sacrococcygeal fistulas. *G Chir*. 1992;13:271–2.

Chapter 15

Role of supportive therapies in anorectal diseases

SUPPOSITORIES

Suppositories are soft, supple, torpedo-like medicaments which are passed into the lower rectum via the anus, where they are melted and absorbed. These act like ointment, but also have the effect of the oral medication. It is said that an ointment has an on-the-spot outcome, whereas suppositories have a lasting result. Nevertheless, suppositories can lead to anal canal trauma and a persistent feeling of defecation. Suppositories for various anorectal ailments are a traditional mode of getting drugs into the body, and suppositories for haemorrhoids are in vogue dating back from Hippocrates, also known as the father of modern medicine, who described a process of utilising reusable suppositories.

The suppositories accessible at the moment are not meant to be reused like the one depicted by Hippocrates. Nevertheless, a huge lot of them gives temporary relief from the ache and distress of the piles. At this time, an assortment of haemorrhoidal suppositories is obtainable over-the-counter. The medication typically comprises antiseptics, anti-inflammatory, anti-pruritus, and local anaesthetics.

Numerous manners are sought for the relief of pain in the anal and perianal areas. An assortment of suppositories and balms are accessible and are being sold all over the world as over-the-counter medicaments and are routinely advocated by family practitioners and specialists. The feeling of pain, tactile sensation, and feelings of extremes of temperature at and in the anal canal region are in particular severe, diffuse, and intense when contrasted with the skin of any other part of the human boy. The sensations on the perianal skin are almost identical to what is felt on the dorsal part of the finger.

Treatment utilising rectal course is an extraordinarily used remedy as part of the act of therapy, particularly in proctological problems; it can be employed as a routine and has good results. Drugs blended with exclusive adjuvants and controlled via the rectal course do provide palatable pharmacokinetics beneficial of local tolerance.

Suppositories are a medicated dosage proposed for insertion into the body openings. The anorectal physiology supplies an active and vast floor zone for medicinal absorption. The large floor field of the anal canal and lower rectum is additionally porous to non-ionised drugs. Suppositories formulations are accessible within the assortment of more than a few ingredients to provide retention and bring down complications.

Suppositories are produced in different shapes and dimensions, and this encourages their smooth insertion and maintenance within the rectal cavity. Adult rectal suppositories weigh somewhere around 1–2 g while those for children are about half that weight. They are available with varieties of compositions either in separate or mixed formulations. The traditionally utilised ones include the following:

Suppositories Containing Local Anaesthetics Agents

The local anaesthetics act by numbing the nerve endings and give brief alleviation from discomfort and pruritus. These work with the aid of bringing on a short block to conduction within the sensory nerves. They are satisfactorily assimilated from the mucous membrane and utilised as surface analgesics. Also, they give considerable alleviation from painful pathologies like strangulated haemorrhoids, fissures, and perianal thrombotic lumps.

Suppositories Containing Steroids

Certain types of glucocorticoids are utilised as a part of rectal suppositories together with hydrocortisone and its subsidiaries, diflucortolone valerate, and prednisolone. These go about as mitigating, decongestant, and anti-pruritic drugs that dispense with inflammation and mucous discharge. It has been found that the affliction-relieving impacts of local anaesthetics may also be drastically delayed by the onset of the discomfort threshold through the anti-inflammatory activities of these steroids.

Suppositories Containing Astringents

Astringent is a substance which spreads along the anal dermal zone to desiccate the perianal skin, offering alleviation from burning and tingling.

Haemorrhoids have swollen veins. The vasoconstricting influences of the astringent medication can support in soothing manifestations of haemorrhoids. On dispersion, these medications intent the vessels to contract, which means diminishing haemorrhoidal varicosities. These astringents are probably incorporated with a mild form of anaesthetic, which helps in assuaging ache and itching.

Passage of a hard and dry stool is the most anxious situation in patients having painful anal pathologies, as it results in the tearing of the sensitive tissues around the anus. This section and splitting can end in bleeding. Likewise, when this soft skin is exposed to fluid or stool, it stimulates the epidermis to itch further and might deliver burning sensations.

Protectants can be used within the form of suppositories to create a physical barrier on the skin that helps in decreasing the ache in depth and the pruritus. These also preserve the damaged epidermis from coming in contact with offending particles within the stool.

Probably the most often used protectants are: glycerine, aluminium hydroxide gel, lanolin, white petrolatum, zinc oxide, aloe vera, and calamine.

On occasions, the chemicals in the suppository can lead to the crumbling of the outer layers of the epidermis and anal canal tissues when applied. This ingredient eventually ensures an efficient infiltration of other medications presents within the suppositories to carry faster relief. The more commonly utilised keratolytic are: resorcinol (1–3%) and aluminium chlorhydroxy allantoinate (0.2–2%).

Calcium dobesilate, a venotonic medicine, is recommended for three major venous ailments—chronic venous disorders, diabetic retinopathy, and symptoms of haemorrhoidal complexities. Alongside calcium dobesilate, the suppositories also contain a local anaesthetic, steroid, and astringent as an adjuvant.

Policresulen coagulates necrotic or pathogenically modified tissue within the anorectum and helps desquamation of such tissues. The natural tissues surrounding the affected area are unaffected. As a local haemostatic, policresulen coagulates blood proteins to actuate compression of the muscle fibres of small vessels and therefore, stops haemorrhage within the anal canal or the perianal region. There is hyperaemia in the affected haemorrhoids which stimulates regeneration and re-epithelisation procedure. It, likewise, has an antimicrobial property that guards towards desquamation and prevents inflammation. Policresulen likewise has astringent property and thus it suppresses bleeding.

A couple of other situations which utilised a suppository for the various anorectal problems include—imiquimod suppository to hinder recurrences of anal warts occurring after ablative surgery; 5-fluorouracil suppository for carcinoma of the rectum before the operation; and suppository combining sodium bicarbonate and potassium bitartrate in a polyethylene glycol base to produce around 175 mL of carbon dioxide. This release expands the rectal ampulla, which accordingly stimulates peristalsis and an ensuing bowel movement to treat constipation. Insertion of a 0.2% glyceryl trinitrate suppository for chronic anal fissure has been found to be worthy in few studies.

HOW TO INSERT A SUPPOSITORY

The regular practice is to embed the suppository with the patient lying on the left lateral side maintaining the right knee folded. The suppositories may be dunked in water before use, as it encourages the insertion of the suppositories readily. They have got to be kept in icy water or icebox about 30 minutes before their use, as the suppositories are excessively supple, making it impossible to be inserted, particularly in a warm climate. Emptying of bowel ought to be demoralised for 60 minutes after its insertion to permit it to be aptly absorbed.

PROBLEMS FOLLOWING USE OF SUPPOSITORIES

Nonetheless, this remedial methodology is not hazard free. Suppositories containing non-steroidal anti-inflammatory medicines are greatly utilised for the alleviation of pain in youngsters, and obstetrical and standard surgical practices. Few reviews are available where these suppositories have brought about complications in the form of rectal and anal ulcerations, rectal stricture, anal stenosis, proctitis, and peri-rectal cellulitis. Systemic absorption of topically applied steroids can arise in kids. Calcium dobesilate is accounted for causing agranulocytosis. Patients utilising diclofenac suppository have reported with a complete recto-anal stenosis and bowel obstruction requiring a permanent colostomy. These patients experienced anal soreness, tenesmus, faecal incontinence, and, in two instances, intestinal obstruction. On examination of the rectum, severe circular narrowing of the distal rectum with shallow ulcerations with stenosis of the anal verge has been observed. Diclofenac suppositories must be utilised with caution in patients with haemorrhoids, rhagades, and anal fissures because it can exert local irritative symptoms leading to haematochezia or an acute attack of haemorrhoids.

Suppositories, when given for alleviation of symptoms in the anal canal, could go away deep in the rectum, where they fall apart, and just a bit of the medicine reaches the anal canal, the place it is required essentially the most. Absorption of medications can be flighty and erratic. A few suppositories spill or are ousted after insertion bringing about a pointless recreation. Suppositories certainly do not keep within the limits of the anal canal and more frequently than not rise up the lower rectum where they can give an emollient impact or just a lubrication to the stools.

It has been postulated that reversed vermicular contractions or stress gradient of the anal canal could have been responsible for this behaviour. It has to be additionally instructed that 'torpedo-moulded' suppositories should be made available which would have a better acceptability and viability.

In any case, within the time of cost containment and alongside the acquired immune deficiency syndrome (AIDS) and other communicable blood-borne illnesses, drug conveyance using suppositories can reveal a practical and feasible option. Suppositories can be looked at as a priceless medicine transportation system in sufferers having anorectal manifestations.

HAEMORRHOID CREAMS

A good wide range of ointments, lotions, and suppositories are on hand for haemorrhoidal application, preferably containing local anaesthetics, mild astringents, or steroids in various mixtures. These agents could also be used to provide quick-term relief from anal discomfort. Nevertheless, there is no available scientific evidence to suggest their preferred use. These remedies have regularly been initiated by the general practitioners before the patient is sent to the colorectal expert. These medicaments do not have any impact on the underlying pathological alterations within the anal cushions, and a long-term application can cause dermatitis and hypersensitivity of the anoderm and, on occasions, rectal absorption leading to systemic side effects. Prolonged topical steroid use can result in dermal atrophy and doctors use these steroid-containing ointments sparingly and for a brief period of time. The role of topical haemorrhoidal preparations is to provide quick-term alleviation from uneasiness, additional control of irritation, provoke shrinkage of the swollen haemorrhoidal tissue, and immediate soothing effects from painful burning, itching, and discomfort.

INSTRUCTION OF APPLICATION

The affected field must be cleaned through patting or blotting with a suitable cleaning tissue, and dried using mopping with toilet tissue or a smooth fabric before applying the cream. The ointment must be applied externally to the affected area no longer than three times daily, chiefly at bedtime, in the morning, and after each bowel motion.

These types of preparations come with a nozzle or dispensing cap, having multiple holes at the tip that is designed to facilitate dispersion of the cream to the affected zone within the lower part of the anal canal. Before applying, the protecting cap should be eliminated from the mouth of the tube. The nozzle is then connected to the tube. The nozzle must be lubricated through squeezing the tube and then it is inserted into the anal canal. The left lateral position is appropriate to do this manoeuvre. After the application, the nozzle should be fully cleansed, and the protective cover is replaced firmly.

One must use these topical preparations with caution in patients with a coronary heart disorder, hypertension, thyroid disease, diabetes, pregnant women or nursing mothers, and sufferers having urinary dysfunction because of an enlarged prostate. The patient should not exceed the advocated daily dosage unless directed. The patient is told to record in case of bleeding or if the situation worsens or does not give relief within seven days. These applications must not be inserted into the rectum by using fingers, with any mechanical device or by an applicator.

Other topical preparations in use incorporate sucralfate and metronidazole, topical nitroglycerin (0.2%) in those with piles and sphincter spasm. Others have steered improvement in such patients with better results using L-arginine and 0.25% oxethacaine chlorhydrate in sphincter hypertonicity. Topical nifedipine or 1% isosorbide dinitrate has additionally been endorsed for the traditional remedy of thrombosed external haemorrhoids. The long-trusted preparation-H has been designed to set off vasoconstriction within haemorrhoid (Pfizer, USA) and includes 0.25% phenylephrine, petrolatum, mild mineral oil, and shark liver oil.

The phenylephrine has special vasoconstrictive effects on the arterial aspect of haemorrhoid and differs from the other agents which could also be considered as protectants. These ingredients may be supplemented with a naturally available combination of honey, olive oil, and beeswax, which have been found useful in the treatment of a few patients with haemorrhoids by obscuring haemorrhage and relieving pruritus with no real threat of side-effects.

Doctors, nonetheless, hardly ever advocate topical medications within the framework of suppositories, creams, enemas, or foams as the remedy to haemorrhoids with most patients volunteering that they are ineffective by the time they have been referred. Other local herbs have also been advocated; these include—*Aesculus hippocastanum, Ruscus aculeatus, Centella asiatica,* and *Hamamelis virginiana,* without any objective trial information about efficacy.

Poorly performed trials, making use of traditional Chinese herbal cures (*Radix sanguisorbae, Gardenia, Radix scutellariae, Fructus sophorae, Cacumen biotae, Radix rehmanniae, Cortex dictamni,* and

Radix sophorae flavescentis), have shown a reduction in haemato-chezia and perianal infection in a record of 1,822 treated patients imparting with symptomatic haemorrhoids derived from nine trials.

SITZ BATH

This mode of treatment is being utilised as a conservative therapy, as post-operative management, or for the prevention of benign anal diseases such as haemorrhoids, fissures-in-ano, and similar others that are in vogue for quite a few centuries. Hot sitz bath means to immerse the anal region in a bowl, filled with warm water at around 40°C for a brief period. One might also use a bidet or a tub. In the past, 20 minutes of a sitz bath used to be recommended; however, seeing that there are potentialities of congestion or prolapse, now shorter bath time is endorsed to avoid congestion or oedema. Warm water sitz bath relieves discomfort via lowering anal pressure, helps to maintain the hygiene of the anus, and improves anal blood circulation that reduces congestion and oedema.

The sitz bath, which is also known as a hip bath, is a type of water treatment where the hips and buttocks are soaked in water or a similar solution. A sitz bath may be used for patients having had a surgical procedure of the rectum to ease the discomfort, or in uterine cramps, in prostate infections, or stipulations with painful ovaries or testicles. It may also be endorsed to alleviate the anguish from inflammatory conditions of the bladder, prostate, or vagina. Inflammatory bowel diseases can also be supplemented with sitz baths.

The particular action of a sitz bath is unknown. The speculation is that pain reduction after the sitz bath might be due to the relaxation of the internal anal sphincter with a resultant diminishment of the rectal neck pressure. A decline in interior sphincter pressure while performing the sitz bath has been observed. It is hypothesised that hot water is known to extend the length of relief of the internal sphincter constriction. It is theorised that the nerves of the interior sphincter muscle intercession by way of tactile perianal epidermal receptors, which get stimulated by using hot water. The lessening of suffering and alleviation is due to the 'thermosphincteric reflex'. It is observed that warm water sitz bath results in relaxation of the internal urethral sphincter also, which in turn produces vesicle contraction and facilitates urination in patients operated for a haemorrhoidectomy.

Sitz baths are frequently advocated but nevertheless, proper directions regarding the right way to perform them are rarely explained to patients. In a real experience, the water is required to cover the perineum and lower pelvis. Submerging various parts of the body in warm water could prompt systemic vasodilatation and diminishing blood flow to the perineal area. Most studies have used inefficient ways to choose controls, more than one related components, and a variety of preparations.

Despite the absence of any rigorous evidence, most of the time the most effective topical remedy for the relief of symptoms comes in the best way of warm (40°C) sitz baths. Soaking time must be restrained (15 minutes) to avoid oedema of the perianal and perineal dermis. The appliance of ice packs to the anal region may also relieve symptoms and the patient should be warned that contact time is not extended. Due to the innocuous nature of this method of treatment, patients must be given particular directions on the best way to effectively take the sitz bath, together with the temperature of the water and the device utilised. Warm sitz baths are one of the crucial advantages and productive strategies to facilitate the pain of haemorrhoids. Sitz bath is likewise useful in lowering the agony associated with genital herpes, uterine spasms, and different agonising conditions within the pelvic zone. A brief period of sitz bath enables in containing infection, constipation, and vaginal discharge. It may be found useful to tone up the muscles in patients with bladder or bowel incontinence.

Ordinarily, a reasonable response is gained with a 'juxtapose sitz bath' making use of cyclic warm and cold baths. This requires a tub of hot water and another one of ice water. The patient has to sit alternatively down in the hot water for 3–4 minutes and then in the cold water tub for around a minute. This has to be repeated 3–5 times and ended with cold water.

If two tubs are not be available, the patient may sit down in a hot water tub up to the navel and afterwards he should stand out of the water. Then, he may pull a cold towel between his legs and over the waist in front and back. The icy towel is kept up for around a minute. Again the patient sits down in the warm water tub and does the same manoeuvre for 3–5 instances, completing with the cold towel.

Additives in the Water Used for Sitz Bath

An assortment of medicaments and supportive components had been attempted and prescribed for various proctological problems. These incorporate anti-infective options like anti-septic lotions, table salt, povidone iodine, potassium permanganate, vinegar, and hydrogen peroxide. Fragrance therapy utilising valuable oils like lavender, neroli, rose, myrrh, orange, grapefruit, mandarin, and Roman chamomile has often been recommended. Notwithstanding, how these delivered materials are beneficial remains a secret.

It has got to be comprehended that the premise of a sitz bath is the utilisation of variable temperature to the ano-perianal area, and different factors account for its effect. It ought to likewise be recalled that the addition of medicaments to the water could be harmful than just right on some events. Local allergies, dermatitis, the disintegration of the sutures of the surgical wound, dispersal of genital herpes, or development of pustules and bullae have been reported on a few occasions.

As a word of warning, the temperature of the water should not be too hot in view that there are few experiences of the gluteal and perineal burns after sitz tub, principally in the paediatric population.

FOOD CONTENTS AND DIET

For the benefit of the patients, use of fluid and fibre intake should be expanded for the stool to be loose and for soft defecation.

Alcohol ingesting should be forbidden to preclude diarrhoea and infection. Also, patients' diet plan must restrict spicy foods and coffee, in the view that such colonic irritants stimulate the intestine and the anal canal.

At the moment, it is given that those who tend to consume plenty of processed meals, meat, and junks of the low-fibre regimen ought to become constipated as the colonic transit time is delayed. Excessive fibre consumption not only curbs haemorrhoids, but can also be of use in restricting the development of symptomatic haemorrhoids. That is why a coloproctologist has to have competencies about fibres.

Dietary fibres are add-ons of vegetation that face up to using human digestive enzymes. They are a non-nutritive substance which is neither digested, nor absorbed. The composition of the fibre can be divided into water-soluble (non-structural) and insoluble (structural) types. The insoluble fibres, which mainly contain cellulose, semi-cellulose, and lignin amount to about 70% of the total fibres consumed, and these are known to increase the bulk of stool and reduce the transit time through the stomach and the intestine.

Cellulose

It is dextrose polymer (exists on the cell wall of crops) that explains probably the most exceptional characteristics of fibre and is rich in wheat bran and apple peel.

Lignin

It exists on the cell wall of timber and is not a carbohydrate.

Hemicellulose

It comprises 15–30% of the cell wall of plants, and pentose-contained polysaccharide in hemicelluloses of wheat bran increases the volume of stool.

Water-Soluble (Non-structural) Fibres

Water-soluble (non-structural) fibres account 30% of the total fibres, which disturb reabsorption of bile acid and have the water-binding capacity. They consist of plant rubber like pectin, guar gum, and Karaya rubber; mucilage like psyllium seed; and algae polysaccharide like agar.

Pectin

It tends to be like a gel and is amply found in citrus fruits, apple, and coats of an onion. It holds the water of the intestinal lumen rapidly.

Plant Rubber (Guar Gum, Karaya Rubber)

It is a kind of bulk-forming laxative, extracted from tropical vegetation and seeds. Guar gum is used in thickening of salads, toothpaste, and different soups.

Mucilage Like Psyllium Seed and Ispaghula

It has hydrophilic substances to preserve water for its seed. Psyllium is rich in mucilage which impacts the traits of volume forming and laxatives of materials.

Algae Polysaccharide (Agar)

It is found best on the cellular wall of seaweed and algae. It has the quality of forming a gel and retaining water.

The composition of dietary fibre has one-of-a-kind structure noticeably both chemically and physically; however, they increase the volume of stool and shorten gastrointestinal transit time. Moreover, for this purpose, their inclusion in the diet is valuable for the relief of constipation as well as prevention and healing of haemorrhoids.

Dietary fibres are fermented variously through microorganism. Fifty per cent of the cellulose is broken down by colonic organisms and is related to the size of its particles (the smaller the particle size, the less complicated the microorganism to access fermentation). Even though the gas, which is formed during the process, could lead to bloating at the beginning, it finally reduces the volume of colonic gas by reducing transit time by way of diminished fermentation time.

Even though patients with haemorrhoids are advised to consume plenty of dietary fibre, bulking agents are most likely being prescribed by the coloproctologist.

Psyllium seed, polycarbophil, artificial polysaccharide, and Karaya rubber are the typical examples of bulking substances. Psyllium does not only absorb water but additionally shortens the colonic transit time through growing the bacterial plenty using bacterial fermentation within the colon. The quantity of bulking agents has to be increased steadily on account that it has a side effect like bloating and belching.

While increasing the amount of fibre intake, one must add a proper amount of grains, fruit, vegetables, and seaweed in the daily diet. When greens are parboiled, it is simpler to consume extra fibre than uncooked vegetables as the water contained within the greens is reduced. Water-soluble fibre increases the quantity of the stool with the aid of absorbing water, but adequate fluid has got to be taken to avoid antagonistic results.

Toilet Training

During the act of defecation, the anal cushion descends downward. If it stays in its prolapsed state for a long time, it cannot be recovered to its original place inflicting prolapse and bleeding. Thus, finishing bowel action within the shortest possible interval is a good idea to avoid haemorrhoids or their complications.

Patients must be urged to complete the bowel movement within three minutes, even if they have got a sense of extra defecation and to set off their defecation after breakfast, if feasible. For the one who has a dependency of defecation immediately after waking up, it is suggested to drink about 200 mL of water to set off gastrocolic reflex. It is prudent to ablute the anus with water rather than using a toilet paper after defecation. If a tissue has to be used, it should be better soaked with water.

Capsicum and different spices have been identified to aggravate signs of anal pathologies. Chillies are believed to be harmful to sufferers with painful anal pathologies like anal fissures and haemorrhoidal disease. Such patients are instructed to take a somewhat bland diet containing little or no spices and chillies. This view is perhaps based on the findings that red chilli powder damages the colonic mucosa. Intragastric insertion of red chilli powder in human volunteers has shown a rise in the deoxyribonucleic acid content of gastric aspirate, inflicting exfoliation of the surface epithelial cells.

There are other advantages of fibre intake for haemorrhoidal patients, including improvement in coronary heart disease, cerebro-vascular disease, hypertension, diabetes, hypercholestaerolemia, and weight problems with gastrointestinal improvement in reflux, peptic ulceration, diverticular disease, and constipation.

The ideal dietary fibre intake for kids and adults are, 14 g 1,000 Kcal, with evidence that the majority of Western population ingests about half of the endorsed dose.

Dietary irregularity or smoking is reportedly held responsible for the progress of haemorrhoids. Meals containing spices and citrus fruits have to be eradicated from the diet in patients with pruritus ani. The addition of dietary fibre nutritional supplements is also useful in the alleviation of constipation, spastic colon, and diverticular sickness.

CLINICAL PEARLS

- Supportive therapies perpetually have a role to play in the treatment of various diseases and proctological disorders should not be an exception to this.
- Rigorous levels of proof do not exist to aid using topical treatment plans, whether physical or pharmacological treatments like sitz baths, anaesthetics, phleboton-ics, corticosteroids, or cooling therapy.
- Pharmaceutical preparations reminiscent of creams, ointments, foams, and suppositories have a somewhat pharmacological cause in the management of anorectal diseases.
- Dietary modification with fibre supplementation (psyllium, methylcellulose, cal-cium polycarbophil) is one of the mainstays of therapy for sufferers of the ano-rectal illness.
- While it is expected that a health practitioner must take a real advantage of these measures along with his acumen and scientific experience, it is usually prudent not to be carried away with the high and panacea-like claims made by the manufacturers of these preparations concerning the efficacy of the products.
- A considered application of these measures would most likely benefit the patients in relieving his agony while at the same time giving a sense of satisfac-tion to the treating doctor.

SUGGESTED READINGS

Alonso-Coello P, Mills E, Heels-Ansdell D, et al. Fiber for the treatment of hemorrhoids complications: a systematic review and meta-analysis. *Am J Gastroenterol*. 2006;101:181–8.

Altomare DF, Giannini I. Pharmacological treatment of hemorrhoids: a narrative review. *Expert Opin Pharmacother*. 2013;14:2343–9.

Chan KK, Arthur JD. External haemorrhoidal thrombosis: evidence for current management. *Tech Coloproctol*. 2013;17:21–5.

Ganz RA. The evaluation and treatment of hemorrhoids: a guide for the gastroenterologist. *Clin Gastroenterol Hepatol*. 2013;11:593–603.

Greenspon J, Williams SB, Young HA, Orkin BA. Thrombosed external hemorrhoids: outcome after conservative or surgical management. *Dis Colon Rectum*. 2004;47:1493–8.

Gupta P. Randomized, controlled study comparing sitz-bath and no-sitz-bath treatments in patients with acute anal fissures. *ANZ J Surg*. 2006;76:718–21.

Gupta PJ. Effects of warm water sitz bath on symptoms in post-anal sphincterotomy in chronic anal fissure—a randomized and controlled study. *World J Surg*. 2007;31:1480–4.

Gupta PJ. Red hot chilli consumption is harmful in patients operated for anal fissure—a randomized, double-blind, controlled study. *Dig Surg*. 2007;24(5):354–7.

Gupta PJ. Supportive therapies in ano-rectal diseases—are they really useful? *Acta Chir Lugosl*. 2010;57(3):83–7.

Gupta PJ. Suppositories in anal disorders: a review. *Eur Rev Med Pharmacol Sci*. 2007;11:165–70.

Gupta PJ. Warm sitz bath does not reduce symptoms in posthaemorrhoidectomy period: a randomized, controlled study. *ANZ J Surg*. 2008; 78(5):398–401.

Johanson JF. Nonsurgical treatment of hemorrhoids. *J Gastrointest Surg*. 2002;6:290–4.

Lohsiriwat V. Hemorrhoids: from basic pathophysiology to clinical management. *World J Gastroenterol*. 2012;18:2009–17.

McConnell EA. Giving your patient a sitz bath. *Nursing*. 1993;23:14.

Menteş BB, Görgül A, Tatlicioğlu E, Ayoğlu F, Unal S. Efficacy of calcium dobesilate in treating acute attacks of hemorrhoidal disease. *Dis Colon Rectum*. 2001;44:1489–95.

Misra MC. Drug treatment of haemorrhoids. *Drugs*. 2005;65:1481–91.

Perrotti P, Antropoli C, Molino D, De Stefano G, Antropoli M. Conservative treatment of acute thrombosed external hemorrhoids with topical nifedipine. *Dis Colon Rectum*. 2001;44:405–9.

Shafik A. Role of warm-water bath in anorectal conditions. The 'thermo-sphincteric reflex'. *J Clin Gastroenterol*. 1993;16:304–8.

Sneider EB, Maykel JA. Diagnosis and management of symptomatic hemorrhoids. *Surg Clin North Am*. 2010;90:17–32.

Song SG, Kim SH. Optimal treatment of symptomatic hemorrhoids. *J Korean Soc Coloproctol*. 2011;27:277–81.

Tjandra JJ, Tan JJ, Lim JF, Murray-Green C, Kennedy ML, Lubowski DZ. Rectogesic (glyceryl trinitrate 0.2%) ointment relieves symptoms of haemorrhoids associated with high resting anal canal pressures. *Colorectal Dis*. 2007;9:457–63.

Chapter 16

Functional anorectal pain

Chronic anorectal pain is a cause of agony for the patient and anguish for the clinician. Anorectal and perineal discomfort are associated with a variety of disease conditions; additionally, they can occur underneath circumstances in which typical motives are absent, and the exact pathophysiology is obscure. The incidence of such pelvic condition in the female populace is estimated to be 3.8%. Although chronic pelvic pain is prevalent in women, it is certainly not limited to the female gender.

In an American survey of clinical gastrointestinal disorders, the incidence of functional anorectal diseases was estimated to be about 11.1% of the male and 12.1% of the female respondents to the survey. The position of the specialist associated with the care of these patients is to rule out intrinsic disorders of the genitourinary and gastrointestinal organs in the pelvis and, if none is found, to deal with this affliction. Variable situations, of which some may be probably life-threatening, should be excluded if one has to make a diagnosis of idiopathic and functional anorectal disease, together with conditions like proctalgia fugax and levator spasm.

Chronic anal or perineal pain may have diverse causes, and a precise and painstaking diagnostic approach is necessary to avoid inadequate and irrational treatments, which may aggravate the situation. Advances in imaging and neurophysiologic testing have improved the ability to diagnose and differentiate coccygodynia, pudendal neuralgia, and the pyriformis muscle syndrome. Most frequently encountered chronic anorectal pains are the levator ani syndrome and proctalgia fugax. These may just typically coexist, but may also be differentiated from each other by the length, frequency, and inherent quality of discomfort.

LEVATOR ANI SYNDROME

The levator ani syndrome has been hypothesised as an outcome of spastic or severely spastic muscles of the pelvic floor. The designated aetiology is obscure. Few studies advocate that levator ani syndrome is more common in people with psychological stress, apprehension, and anxiety. That is additionally termed as levator spasm, extended syndrome, puborectalis syndrome, chronic proctalgia, and pelvic tension myalgia. The agony is better described as a vague or dull discomfort with pressure sensation noticed within the rectum that exacerbates with sitting or lying down and which lasts for hours to days. Levator ani syndrome is outlined as a symptom complex associated which recurrent or persistent distressing suffering, with a sense of pressure or pain in the region of the rectum, sacrum, and coccyx, and can extend up to the gluteal area or thighs. No organic pathology is detected clinically.

These diagnoses must be entertained only after excluding the presence of an organic ailment with a careful physical examination, endoscopy, and ancillary diagnostic evaluation by defecography, ultrasound, CT scan, or MRI. The utility of electromyography, anal manometry, and pudendal nerve studies has not been proven sans doubt. No consistent abnormalities in any of this investigation had been established in the majority of patients. Probably, the most rational mechanism explaining this pathology is the spasm of the levator ani muscular tissues. The discomfort of the levator ani syndrome is also exacerbated via stress, trauma from sitting for hours and in the same position, parturition, few surgical procedures like herniated lumbar disc, low anterior resection, hysterectomy, sexual encounters, and defecation.

Another thought is that the pathogenesis of proctalgia fugax is neuralgia of the pudendal nerves. The diagnosis is mostly established on clear manifestations plus the absence of any definitive pathological origin of pain. Physical examination, rectoscopy, and anoscopy are normal in these patients. Endoanal ultrasonography or magnetic resonance imaging scans are otherwise normal, but sometimes one may find an unexpected hypertrophy of the internal sphincter; in such cases, an internal anal sphincterotomy may be of help. Anorectal manometry demonstrates an increased internal anal sphincter pressure with a paroxysmal inability to relax in some instances.

The differential diagnosis of anorectal pain should include common organic lesions such as haemorrhoids, perineal fistula and sepsis, anal fissure, carcinoma, compression of sacral nerves, and gynaecological disease.

Treatment

At the outset, the patient should be assured that these attacks are innocuous and not in any way heading for cancer or another serious illness. A bag of treatment options is available. Grant et al. used 2–3 massages over a gap of 2–3 weeks, mixed with the heat and diazepam, and had reported satisfactory results in 68% of the sufferers and marginal improvement in 19%. Kang et al. described a sequence of 104 patients in which transanal injection of triamcinolone gave 37% of patients a freedom from pain. Biofeedback has also shown some success. Electrical sacral nerve stimulation, which is recommended for voiding disorders and faecal incontinence, has additionally effectually decreased the severity of discomfort in patients who had been characterised as having a persistent pelvic ache.

Apprehension and gloomy mood were related to chronic pelvic pain syndrome, and these conditions will have to be regarded in the comprehensive approach while dealing with the patients having functional pelvic pain. The treatment plan is aimed at reducing pressure on the levator ani muscles, by way of sitz baths; use of muscle relaxants like methocarbamol, diazepam, and cyclobenzaprine; electro-galvanic stimulation; and biofeedback training. However, this approach is not a 'fit for all' type as the results are variable in different patients. Massaging of the levator ani muscles by finger passing from anterior to posterior, in a consistent manner till the patient can tolerate is beneficial and should be done at three to four weeks' intervals.

The affected site, if one-sided, or both if two-sided, ought to be massaged up to 50 times contingent upon the patient's resilience. The most usual cause behind an insufficient rub is the inability to achieve sufficiently high digitation in the rectum to palpate the levator. The convenience of sitz baths in levator ani syndrome (LAS) is dubious; yet, they have no unsafe impact. Since spasm of the levator ani muscles is in all likelihood the reason for LAS, electro-galvanic stimulation is proposed. The mechanism acting behind this relief of pain is because of the institution of convulsive muscle fasciculation leading to muscle fatigue by rehashing, use of a direct electrical current through an intra-anal probe. It has been demonstrated that galvanic current could accomplish pain relief in 40–91% of patients experiencing LAS.

Biofeedback as a treatment methodology is attempting to tune the psyches of patients with LAS to unwind their affected muscles, subsequently breaking the spastic cycle. No unwarranted symptoms of electro-galvanic stimulation and biofeedback have been recorded. Injecting a blend of triamcinolone acetonide and lidocaine into the zone of highest tenderness in the Arcus tendon of the levator muscles has additionally been attempted. The unrivalled result in the short term with this infusion treatment recommends that inflammation of the Arcus tendon of the levator ani muscles (tendinitis hypothesis) may likewise have some role to play in causing of the LAS. As proposed by few, the surgical division of the puborectalis muscle had brought about noteworthy frequencies of incontinence for fluid or gas, and, along these lines, this surgical treatment ought not to be attempted.

PROCTALGIA FUGAX

Proctalgia fugax, as the name infers, is a sudden pain in the vicinity of the rectum, which could be so extreme as to be debilitating. The attack of pain is severe, paroxysmal, and mostly occurs at night to last for 10–20 minutes. Another characteristic is that it usually only happens 3–4 times a year and for many years in continuity. Very sparse knowledge is available about the aetiology of this pain except that some have claimed to have examined a patient during an attack and found intense spasm of the puborectalis and pubococcygeus muscles which they have interpreted as being like a tetanic cramp. Presumably, it is secondary to spasm of the rectum itself or muscular components of the pelvic floor. The patient may learn methods of relieving the pain before its spontaneous cessation. A passage of wind, digital manipulation of the anal canal, or the insertion of a glycerine suppository may give rapid relief. The condition disturbs the patient mostly because of fears as to its cause rather than because of the pain itself, which is infrequent and transient. The role of the physician in these cases is mainly to assure the patient that this is not a symptom of some fatal disorder. Once reassured, he may well not wish any active therapy.

The diagnosis of proctalgia fugax should only be made when the story is characteristic, when the attacks are infrequent, and when they are relieved by simple measures. It is only too easy to make this diagnosis, which involves no further investigation or treatment, when in fact, a definitive abnormality is present. Conditions which tend to be given this label are anal fissures, mucosal prolapse, anal fistula, and even more severe pathologies like carcinoma of the anorectal region or prostate. Careful history taking and examination will avoid such errors. Psychological testing indicates that many patients are perfectionists, anxious, and hypochondriacal.

Treatment

In most patients, episodes of pain are so brief that treatment consists only of reassurance and explanation. However, a small group of patients has proctalgia fugax on a frequent basis. Many treatments have been attempted with different success rates, namely cholinergic drugs, calcium antagonists, botulinum A toxin, adrenergic drugs such as salbutamol inhalations during episodes, intravenous lidocaine, hip-baths, topical nitroglycerin ointment, biofeedback techniques, anal dilatation, lateral internal sphincterotomy when internal anal sphincter (IAS) hypertrophy is demonstrated, and psychotherapy. Most of the symptoms can be partly relieved and the rate of episodes reduced. The very basic fact in the management of proctalgia fugax is to reassure patients about the disease to enable them to learn to cope with the pain and tolerate it better. The use of perineal nifedipine in the same doses and method as for anal fissure and hypertrophic internal anal sphincter may be of benefit.

PUDENDAL NERVE ENTRAPMENT

Pudendal neuralgia is a syndrome like entity, which is shown by persistent pelvic/perineal agony in the distribution of one or both pudendal nerves. It might be apparent as vulvodynia, orchalgia, proctalgia, or prostatodynia. The pain is a blend with those of levator syndrome, coccydynia, and urethral disorder. It is owing to pressure or entrapment of the pudendal nerve, and is frequently positional in nature. This finding ought to be entertained if there is a background marked by injury, either a particular episode or constant perineal injury; for example, found in cyclists or rowers. The two recorded sites of pudendal nerve entrapment are between the sacrotuberous and sacrospinous ligament and in the Alcock's canal.

The diagnosis of pudendal neuralgia is upheld by the generation of the pain with pressure on the ischial spine despite the fact that this is not a consistent finding. Pudendal nerve latency is frequently noticed on examination. Nerve block under CT scan or ultrasound guidance has been utilised to deal with those patients who might likely be benefitted by neurolysis.

VULVODYNIA

It is the discomfort felt in the vulvar region and might be connected with stress urinary incontinence and dyschezia. This is a disorder of unexplained vulvar pain, sexual disability, and mental incapacity.

Perineal and vulvar hypoesthesia, weak anal reflex, and decreased electromyography (EMG) activity of the external anal sphincter, urethral sphincter, and the levator ani muscle are few of the clinical findings. There is a noteworthy increment of the pudendal nerve terminal motor latency in every such patient.

COCCYGODYNIA

The term coccygodynia has been connected to pain in the area of the coccyx. It has likewise been termed as piriformis disorder, puborectalis disorder, diaphragma pelvis spastica, and pelvic tension myalgia. Grant et al., in one of the biggest and the recent series of cases, depicted it as uneasiness in the area of the rectum and sacro-coccygeal region that might be connected with pain in the gluteal area and thighs. The pervasiveness of this manifestation in the general community is roughly 6%. It is more commonly seen in females.

In most of the patients, excessive mobility is perceived on both standing and seated radiographs, despite the fact that the reason for pain could not be located for other patients. Inflammation and oedema might be seen on bone scan and MRI. Nonetheless, neither of these techniques is as accurate as dynamic radiography. Treatment for patients with extreme pain should start with an injection of local anaesthetics and corticosteroid into the painful area. Rubbing the coccyx or stretching of the levator ani muscle can provide some relief. Coccygectomy is recommended when non-surgical treatment does not give adequate relief. Coccygectomy is effective in a couple of precisely chosen patients, with the best results in those who radiographically show irregularities of coccygeal mobility. In spite of the fact that coccygectomy was routinely performed at one time, as of late, it has been viewed as half-baked by the surgeon.

PIRIFORMIS SYNDROME

It is a neuromuscular condition manifested in the form of hip and buttock pain. The sciatic nerve is compacted inside the butt cheek by the piriformis muscle, creating pelvic pain, which is exacerbated by muscular contraction, palpation, or persistent sitting. This disorder is often neglected in clinical settings since its presentation might be like that of lumbar radiculopathy. A comprehensive way to diagnosis requires a detailed neurological history and physical appraisal of the patient, which depends on the pathologic characteristic of piriformis syndrome.

Diagnosis is accomplished by rectal palpation of myofascial trigger points within the piriformis muscle, also pain and weakness on the resistant abduction-external rotation of the thigh. The simplest therapy is the injection of a local anaesthetic or a small dose of corticoid into the exact focal point of hyperirritability deep in the belly of the muscle. The treatment gives a long-lasting effect with minimum chances of recurrences.

OBTURATOR INTERNUS SYNDROME

Hypertonicity of the gluteal part of the obturator internus muscle may bring about a persistent pain in the perineal regions. The diagnosis can be affirmed by evoking pain on deep pressure over the ischial tuberosity.

PERINEAL NERVE SYNDROME

The inferior perineal nerve can produce pain on the posterior aspect of the thigh and behind the buttock.

SACRAL NERVE IRRITATION

This occurs due to compression or irritation of the cauda equina or sacral plexus. Loss of perineal sensation and difficulty in micturition or defecation are the principal clinical features. MRI of the spine can help in the diagnosis of this condition.

HEREDITARY SPHINCTER MYOPATHY

Hereditary anal sphincter myopathy is rare. It may be associated with proctalgia fugax, constipation, and internal anal sphincter hypertrophy. This condition is characterised by an isolated IAS myopathy, which is a variant of polysaccharide storage disease. This situation requires a specific surgical therapy with specimen preservation and ultrastructural examination for optimal characterisation and treatment.

ESSENTIAL PROCTALGIA

The aetiology of essential proctalgia is unclear, but functional disorders of the pelvic floor and sphincter muscles, along with an altered perineal stasis and pudendal conditions, have been found to be responsible. It was found that puborectalis syndrome, external sphincter spasm, and perineal descent are involved in over 70% of cases with chronic anorectal pain. Defecography is diagnostic as it permits diagnosis of abnormal anorectal morphology, and of the sphincter and puborectalis muscle dysfunctions.

BIOFEEDBACK

Though biofeedback has been described as a useful therapeutic intervention in patients with pelvic floor disorders like incontinence or constipation, it will not be inappropriate to discuss it in this chapter as few functional anal pains like the levator ani syndrome have been found to be relieved with biofeedback therapy.

The concept of biofeedback is that patients with disordered defecation are unable to respond appropriately to the stimulus of rectal distension. With incontinence, contraction of the external anal sphincter (EAS) is impaired, and with obstructive defecation, relaxation of the EAS is impaired. To defecate properly, patients must relearn the sensation of rectal distension and how to respond appropriately. During biofeedback therapy, a rectal balloon is used to mimic the sensation of rectal filling. Electrodes on an anal plug record the motor units of the EAS contraction and convey this information to the patient in the form of visual or auditory feedback. The balloon is expanded, and the patient is trained to achieve maximal external anal sphincter contraction in response to the balloon stimulus in the case of incontinence or to relax the EAS in the event of constipation.

For a successful biofeedback, there must be some degree of rectal sensation and ability to voluntarily contract the EAS.

Patients are made to learn to use the machine independently and then perform sessions at home. With time, the rectal sensation is heightened, external anal sphincter strength increased, and the coordination between rectal distension and EAS contraction improved. Biofeedback is useful to train the minds of patients with levator ani syndrome to relax their levator ani muscles and break the spastic cycle. A study has claimed that after biofeedback, the pain score and analgesic requirements were significantly reduced in patients with levator ani syndrome. There were no remarkable changes in the anorectal physiology, and there have been no side effects.

If the patient has obstructive defecation-related to anismus, biofeedback is very likely to improve his symptoms. A small degree of success has been reported in patients with combined pelvic floor disorders and slow transit time. One can expect improvement of symptoms after biofeedback training, sustaining for several years, and can be useful regardless of the patient's age. In elderly patients with limited mobility, home exercise has been shown to be a useful alternative option.

CLINICAL PEARLS

- Functional anorectal pain is experienced in the practice of gastroenterologists, gynaecologists, and colorectal specialists.
- The assessment of this issue has made some incredible progress in the development of more up to date symptomatic tests, including anal manometry, endoanal sonography, static and dynamic pelvic imaging, and electromyography.
- Until as of late, the approach to these disorders has been to a great extent narrative. Nonetheless, with the extension of different pharmacological formulations such as nitrates, calcium channel blockers, and botulinum toxins, the treatment scenario has been radically altered.
- This has been supplemented with the advancement of novel procedures; for example, sacral nerve stimulation and biofeedback training.

SUGGESTED READINGS

Beer-Gabel M, Carter D, Venturero M, Zamora O, Zbar AP. Ultrasonographic assessment of patients referred with chronic anal pain to a tertiary referral centre. *Tech Coloproctol*. 2010;14:107–12.

Bharucha AE, Trabuco E. Functional and chronic anorectal and pelvic pain disorders. *Gastroenterol Clin North Am*. 2008;37:685–96.

Bharucha AE, Wald A, Enck P, Rao S. Functional anorectal disorders. *Gastroenterology*. 2006;130:1510–8.

Chiarioni G, Asteria C, Whitehead WE. Chronic proctalgia and chronic pelvic pain syndromes: new etiologic insights and treatment options. *World J Gastroenterol*. 2011;17:4447–55.

Chiarioni G, Nardo A, Vantini I, Romito A, Whitehead WE. Biofeedback is superior to electrogalvanic stimulation and massage for treatment of levator ani syndrome. *Gastroenterol*. 2010;138:1321–9.

García-Montes MJ, Argüelles-Arias F, Jiménez-Contreras S, Sánchez-Gey S, Pellicer-Bautista F, Herrerías-Gutiérrez JM. Should anorectal ultrasonography be included as a diagnostic tool for chronic anal pain? *Rev Esp Enferm Dig*. 2010;102:7–14.

Grant SR, Salvati EP, Rubin RJ. Levator syndrome: an analysis of 316 cases. *Dis Colon Rectum*. 1975;18(2):161–3.

Grimaud JC, Bouvier M, Naudy B, Guien C, Salducci J. Manometric and radiologic investigations and biofeedback treatment of chronic idiopathic anal pain. *Dis Colon Rectum*. 1991;34:690–5.

Hompes R, Jones OM, Cunningham C, Lindsey I. What causes chronic idiopathic perineal pain? *Colorectal Dis*. 2011;13:1035–9.

Kang YS, Jeong SY, Cho HJ, Kim DS, Lee DH, Kim TS. Transanally injected triamcinolone acetonide in levator syndrome. *Dis Colon Rectum*. 2000;43(9):1288–91.

Longstreth GF, Thompson WG, Chey WD, Houghton LA, Mearin F, Spiller RC. Functional bowel disorders. *Gastroenterol*. 2006;130:1480–91.

Pascual I, García-Olmo D, Martínez-Puente C, Pascual-Montero JA. Ultrasound findings in spontaneous and postoperative anal pain. *RevEsp Enferm Dig*. 2008;100:764–7.

Renzi C, Pescatori M. Psychologic aspects in proctalgia. *Dis Colon Rectum*. 2000;43:535–9.

Tu FF, Holt J, Gonzales J, Fitzgerald CM. Physical therapy evaluation of patients with chronic pelvic pain: a controlled study. *Am J Obstet Gynecol*. 2008;198:272.e1–272.e7.

Vieira AM, Castro-Poças F, Lago P, et al. The importance of ultrasound findings in the study of anal pain. *Rev Esp Enferm Dig*. 2010;102:308–13.

Wald A, Bharucha AE, Enck P, et al. Functional anorectal disorders. In: *Rome III: The Functional Gastrointestinal Disorders* 3rd ed. Drossman DA, Corazzairi E, Delvaux M, et al. (eds). McLean: Degnon Associates; 2006:639–85.

Whitehead WE, Bharucha AE. Diagnosis and treatment of pelvic floor disorders: what's new and what to do. *Gastroenterol*. 2010;138:1231–5.

Chapter 17

Quackery in proctology

It is quite natural that a human will do nearly anything to draw out his presence or get mitigated himself from the affliction of a disease. For this, someone will count on this human nature to misuse these desires by offering what he claims to be a panacea or otherworldly solutions for all his sufferings, even for the incurable ones. The culprits cut over the entire strata of medicinal and well-being specialists. These alternative therapeutic systems and natural health practices have mainly assumed great fame disregarding that they are false, generally fake treatment cures. Quacks are a class of professionals or country doctors who utilise, as far as anyone knows, irrational medications after working as a clinical assistant or medicine dispensing attendant under a qualified doctor for few months and label themselves as a doctor with a fake qualification.

A quack is one who practices some form of the medicinal system without required capability, formal preparing, and enrolment from the suitable therapeutic board or authority. These experts effectively advance their asserted therapeutic and surgical capacities and their solutions to a gullible public. While most of them may be innocuous, others are potentially dangerous and risky. Non-customary treatment systems have reliably had an interest for a group of people from the gathering, and this allurement has even continued into the twenty-first century.

The quacks can practise any and each field of medicine, the field of surgery being no exception. As regards the surgical field, for the most part, it spins around the treatment of anal canal diseases, that is, piles, fistula-in-ano, fissure-in-ano, and so forth. Quacks here frequently draw in individuals more than the customary experts in light of their eye-getting promotions, billboards, and workplaces in each township. They have neither a perceived degree, nor a permit to practice medication, but then a few quacks are running their 'dispensaries' with the exemption in all parts of the globe. This is a result of the absence of an administrative and supervisory system set up. The expense of the treatment is likewise a contributory component in the expansion of such quackery. The majority of them have one-room centres. They claim to be specialists and even write down prescriptions on their letterheads with unrecognised degrees under their names. With their verbal ability and organisational skills, they can overcome even a qualified one from the territory of their operations.

Quacks are additionally found to draw in individuals promising home-grown cures given claimed customary information of herbs and roots. Many numbers of patients from all walks of life and different cross-segments of society routinely go to these fake doctors for their anal and perianal issues. Of them, some are satisfied as well and pronounce that their illnesses were cured. However, most of them have to repent for life; mainly, because there is only a superfluous relief while the original problem is compounded and complicated. The patients need to endure and bring about a substantial cost to get rid of such inconveniences. Most quacks brag to be super-specialists in their fields of aptitude.

A unique segment of the fake case to treat haemorrhoids within an hour with a 'charm wand' and people, especially from the lower strata of society, transform into a prey to such traps. Additionally, to demonstrate this mystical cure working in 60 minutes, these quacks impart different corrosives directly into the pile mass which results in extreme aggravation and additional severe agony to the patient. Mostly, a single needle is utilised for injecting the haemorrhoids in numerous patients. This can bring about the higher frequency of blood-borne contaminations like hepatitis and acquired immune deficiency syndrome (AIDS) in patients visiting them. While quacks are guaranteeing to treat piles at each niche and corner of the globe, on the whole, the Ayurvedic, Unani, and Homoeopathic experts likewise go about as specialists and handle all of the anorectal problems including malignancy.

These quack set up clinics and offer 'cash-back insurance'. They shamelessly make announcements close to big hospitals. These quacks case to practise some conventional herbal medicinal treatment. Be that as it may, in a real sense, they treat the anal afflictions of the patients utilising different harmful chemicals and acids, and afterwards attempt to adjust the resultant inflammation by a large spectrum of anti-microbial and analgesics otherwise used as a part of veterinary practice. Most of the casualties wind up with fibrosis and lifetime suffering. The anorectal illnesses are considered as some impressive condemnation, forbidden, and a matter of disgrace. Ladies, specifically, are hesitant to unveil and concede that they experience the ill-effects of an anorectal issue. They undergo some home cures that in time result in worsening of the problem. The victims of such pretenders, consequently, suffer in silence. Even the learned and people from affluent class visit these quacks because either the treatment from their doctors could not have been up to their expectations as regards efficacy and relief with haemorrhoids, fistula, and fissure, or they are excessively shy, not allowing to examine the illness by their family doctor or companions.

The possible purposes behind the patients going to quacks could charm consideration creations like stating speedier, less costly, and cure without question. Interestingly, the general or family practitioners are less eager about treating these illnesses. Confusion in patient's mind makes him think that surgery for anorectal diseases is trailed by a considerable amount of torment, incontinence, bleeding, and so on. The other factors that take people to quacks are minimal cost of treatment, the guarantee of a lifetime by the quacks (some of them even issue a lifetime guarantee card mentioning that the patient would be provided with free treatment throughout his life for the ailment he has undergone the said treatment), and a false conviction that treatment by quack was only a 'treatment' involving no surgical intercession.

Perceptions and involvement in this field have demonstrated that quacks are treating fissures and sentinel piles escape without numerous intricacies. Issues emerge when they set out on treating fistulas, haemorrhoids, or anorectal neoplasms. The entanglements are made because of the absence of scientific knowledge and lack of careful asepsis. The majority of these quacks are most likely previous assistants or relatives of a senior quack proctologist. In the wake of watching the proctological surgery from their seniors, they impersonate the system; however, for the need of formal medical education, they remain technicians and create complications mishandling the cases or handling them in wrong circumstances.

In the subsequent paragraphs, a brief treatise from the author's personal experience is given about the different strategies adopted by the quacks to manage anorectal diseases and the resultant complications emerging out of them.

WRONG INJECTIONS IN WRONG PLACE

Injection sclerotherapy is mainstream in many parts of the world to treat first- and second-degree haemorrhoids by making a submucous fibrosis of the haemorrhoidal tissue. The utilisation of injection sclerotherapy began a century earlier and ever through its progression, particular sclerosants have been used. The most satisfactory sclerosant used is 5% phenol solution in oil. The ease of injection sclerotherapy and the simplicity with which it can be regulated by a sole administrator in an outpatient setting have added to its prominence. The methodology is considered safe.

All things considered, the method of injection needs learning of the basic structure and anatomy of the region and the prudence to inject the medication in the dose, depth, and direction of the targetted haemorrhoidal tissue. Technically, the injection is to be ingrained in the submucosa which creates an aseptic inflammation which upon healing, induces fibrosis, which obscures the pathological vascular enlargement of haemorrhoid that is responsible for most haemorrhoidal symptoms.

In any case, the quacks know minimal about these anatomical actualities and in this manner instil the solution even in spots other than where it is required. Misapplication of this injection results in it being either excessively superficial, that is, in the mucosa bringing about ulceration or bleeding, or too deep in the muscles or underlying tissue to create various septic complications. Such complications include severe pain, injection-site haemorrhage, and ulceration.

Urological complications are also likely to result from an anteriorly misdirected injection into the prostate, urethra, or the peri-prostatic venous plexus. The difficulties incorporate haematuria, oliguria, urinary retention, urethral stricture, epididymitis, prostatic abscess, and impotence. As the most commonly found haemorrhoidal spot is in right anterior position (11 o'clock position), the odds of an event of this intricacy are moderately high.

Correspondingly, the phenol in oil solution is to be set up under strict aseptic conditions and ought to be infused with every single aseptic measure. Every patient must be tested for HIV and Australia antigen before being subjected to any surgical manoeuvres. Immunologically compromised patients represent an extra hazard in such circumstances. The amount of phenol to be infused must be circumspectly measured, as there is a potential for phenol to be absorbed systemically with dire consequences.

Odds of a consequent putrefaction of the underlying tissues creating rectal perforation and retroperitoneal abscess requiring emergency laparotomy and defunctioning colostomy pose a potential threat. Extreme local reactions, necrosis followed by haemorrhage and allergic reactions, external haemorrhoid thrombosis, and delayed haemorrhage are some of the other complications. Notwithstanding, the quacks barely take any such safety measures before injecting the haemorrhoids.

QUACKS AND THE FISTULOUS TRACT

Quacks inject various corrosives and unknown chemicals in the fistula tract, which induces inflammation and necrosis, which when heals, leads to excessive fibrosis and in the end, the closure of the fistula tract. A significant number of the patients do not attain a reasonable cure and land up with various issues like necrotising fasciitis of the anorectum, perianal region, and scrotum, which requires immediate debridement and defunctioning colostomy. Few fortunate are lucky enough to have their tract getting obliterated. Septicaemia and renal failure can occur because of absorption of the toxic material and will require expensive treatment and an expanded hospital stay (Figure 17.1).

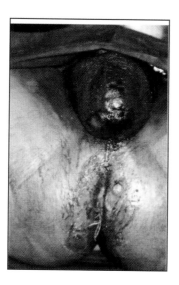

Figure 17.1 Fournier's gangrene due to infected threads in the anal fistula.
Courtesy: Pravin Jaiprakash Gupta.

For treating anal fistula, the 'Kshara-Sutra treatment' (medicated seton insertion) that has its birthplace in the age-old Ayurveda atypical to India, seems to have picked up prominence. In this technique, the doctor utilises a medicated string, to be inserted through the tract of anal fistula repeatedly soaked in a medicated solution and allowed to dry up. One of the ends of this thread is embedded from the outer opening to bring it out of the internal opening of the anal canal utilising a probe with an eye. The two ends of this string are then tied and after that fixed at the external opening with three knots. This methodology is rehashed each week, extending between 15 and 50 sittings until it slices through the fistulous tract. This synchronous procedure of dividing through the tract towards the edges, and recovering the wound thus created, finally, winds up in slitting open the entire tract during recuperation of the injury.

This is an established and proven therapy provided the treating doctor be well versed in the anatomy and basics of anal fistula pathology. The quacks, unfortunately, lack both these primary essentials and just either put the thread in a wrong place creating a false passage or keep the thread too loose to achieve slitting of the tract (Figure 17.2).

The process of changing the thread is excruciatingly painful. Often the patient would not allow the doctor to insert the thread in proper position due to the unbearable pain; and with the lack of adequate pressure and tension, the very basic role of cutting the tract due to pressure necrosis could not take place. A sizable number of such patients are seen attending the proctologists with the strings in place around the fistula fraught with foul-smelling discharge, suppuration with excoriated skin, intolerable pain, and induration in that region.

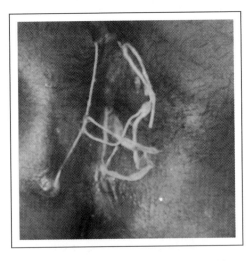

Figure 17.2 Multiple threads in the fistulous openings, with some even in false openings.

Courtesy: Pravin Jaiprakash Gupta.

In a patient having multiple fistulas, the proximal opening close to the anal verge can be threaded with relative ease, while the distally placed openings (which ideally should be treated first) are left as it is for want of difficulty in probing them in the correct direction. In this way, the tract persists requiring months of treatment and sufferance for a considerable length of time.

In such circumstances, it is ideal to expel the culpable string and clean the wound completely. If any necrotic or suppurative cavity is discovered, it ought to be debrided. Anti-infection agents and the anti-inflammatory drug would help in mitigating the torment and discharge. Once the state of crisis is over, appropriate surgical choices could be adjusted to treat such fistula.

THROTTLING HAEMORRHOIDS OR THE PATIENT?

The way quacks treat large prolapsing, or interno-external haemorrhoids, is based on the essential standard, throttling the mass to obstruct the blood supply, making it die and subsequent sloughing of the pile mass from its pedicle. Different strings, ligatures, and banding materials are utilised to complete this move (Figure 17.3). In any case, the patient needs to go through a nightmare of extreme torment, thrombotic protuberance at their butt, bleeding, and other septic side effects. Few may get mitigated once the mass is sloughed off. However, it deserts a substantial injury, which takes a month to recuperate with consequent anal stenosis or stricture.

The difficulties of such *en masse* haemorrhoidal ligation include bacterial septicaemia or toxaemia, bleeding and thrombosis, supra-levator abscess, delayed massive rectal bleeding, perianal abscess, perianal fistula (Figure 17.4), and painful priapism. Numerous patients have reported with pelvic cellulitis with movement to shock and death.

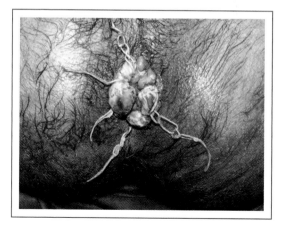

Figure 17.3   Threads tied on the external haemorrhoids.
Courtesy: Pravin Jaiprakash Gupta.

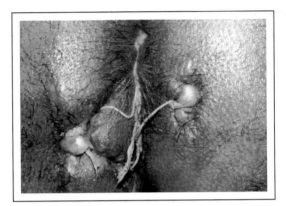

Figure 17.4   Threads in multiple fistulous openings with gross scarring.
Courtesy: Pravin Jaiprakash Gupta.

THE PROBLEM OF QUACKERY

Despite the fact that a modern quack still mouths the same old guarantees, his way and style have changed. He has turned out to be more sophisticated in his way to deal with the affected individuals. He quotes or misrepresents exploratory references, and sprinkles his discussion with medicinal terms in managing future patients. In addition, modern quackery has turned into an innovative and influential method to lure more and more people in the more convincible way. In any case, quacks barely speak of the negatives of their medicinal practice. They tout it as one of the methods for social services.

Numerous patients visit quacks for anal canal ailment in the trust of ease, an operation-less cure. A significant portion of them face rough, irrational, and idiotic treatment which continues with the ill effects of prolonged morbidity. They are modest to approach to advice about these entanglements and counsel appropriate specialists until they are in a hopeless circumstance.

Tall claims are made by quacks about the curative powers of their medication and therapies. These claims are rarely supported by clinical research or any systematic study of the drug. The safety and efficacy of these drugs are always a suspect.

Ironically, individuals who approach quacks because of lower charges, in any case, end up paying more due to the wrong treatment they experience. The innocent patient is effortlessly taken for a ride because of simple access to such quacks and the guarantee to early relief. The masses needs to be made aware of the perils of being dealt with by the quacks. The medical societies and lawmakers are required to manage these vainglorious frauds offering quack cures, with iron hands.

The pretence is not constrained to persons posing as physicians and surgeons. It rises above into the domain of over-the-counter prescriptions. Tall claims are made about the remedial forces of these medications. These claims are not supported by clinical research or any systematic study of the drug. The safety and usefulness of these drugs are always doubtful.

While there are stringent and strict laws insuring patients against such quacks and otherworldly cures, they are hardly exercised by the victims. Hence, quacks keep on prospering uncontrolled and unabated.

CLINICAL PEARLS

- Patients treated by quacks land up with a various life-threatening complications like urinary difficulties, fever, severe pain, septic shock, and leucocytosis.
- The absence of mindfulness among the general population and lack of concern for enforcement agencies have resulted in a situation where quacks are flourishing admirably.
- To recognise quacks from enlisted specialists, the qualified experts ought to show their endorsements in their centres.
- Serious sepsis can happen post-treatment by such acts and all specialists who treat such patients ought to know about these potential complications and recognise them at their earliest.
- If they present early and having no evidence of tissue necrosis, they can well be managed conservatively, but the sad story is that by and large, surgical intervention is what is needed.
- A good deal of public education is important to create awareness about anal canal diseases and their logical treatment and new short stay, curative, and patient-friendly surgical choices.

SUGGESTED READINGS

Gupta PJ. Quacks in anorectal practice in India. *Indian J Med Ethics*. 2010;7(2):125.

Gupta PJ. The role of quacks in the practice of proctology. *Eur Rev Med Pharmacol Sci*. 2010;14(9):795–8.

Hammerschmidt DE. The quack doctor. *J Lab Clin Med*. 2005;146:352–3.

Kulkarni ND. Price of visiting a quack—case reports. *Indian J Med Sci*. 2000;54:290–2.

Pray WS. Ethical, scientific, and educational concerns with unproven medications. *Am J Pharm Educ*. 2006;70:141.

Ramesh G. Quackery—a feedback discussion. *J Indian Med Assoc*. 2007; 105:656.

Umre GA. Quackery—a burning threat of human health. *J Indian Med Assoc*. 2007;105:423.

Verma S. Proposal to ban quackery. *J Indian Med Assoc*. 1987;85:60–1.

Index

(Page numbers followed by *f* indicate figures; and those followed by *t* indicate tables.)